Biological Amplification Systems in Immunology

Comprehensive Immunology

Series Editors: ROBERT A. GOOD and STACEY B. DAY
Sloan-Kettering Institute for Cancer Research
New York, New York

Biological Amplification Systems in Immunology

Edited by
NOORBIBI K. DAY

and
ROBERT A. GOOD

Sloan-Kettering Institute for Cancer Research
New York, New York

PLENUM MEDICAL BOOK COMPANY
New York and London

Library of Congress Cataloging in Publication Data

Main entry under title:

Biological amplifications systems in immunology.

   (Comprehensive immunology; v. 2)
   Includes bibliographies and index.
   1. Complement deficiency. 2. Complement (Immunology) 3. Complement fixation. 4.
Immunology. I. Day, Noorbibi K. II. Good, Robert A., 1922-   III. Series.
RC582.2.B56   616.07'9   76-56828
ISBN 0-306-33102-0

©1977 Plenum Publishing Corporation
227 West 17th Street, New York, N. Y. 10011

Plenum Medical Book Company is an imprint of
Plenum Publishing Corporation

Printed in the United States of America

Contributors

Mark Ballow   Department of Pediatrics, UConn Health Center, Farmington, Connecticut

Celso Bianco   The Rockefeller University, New York, New York

Tibor Borsos   Laboratory of Immunobiology, National Cancer Institute, National Institutes of Health, Bethesda, Maryland

Charles G. Cochrane   Department of Immunopathology, Scripps Clinic and Research Foundation, La Jolla, California

Harvey R. Colten   Division of Allergy, Department of Medicine, Children's Hospital Medical Center and Department of Pediatrics, Harvard Medical School, Boston, Massachusetts

Noorbibi K. Day   Sloan-Kettering Institute for Cancer Research, New York, New York

Jack S. C. Fong   Department of Pediatrics, McGill University, Montreal, Quebec, Canada

Hartmut Geiger   Universitäts-Kinderklinik, Heidelberg, Germany

Henry Gewurz   Department of Immunology, Rush Medical College, Chicago, Illinois

Irma Gigli   Departments of Dermatology and Medicine, New York University Medical Center, New York, New York

Frank M. Griffin, Jr.   The Rockefeller University, New York, New York

Robert A. Good   Sloan-Kettering Institute for Cancer Research, New York, New York

William D. Hardy, Jr.   Sloan-Kettering Institute for Cancer Research, New York, New York

Casper Jersild   Tissue Typing Laboratory, Blood Bank and Blood Grouping Department, University Hospital (Rigshospitalet), Copenhagen, Denmark

Robert L. Kassel   Sloan-Kettering Institute for Cancer Research, New York, New York

Thomas F. Lint   Department of Immunology, Rush Medical College, Chicago, Illinois

B. Moncada   Universidad Autonoma de San Luis Potosi, San Luis Potosi, S. L. P., Mexico

Louis H. Muschel   Research Department, American Cancer Society, New York, New York

Sarkis H. Ohanian Laboratory of Immunobiology, National Cancer Institute, National Institutes of Health, Bethesda, Maryland

W. Opferkuch Institute for Medical Microbiology, Ruhr-University Bochum, Bochum, Germany

Marilyn Pike Department of Medicine, Duke University Medical Center, Durham, North Carolina

Pablo Rubinstein Kimball Research Institute of the New York Blood Center, New York, New York

M. Segerling Institute for Medical Microbiology, Ruhr-University Bochum, Bochum, Germany

Ralph Snyderman Division of Rheumatic and Genetic Diseases, Duke University Medical Center, Durham, North Carolina

Richard J. Ulevitch Department of Immunopathology, Scripps Clinic and Research Foundation, La Jolla, California

Foreword

Interest in complement developed at the end of the nineteenth century from observations on cellular and humoral defense mechanisms against bacteria. It was recognized at that time that there were factors in body fluids of animals and man that were capable of killing and lysing bacteria in the absence of cellular factors. Due to the efforts of two of the founders of immunology, Bordet and Ehrlich, and their colleagues, by 1912 the multicomponent nature of complement action was well recognized, the sequence of reaction of the components in the lysis of erythrocytes was defined, complement fixation as a major tool for studying antibody–antigen interaction was well established, and studies on the physicochemical properties of the components had been started. Yet, with a few notable exceptions, research on complement was largely abandoned by most "mainstream" immunologists for the following two or three decades. When one looks at the contents of the present volume, it is hard to imagine that as recently as 20 years ago, there were probably fewer than ten major laboratories where complement research was the primary theme. The contents attest to the fact that there are today dozens of laboratories on three continents where research on complement is pursued in depth.

It is not easy to point to all the advances that have occurred in complement research during the past few years. The chapters in this book, however, offer a wide selection from the vast subject of complement research representing some of these advances. Our knowledge of complement action was put on a molecular basis by the analysis of the steps leading from the interaction of sheep red cells with antibody to the lysis of the cells due to complement action; from these studies we have progressed so that presently hemolytic activity can be defined on a molecular basis, activation and interaction are interpretable on a biochemical basis, and the physicochemical, biochemical, and biological consequences of these interactions have become amenable to chemical analysis.

It is now understood that the classical complement cascade consists of nine proteins, each existing in serum in a precursor form; the individual components are either activable to a specific enzyme or become part of a multimolecular complex with enzyme activity. The enzymes of the classical pathway are esterases and/or proteases and under certain conditions some can be replaced by trypsin and other common proteases. Thus the activation of a substrate component by the previously activated component in the sequence is usually accompanied by splitting of the substrate into two or more fragments. The various fragments have specific biological properties and most of these properties are discussed in various chapters.

Some of the biological functions link the cellular and humoral compartments of the immune system. For example, a fragment of C5 serves as a positive chemotactic agent for monocytes and granulocytes; monocytes and macrophages have surface receptors for fragments of C3; and there is some evidence that a functional C system in some instances is needed for induction of antibody production.

Ever since it was shown that complement causes injury to cells, investigators have postulated that cells can resist the cytotoxic action of complement. Studies on the cytotoxic effect of complement on nucleated cells now furnish evidence for an active defense mechanism of cells against immune attack. The *in vivo* activation of complement can lead in some instances to self-injury; often *in vivo* activation is accompanied by a drastic reduction in serum levels of certain components. In addition to pathological changes, components may be reduced or absent from serum for genetic reasons. The genetic lack of a component may be associated with pathological changes; however, this is not always the case. Problems concerning the significance of complement in clinical states are being intensively investigated and clarification of many of them is only a matter of time.

The recent revival of the properdin or alternative pathway demonstrates that there are several pathways within the complement system designed to permit activation of the various functions; such backup systems testify to the importance of complement in the preservation of the species; the ubiquity of complement among vertebrates also testifies to the evolutionary significance of complement. Complement seems so important in the individual that, at birth, most animals have a functional complement system. Studies in phylogeny and ontogeny of complement have raised questions of the genetic control and origin of complement. A new and exciting area of research is the genetic mapping of linkages of complement components; such studies may cast some light on the molecular evolution of complement.

During the last decade, we have also learned much about where complement is produced. Not only is the organ site of synthesis known for many of the components, but even the cell types producing complement have been identified in many cases.

On the biochemical side, the molecular structure of several components is being determined. In some instances, polypeptide chains have been identified and amino acid sequencing studies have been initiated. Without doubt such studies will be performed for most if not all components during the next decade.

It should be evident to the reader that even a book of this type cannot cover all that is known about complement. The treatment of the subject is necessarily weighted according to the points of view and special concerns of the individual authors. Thus omissions may have occurred. All in all, however, the editors have gathered together much new material in easily readable chapters that should make an exciting and adventurous journey through the complement system.

Tibor Borsos
National Cancer Institute, NIH
Bethesda

Contents

Chapter 8
Biologic Aspects of Leukocyte Chemotaxis   159
Ralph Snyderman and Marilyn Pike

Chapter 9
Phylogenetics and Ontogenetics of the Complement Systems   183
Mark Ballow

Chapter 10
The Chemistry and Biology of the Proteins of the Hageman Factor-Activated Pathways   205
Richard J. Ulevitch and Charles G. Cochrane

1

Biochemistry and Biology of Complement Activation

W. OPFERKUCH and M. SEGERLING

1. Introduction

The immunological response of the organism to a foreign antigen involves both the humoral and cellular immune system. When antigen is recognized by humoral antibodies, this recognition step is the trigger of a biological reaction mediated by the complement system. The complement system, therefore, may be considered as the effector and amplification system of the humoral immune reaction.

The complement system consists of eleven distinct components, and thus far, seven inhibitors of single components have been described (Austen, 1974; Lepow, 1971; Mayer, 1973; Müller-Eberhard, 1974; Nelson, 1974; Rapp and Borsos, 1970) (see Section 3).

The single components exist in serum in an inactive precursor form. When activated, they react with each other in a certain sequence, during which various biological activities are generated. It is now well established that the complement system not only represents an important part of the host's defense mechanisms, but is also involved in various pathological processes.

Most of the biochemical events in each individual activation step and the interactions of the single components have been elucidated. The study of the immune hemolysis by antibody and complement has proved to be a fruitful model in these investigations. However, although observations made *in vitro* probably reflect what is happening biologically *in vivo,* one should be aware that *in vitro* observations may represent only a narrow section of the total complement activity *in vivo*. The latter is of complex nature and comprises not only the interactions of the eleven components, but also the influence of the inhibitory mechanisms by

W. OPFERKUCH and M. SEGERLING • Institute for Medical Microbiology, Ruhr-University Bochum, Postfach 2148, D-4630 Bochum, Germany

1

which it is balanced and moderated. In addition, the complement system is also connected in a poorly understood manner with other serum protein systems. e.g., with the blood-clotting, kinin, and plasmin systems (Kaplan and Vogt, 1974). Therefore, complement activity *in vivo* does not necessarily imply that the final step, the lysis of an invading parasite or other target cells, will be reached. Already, early events during the activation of complement in connection with the other serum protein systems cause considerable biological activities, amplifying the inflammatory processes in a beneficial or deleterious way.

This chapter will discuss the action and biochemistry of complement, obtained from *in vitro* experiments, in regard to possible concepts and aspects of its mode of action *in vivo*.

2. Biochemistry of Complement Activation

Biochemical data and the concentrations in human serum of each of the eleven known complement components are listed in Table 1. If the reaction sequence is started by immune complexes, it is called the *classical pathway* of complement activation. In addition to this pathway, a so-called alternative pathway is known, in which activation of the complement sequence starts when the third component becomes activated by the properdin system (Pillemer *et al.*, 1954) (see Chapter 2). Once activation is initiated, the components react sequentially in a cascade-like manner, by which some of them gain enzymatic activity (see Figure 1). Immune complexes normally initiate the activation of the complement sequence by binding to, and thus activating, the first component. In general, immune complexes consisting of IgG or IgM antibodies are effective in binding the first component of complement (Ishizaka *et al.*, 1966). Of sublasses of human IgG, γ_1 and γ_2 bind and activate C1 readily, γ_3 binds poorly (Ishizaka *et al.*, 1967), and γ_4 cannot bind at all (Augener *et al.*, 1971). IgA, IgD, and IgE have no complement-binding capacity (Ishizaka *et al.*, 1970). The chemical structure of the antibody molecule reacting with C1q is located on the Fc portion (Kehoe and Fougereau, 1969). This part of the molecule is exposed when the antibody has reacted with its corresponding antigen (Valentine and Green, 1967).

TABLE 1.   Proteins of the Classical Human Complement System[a]

Protein	Serum concentration (μg/ml)	Sedimentation coefficient (S)	Molecular weight	Relative electrophoretic mobility	Number of chains
C1q	180	11,1	400,000	γ_2	18
C1r	—	7,5	180,000	β	2
C1s	110	4,5	86,000	α	1
C2	25	4,5	117,000	β_1	—
C3	1600	9,5	180,000	β_2	2
C4	640	10,0	206,000	β_1	3
C5	80	8,7	180,000	β_1	2
C6	75	5,5	95,000	β_2	1
C7	55	6,0	110,000	β_2	1
C8	80	8,0	163,000	γ_1	3
C9	230	4,5	79,000	α	—

[a]Reprinted from Müller-Eberhard, H. J., 1975, *Ann. Rev. Biochem.* **44**:697.

Dose–response experiments have shown that a single IgM molecule can fix C1, whereas two closely spaced IgG molecules (doublet) are required (Borsos and Rapp, 1965).

C1 is a macromolecule consisting of three distinct subunits: C1q, C1r, and C1s (Lepow *et al.*, 1963). Their molecular weights are listed in Table 1. The integrity of the molecule is calcium ion–dependent, and the subunits can be dissociated by chelating agents (Lepow *et al.*, 1963) and high ionic strength (Colten *et al.*, 1968). Both processes are reversible. Present evidence suggests that the activation of C1 is an internal step within the macromolecule, which is dependent on time and temperature. The subunit C1q is attached to the antibody of the immune complex (Calcott and Müller-Eberhard, 1972) and after it has been fixed, it converts C1r into a peptidase-like enzyme (C1̄r̄) (Valet and Cooper, 1974a). The biochemical event leading to C1r activation is still unknown. C1s is a proesterase and is activated by C1̄r̄ to become an active esterase (Naff and Ratnoff, 1968; de Bracco and Stroud, 1971; Valet and Cooper, 1974b). The activation of C1s results in the cleavage of its polypeptide chain (Sakai and Stroud, 1973).

Studies of the behavior of the C1 molecule by different chemical treatments and various purification methods suggested that C1q may consist of at least three different polypeptide chains (Opferkuch, 1967). This view was supported by the finding that C1 activity after ultracentrifugation at high ionic strength was recovered in the same region as serum albumin (Colten *et al.*, 1968), revealing that the C1q molecule consists of different noncovalently linked polypeptide chains. Structural

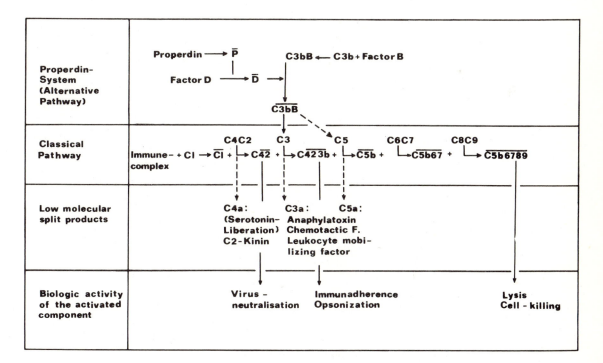

Figure 1. Diagrammatic representation of the classical and alternative pathways of complement activation.

analysis and electron microscopy of purified C1q led to the development of two models. The first one proposes that C1q is composed of six identical noncovalently bound subunits, and the second one assumes the existence of two different polypeptide chains (Shelton *et al.*, 1972; Calcott and Müller-Eberhard, 1972). The nonlinear dose–response curve of serum C1 indicates the existence of a hitherto unrecognized factor, which influences the activation of the C1 molecule (Loos *et al.*, 1973). A similar observation was made when a kinin fragment was added during C1 titration (Gigli *et al.*, 1971). Recently, Assimeh and Painter (1975) have presented evidence for the existence of a fourth subcomponent of C1, C1t.

2.2. Generation of the $\overline{42}$ Enzyme (C3-Convertase)

The natural substrates of the C1-esterase are the components C4 and C2 (Becker, 1956; Lepow *et al.*, 1956a; Lepow *et al.*, 1956b). Both are split into two fragments: a major one, which represents the activated component, and a small polypeptide fragment, which can be detected in the fluid phase. The C4 molecule consists of three polypeptide chains (α, β, and γ) that are linked by disulfide bonds (Schreiber and Müller-Eberhard, 1974). During activation of C4, a small polypeptide fragment called C4a (6000–7000 daltons mol. wt.), is cleaved from the α chain by C1s (Patrick *et al.*, 1970; Budzko and Müller-Eberhard, 1970), thus uncovering the binding site of activated C4, C4b. Simultaneously, a second functional area is exposed, which represents a very stable binding site for C2 (Müller-Eberhard *et al.*, 1967). Recent studies (Cooper, 1975) showed that this binding site might be located on the α chain. C4b molecules, bearing oxidized human C2, were not accessible to a C4b inhibitor that splits the α chain into the α_2 and α_3 fragments (Cooper, 1975). The combining site of the C4 molecule has a very short half-life and undergoes rapid decay unless it becomes bound to its corresponding receptor.

Due to the short half-life of its membrane binding capacity, only about 10% of activated C4b is actually bound to the cell membrane, whereas 90% can be detected in a hemolytically inactive state in the supernatant (Polley and Müller-Eberhard, 1966). Nevertheless, the activation of C4 has an amplifying effect on the further complement reaction. The high serum level of C4 enables a single activated, bound C1 molecule to assemble at least 200 molecules of C4b around its hemolytic site, which could be shown by the uptake of radioactively labeled C4 (Cooper and Müller-Eberhard, 1968) and by hemolytic analysis of the SAC$\overline{42}$ intermediate (Opferkuch *et al.*, 1971a; Borsos and Opferkuch, 1970).

It has been reported that in the presence of magnesium ions, the native C2 molecule and activated C4 can form a loose inactive complex either in the fluid phase or in a cell-bound state (Sitomer *et al.*, 1966). Interaction of the C$\overline{1s}$ esterase with C2 results in splitting of the C2 molecule into two fragments. The larger one, C2a, remains bound to the C4b, thus representing the activated $\overline{42}$ enzyme or C3-convertase (Polley and Müller-Eberhard, 1968). The molecular weight of activated C2 (C2a) is about 33,000 daltons less than that of the native molecule. The polypeptide which is split from the C2 molecule could not be isolated, and little is known as to whether the C2b fragments consist of single polypeptide chains or whether they are even split further into more pieces (Mayer *et al.*, 1967; Polley and Müller-Eberhard, 1968). The $\overline{42}$ enzyme has proteolytic activity and its natural substrates are C3 and C5 (Müller-Eberhard *et al.*, 1967; Shin and Mayer, 1968; Shin *et al.*, 1968).

Treatment of human C2 with critical amounts of iodine results in a marked increase of hemolytic activity and a prolonged half-life stability of the activated $\overline{C42}$ enzyme (Polley and Müller-Eberhard, 1967). It is assumed that the C2 molecule undergoes a chemical modification after iodine treatment, which is supported by the following observations: Inactivation of C2 by binding of p-chloromercuribenzoate (p-CMB) indicates the presence of free, reactive SH groups (Leon, 1965). Upon iodination, the SH groups are oxidized and form intramolecular disulfide bonds, and the C2 molecule is no longer accessible to the binding and inactivation of p-CMB. However, after mild chemical reduction of the iodinated C2, both increased hemolytic activity and prolonged enzymatic stability return to values of native, untreated C2, and hemolytic activity can be inactivated by p-CMB (Polley and Müller-Eberhard, 1967).

The $\overline{C42}$ enzyme is unstable and undergoes a time- and temperature-dependent inactivation (Mayer *et al.*, 1964; Borsos *et al.*, 1961b). During this process, activated C2a is converted into the inactive form C2d (Stroud *et al.*, 1966), which is released from the C4b molecule into the fluid phase. The activity of the $\overline{C42}$ enzyme can be restored when another activated C2a molecule is bound to its receptor on the C4b molecule. Recently it could be shown that a cell-membrane (Hoffmann, 1969a,b) and a serum-associated factor (Opferkuch *et al.*, 1971a) accelerate the natural inactivation of C2a. These factors are probably the reason for the natural decay.

2.3. Activation of the C3 Molecule and Its Antigenic Properties

The C3 molecule consists of two polypeptides (α and β chain), which are linked by disulfide bonds (Nilsson *et al.*, 1975). When C3 is activated by the $\overline{42}$ enzyme (C3-convertase), a small fragment, C3a (about 9000 daltons mol. wt.) (Bokisch *et al.*, 1969), is split off the N-terminal part of the α chain (Nilsson and Mapes, 1973). The larger fragment, C3b, represents the activated component, which in its nascent state forms a triple complex with the C3-convertase, the $\overline{423b}$ enzyme; and C3b becomes firmly bound to the cell membrane (Müller-Eberhard *et al.*, 1966).

Once C3b is activated and bound to the cell membrane, its hemolytic activity is very stable. C3b fulfills important biological functions in phagocytosis and possibly in the humoral immune response (see Section 4.3).

C3b can be enzymatically degraded by a naturally occurring inactivator (C3b inactivator), as will be discussed later. The resulting fragments are C3c and C3d (Ruddy and Austen, 1971). C3d remains bound to the cell surface and consists of polypeptides that were originally part of the α chain. The second split product, C3c, can be recovered from the supernatant and is composed of the β chain and parts of the α chain. All these split products—C3a, C3b, C3c, and C3d—bear distinct antigenic determinants, against which specific antisera have been raised (Pondman and Rother, 1972; Molenaar *et al.*, 1974).

2.4. The Role of Activated C5 and the Formation of a C5b6789 Complex

Similar to the C3 molecule, C5 is composed of two polypeptide chains (α and β), which are linked by disulfide bonds (Nilsson *et al.*, 1975). The $\overline{C423b}$ enzyme splits a polypeptide of molecular weight of between 9000–15,000 daltons from the N-terminal part of the α chain (Shin *et al.*, 1968; Cochrane and Müller-Eberhard,

1968). This polypeptide is called C5a, while the remaining larger molecule (C5b) represents the activated component. As far as it is known, activation of C5 is the last occurring enzymatic step in the complement sequence. Activated C5b is bound to the cell membrane, distinct from the $\overline{423b}$ complex. The functional activity of C5b undergoes a rapid decay, similar to that of the $\overline{42}$ enzyme (Cooper and Müller-Eberhard, 1971). In contrast to the $\overline{42}$ enzyme, C5b decay is apparently not accompanied by the loss of radioactively labeled C5b from the cell membrane (Cooper and Müller-Eberhard, 1971).

C5b, either cell-bound or in the fluid phase, initiates the generation of a complex of the components C6 and C7 (Arroyave and Müller-Eberhard, 1973). C5b reacts with C6 in the fluid phase. By further uptake of C7, a triple complex is formed. The C5b67 complex can react with the membranes of unsensitized cells, which is the basis for "reactive" (Lachmann and Thompson, 1970) or "deviated" lysis (Rother *et al.,* 1974). After the complex is bound to the cell membrane either in immune or reactive lysis, the complement sequence can be completed by the uptake of one molecule of C8 and up to six molecules of C9. The binding of C9 finally completes the cell attack mechanism (Kolb and Müller-Eberhard, 1973).

The biochemical events that lead to lysis of cell membranes are still unexplained. The original hypothesis suggested that the complement reaction causes osmotic swelling of the target cells, leading to an extrusion of the cellular contents (Green *et al.,* 1959). It was discussed that the late-acting complement components might damage the cells by a phospholipase-like activity (Fischer, 1965). These enzymatic activities supposedly cause a leaky patch in the membrane. A variety in the size of these lesions should be expected. However, in negative-staining electron microscopy, uniform lesions ("holes") were observed on the cell membrane (Borsos *et al.,* 1964). These findings did not fit the leaky patch model. The incongruity between the leaky-patch hypothesis and the observed "holes" led to the assumption (doughnut theory) that the late-acting components stabilize the lesion by forming a rigid channel in the cell membrane (Mayer, 1972). Models based on freeze-etching electron-microscopic pictures apparently support this hypothesis (Iles *et al.,* 1973).

Recent studies on volume changes of cells lysed by complement provided some new insight into the events of the lytic mechanism (Valet and Opferkuch, 1975). It was found that the volumes of osmotically and complement-lysed cells differ remarkably in size. In addition, it could be shown that the volumes of osmotically induced ghosts were enlarged by the action of complement under conditions where osmotic forces have been avoided. The action of C9—regardless of the osmotic conditions—led to a remarkable swelling of cells, indicating a profound alteration in the membrane structure. Not only "holes" but also a conspicuous thickening of the cell membrane could be observed in thin-layer electron microscopy (Humphrey and Dourmashkin, 1969). In scanning electron microscopy, both types of membrane alteration were seen (Morgenroth and Opferkuch, unpublished data); see Figure 2. Whereas "holes" might be interpreted as "protrusions," a cloudy disintegration of the whole cell membrane can be observed. The biochemical mechanism of these membrane changes is still unknown.

Kinetic studies on the events and the extent of immune hemolysis led to the formulation and introduction of the *one-hit theory,* which states that a single hit, or the reaction of all components of a single site of a red cell, is sufficient for lysis

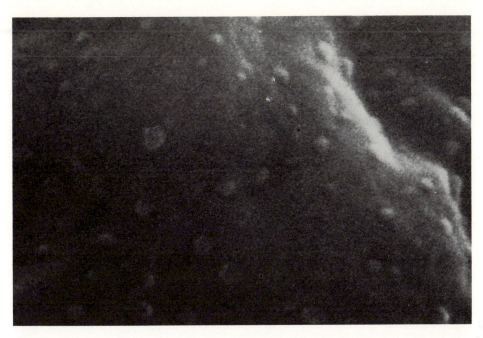

Figure 2. Scanning electron-microscopic picture of the membrane of a sheep erythrocyte lysed by anti-body and guinea pig complement 1:20. × 50,000. Multiple protrusions can be seen, as well as a cloudy disintegration of the surface. The diameter of the protrusions is approximately 100 Å. The above-mentioned changes of the membrane could not be observed either on untreated or on osmotically lysed red cells.

(Mayer, 1960). Experimental and theoretical data substantiated the one-hit theory. Titration curves of single components (Hoffman, L. G., 1960; Borsos *et al.*, 1961a) fit the theoretical response curves calculated from binominal probability distribution curves for threshold values (Figure 3), and it could be demonstrated that a single molecule of at least one of the complement components is sufficient for cell lysis. The one-hit theory is the basis for titration of the hemolytic activity of individual components on a molecular basis, for which the following conditions must be fulfilled (Borsos *et al.*, 1961a). (1) The number of receptor sites on the cell surface that are capable of reacting with the components to be assayed must be large enough so that the kinetics of the reaction will be of pseudo-first order. (2) The rate and extent of lysis must be a function only of the particular component to be assayed. (3) All other components must be supplied in such an amount that an increase in their concentration would have a negligible effect on the rate and extent of lysis.

Under these conditions, the degree of hemolysis, or the average number of lytic lesions per cell, is a linear response to the concentration of the component to be assayed, which can be expressed algebraically by the Poisson distribution curve. In its convenient equation, $z = -\ln/(1 - y)$, where z is the average number of lesions per cell and y is the degree of hemolysis, it can be applied to the calculation of the number of hemolytically effective molecules of a given component. At the present, these conditions can only be fulfilled for the early-acting components, namely C1, C4, and C2.

W. OPFERKUCH AND
M. SEGERLING

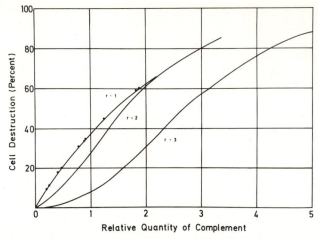

Figure 3. Theoretical curves for the one-hit theory (which states that complement needs to produce only one lesion in the cell membrane in order to destroy the cell) and the multihit theory (which states that two or more lesions are required) of immune hemolysis. The curves were calculated from the binomial probability distribution for threshold values of $r = 1$, $r = 2$, and $r = 3$. Measurements were then made of the number of cells destroyed by complement reaction in which the amount of complement protein C1, C2, or C4 was varied. The results (black dots) fit the one-hit curve. Reprinted from Mayer, M. M., 1973, The complement system, *Sci. Amer.* **223**.

So far, the one-hit theory has been shown to be valid for the immune hemolysis of red blood cells; no data are available that indicate that it can also be applied to other eukaryotic or prokaryotic cells.

3. Regulation Mechanisms of the Complement Reaction

Both the extent of activation and the reaction of individual components are under biological control by different inhibitors and inactivators (see Table 2), thus guaranteeing the limitation and balance of the complement reaction.

TABLE 2. Inhibitors and Inactivators of the Complement System

	Electrophoretic mobility	Sedimentation rate	Molecular weight	Remarks
Clq	—	—	—	—
C$\bar{1}$-INH	α_2	4.5S	90,000	20–30 μg/ml human serum; neuroaminoglycoprotein; inhibition of C$\bar{1}$r, C$\bar{1}$s, kallilrein, plasmin, Hageman factor, and PTA
C2-DAF derived from				
(a) serum	α_1	5S	70,000	
(b) erythrocyte membranes		7.3S	Unknown	Accelerates the decay of the $\overline{42}$-enzyme
C3b-INA	β_1	5.5–6S	100,000	25 μg/ml human serum, splits C3b in C3c + C3d
C3a-INA anaphylatoxin-INA	α_1	9.5S	310,000	Carboxypeptidase B-like enzyme
C6-INA	β_2	6.6S	Unknown	Inactivates cell-bound C6
C7-INA	—	—	—	From patient study

There are different mechanisms by which inhibitors can exert their biological functions. The C1 inactivator (Levy and Lepow, 1959) is a natural substrate of the C1 esterase and interacts stoichiometrically with the activated enzyme (Gigli *et al.*, 1968), thus interfering with the reaction of the other natural substrates, C4 and C2. Because of the irreversibility of the reaction between C1s and the C1 inactivator, it can be assumed that the inhibition is not simply a competitive one (Loos *et al.*, 1972).

Recently, a C4b inactivator was isolated from human serum (Cooper, 1975) which abrogates the biological functions of C4b by cleaving the α polypeptide chain of the molecule into two fragments, C4c and C4d. The C4b inactivator is a β-globulin with an approximate molecular weight of 88,000 daltons. At the present time, it is not possible to determine whether the C4b inactivator is identical with the C3b inactivator, but both inactivators seem to have the same physicochemical properties.

The inactivation of C3b (Tamura and Nelson, 1967) by C3b inactivator is a proteolytic degradation (Lachmann and Müller-Eberhard, 1968) that leads to cleavage of C3b into two fragments, C3c and C3d (Ruddy and Austen, 1971). Similarly, C3a is inactivated by a carboxypeptidase B-like activity, which splits the C-terminal arginine residue of the polypeptide chain (Bokisch and Müller-Eberhard, 1970). The biochemistry of the C6 inhibitor is unknown (Tamura and Nelson, 1967). Besides these well-established inhibitors, a C7 inactivating principle was found in a patient with hereditary deficiency of C7 (Wellek and Opferkuch, 1975), and an inhibitor of Clq has recently been described by Conradie *et al.* (1975). Another control mechanism of the complement reaction is the so-called "natural" decay of activated C2 and C5 (Mayer *et al.*, 1954; Cooper and Müller-Eberhard, 1968). The decay is a temperature-dependent loss of hemolytic activity. A possible explanation for the decay mechanism of C2 was offered by the detection of membrane- and serum-derived decay accelerating factors (Hoffmann, 1969; Opferkuch *et al.*, 1971a).

The complement reaction may be further balanced in itself: First, it is known that C4 and C2 are the natural substrates of the activated C1 esterase. Therefore it is not surprising that the interaction between C1 and C4 can be blocked competitively by C2 or vice versa (Gigli and Austen, 1969). The second mechanism is induced by the activation of the properdin system and the resulting generation of fluid-phase complexes of the late-acting components. These complexes are able to interact with activated or native late-acting components to render them functionally inactive (Koethe *et al.*, 1973).

4. Biological Activities Generated during Complement Activation

In the course of complement activation, various biological activities are present by which the effect of the humoral response is expressed. In general, four different reactions can be distinguished: (1) the inflammatory reaction, caused by low-molecular polypeptides, which are split products, generated during activation of the components C4, C3, and C5; (2) biological reactions, which are mediated by the activated component itself; (3) cytolytic reactions induced by the activation of the late-acting components C5–C9; (4) reactions, caused by the interaction of activated complement components with other serum protein systems.

One should always be aware that activation of the complement system does not necessarily result in lysis of the target cell. However, each activation step of the complement sequence can be interrupted at various stages by the inactivating mechanisms, described in the following pages. The quality of the biological activities and the extent to which they are generated depend on how far the complement activation has proceeded. The interference of inhibitory mechanisms may depend on conditions under which the complement activation is initiated. For example, it is known that at elevated temperatures with human or guinea pig complement, so-called unfruitful $\overline{C42}$ sites are generated that are unable to complete the complement sequence to lysis. The reason might be due to inhibitory mechanisms of the late-acting components in the homologous system. By using late-acting components from the rat, it can be shown that these $\overline{C42}$ sites are highly hemolytically active (Miyakawa *et al.*, 1969, Opferkuch *et al.*, 1971c).

The scope of this discussion will be a description of biological activities that are generated during each individual step of activation of the complement cascade.

4.1. The C1 Activation Step

In the classical pathway, C1 is activated by immune complexes. However, *in vivo*—as observed in hereditary angioneurotic edema—spontaneous activation of C1 can occur (Donaldson and Evans, 1963). The reason for this is a deficiency of the C1 inactivator, causing the activation of fluid phase C4 and C2. Furthermore, it is known that the C1 inactivator is also active against kallikrein, activated Hagemann factor, and plasmin (Ratnoff *et al.*, 1969). Therefore lack of C1 inactivator not only promotes partial activation of complement, but it also promotes kinin and blood-clotting systems as well. An additional possibility for C1 activation exists in the action of proteolytic enzymes like plasmin, showing the close interrelationship between the complement system and other plasma–protein systems.

4.2. The $\overline{42}$ Activation Step

Little is known about biological activities generated during the activation of C4 and C2. There is some evidence that the smaller split product of C4, C4a, leads to serotonin liberation (Budzko and Müller-Eberhard, 1970) and the fragments that are derived from C2—called C2b—have kinin-like activity (Klemperer *et al.*, 1969; Donaldson *et al.*, 1970). The activated cell-bound fourth component (C4b) causes immune adherence (Cooper, 1969), which is the ability of particles that have reacted with certain complement components to attach to membrane receptors found on different mammalian cells (Nelson, 1962). Furthermore, under conditions of limited amounts of antibodies, the uptake of C4 and C2 results in neutralization of viruses (Daniels *et al.*, 1970).

4.3. The Activation Step of C3 and C5

The key role in the biological significance of the complement system may be ascribed to the activation step of C3 and C5. Both components are split—as already described—into a small and a large fragment. The smaller split products C3a and C5a induce the inflammatory process due to their anaphylatoxic-, chemotactic-, and leukocyte-mobilizing activity and cause widening of capillary vessels, release of edematous fluids, and the local assembling of phagocytic mononuclear and poly-morphonuclear cells. This inflammatory process by itself is not sufficient to eliminate the nocuous agent. There is now evidence that particles that have reacted with C3b become bound to certain cells that bear a C3b receptor on their membranes. Therefore, it can be said that C3b acts as a linkage between the antigen and the receptor cell. Various C3b-receptor-bearing cells with different biological activities have been identified. The most important receptor cells are granulocytes and mononuclear phagocytes. If a particle (e.g., a bacterium) has reacted with C3b, it is fixed to the C3b-receptor-bearing cell and is thus accessible to enhanced phagocytosis. This process is called *opsonization*.

Recently, it was shown that mononuclear phagocytes can also react with C3d, which is a degradation product of the C3b inactivator (Wellek *et al.,* 1975). A C3b receptor has also been found in the membrane of other mammalian cells. Predominantly human red blood cells and thrombocytes have been investigated. These cells react in the immune adherence phenomenon with C3b carrying particles (Nelson, 1962). Aggregation of thrombocytes due to the uptake of C3b leads to the release of biologically active substances of the cell content (Henson, 1972). Recently, a possible participation of C3b in antibody formation has been discussed (Pepys, 1974). This hypothesis states that antigen is fixed in the lymphoid follicles by means of C3b to a cell type thus far unspecified.

The biological reactions generated by C3a, C5a, and C3b may cause the elimination of invading cells and thus are beneficial. On the other hand, they can also lead to serious immunopathological tissue damage. (For a more detailed discussion, see Rother, 1974.)

4.4. The C6 Activation Step

In C6-deficient rabbit serum, the clotting time is prolonged as compared to that of normal rabbits. The substitution of either purified human or rabbit C6 reduced the clotting time to normal. The prolongated clotting time could not be correlated to any one of the known clotting factors (Zimmermann *et al.,* 1971). At the present time, it is not clear if this observation with rabbits can also be transferred to other species. Indeed, evidence from studies of C6-deficient humans and hamsters indicates that this association is not a general case.

4.5. The C8 Activation Step

It is still controversial whether cells that have reacted with the first seven complement components can be lysed in the presence of C8 or if the further uptake of C9 is necessary for lysis (Stolfi, 1968). It has been discussed that C9 may only act as an enhancing and accelerating factor (Manni and Müller-Eberhard, 1969). In addition, cells that have reacted with C1–C8 are lysed by macrophages or lymphocytes (Perlman *et al.,* 1969). Although this finding seems to rule out C9, another explanation has been offered by the suggestion that the lytic cells might produce C9 (Perlmann and Holm, 1969).

4.6. The Lytic Mechanism of Complement Action

A great variety of cells has been investigated for sensitivity to the action of complement. Of special interest is the lysis of some classes of pathogenic viruses, the envelopes of which contain lipoproteins (Almeida and Waterson, 1969). Some species of bacteria, e.g., vibrios and mycoplasma, are very susceptible to complement action. Others (some gram-negative rods and *Treponema pallidum*) are killed only by the combined action of complement and lysozyme (Muschel, 1965; Davis *et al.*, 1972, Müller *et al.*, 1973). However, gram-positive cocci are not susceptible to the action of complement. Red blood cells and thrombocytes are readily lysed by complement. Tumor cells of mammalian origin, on the other hand, show poor reactions to tumor-specific antibody and complement. Recently, it was shown that tumor cells could be rendered more susceptible to complement-dependent lysis when they were pretreated with metabolic inhibitors and chemotherapeutic agents such as are currently used in cancer therapy (Segerling *et al.*, 1975). From what is known so far, it may be concluded that the lytic action of complement on cell membranes depends on (1) intrinsic properties of the cell membrane; (2) the surface area, where the complement reaction is initiated; (3) possible repair mechanisms of the cell membrane; and (4) the source of complement.

5. Conclusion

The aim of this chapter has been to provide a brief summary of complement activation and the variety of biological processes induced by that activation. Since complement acts as one of the effector systems in humoral immunity, it also participates in certain autoimmunological processes. The detailed knowledge of complement reactions will lead to a better understanding of immunity, in general, and the underlying pathophysiological events in these diseases.

References

Almeida, J. D., and Waterson, A. P., 1969, The morphology of virus–antibody interaction, *Adv. Virus Res.* **15**:307.

Arroyave, C. M., and Müller-Eberhard, H. J., 1973, Interactions between human C5, C6 and C7 and their functional significance in complement-dependent cytolysis, *J. Immunol.* **111**:536.

Assimeh, S., and Painter, R. H., 1975, The identification of a previously unrecognized subcomponent of the first component of complement, *J. Immunol.* **115**:482–487.

Augener, W., Grey, H. N., Cooper, N. R., and Müller-Eberhard, H. J., 1971, The reaction of monomeric and aggregated immunoglobulins with C1, *Immunochemistry* **8**:1111.

Austen, K. F., ed., 1974, The immunobiology of complement, *Transpl. Proc.* **6**:1.

Becker, E. L., 1956, Concerning the mechanism of complement action. II. The nature of the first component of guinea pig complement, *J. Immunol.* **77**:469.

Bokisch, V. A., and Müller-Eberhard, H. J., 1970, Anaphylatoxin inactivator of human plasma: its isolation and characterization as a carboxypeptidase, *J. Clin. Invest.* **49**:2427.

Bokisch, V. A., Cochrane, C. G., and Müller-Eberhard, H. J., 1969, Isolation of a fragment (C3a) of the third component of human complement containing anaphylatoxin and chemotactic activity and description of an anaphylatoxin inactivator of human serum, *J. Exp. Med.* **129**:1109.

Borsos, T., and Opferkuch, W., 1970, Kinetics and assay of complement components; clustering and hemolytic competence of $\overline{42}$-complexes at a single site, in: *Biologic Activities of Complement,* Fifth International Symposium of the Canadian Society for Immunology, Guelph 1970 (D. G. Ingram, ed.), pp. 27–38, Karger, Basel.

Borsos, T., and Rapp, H. J., 1965, Complement fixation on cell surfaces by 19S and 7S antibodies, *J. Science* **150**:505.

Borsos, T., Rapp, H. J., and Mayer, M. M., 1961a, Studies on the second component of complement. I. The reaction between EAC14 and C2: evidence on the single site mechanism of immune hemolysis and determination of C2 on a molecular basis, *J. Immunol.* **87**:310.

Borsos, T., Rapp, H. J., and Mayer, M. M., 1961b, Studies on the second component of complement. II. The nature of the decay of EAC 1, 4, 22, *J. Immunol.* **87**:326–329.

Borsos, T., Dormashkin, R. R., and Humphrey, J. H., 1964, Lesions in erythrocyte membranes caused by immune haemolysis, *Nature* **4929**:251.

de Bracco, M. M. E., and Stroud, R. M., 1971, C1r, subunit of the first complement component: purification, properties and assay based on its linking role, *J. Clin. Invest.* **50**:838.

Budzko, D. B., and Müller-Eberhard, H. J., 1970, Cleavage of the fourth component of human complement (C4) by C1 esterase: isolation and characterization of the low molecular weight product, *Immunochemistry* **7**:228.

Calcott, M. A., and Müller-Eberhard, H. J., 1972, C1q protein of human complement, *Biochemistry* **11**:3443.

Cochrane, C. G., and Müller-Eberhard, H. J., 1968, The derivation of two distinct anaphylatoxin activities from the third and fifth component of human complement *J. Exp. Med.* **127**:371.

Colten, H. R., Borsos, T., and Rapp, H. J., 1968, Ultracentrifugation of the first component of complement: effects of ionic strength, *J. Immunol.* **1**)):808.

Conradie, J. D., Volanakis, J. E., and Stroud, R. M., 1975, Evidence for a serum inhibitor of C1q, *Immunochemistry* **12**:967–971.

Cooper, N. R., 1969, Immune adherence by the fourth component of complement, *Science* **165**:396.

Cooper, N. R., 1975, Isolation and analysis of the mechanism of action of an inactivator of C4b in normal human serum, *J. Exp. Med.* **141**:890.

Cooper, N. R., and Müller-Eberhard, H. J., 1968, A comparison of methods for the molecular quantitation of the fourth component of human complement, *Immunochemistry* **5**:155.

Cooper, N. R., and Müller-Eberhard, H. J., 1971, The reaction mechanism of human C5 in immune hemolysis, *J. Exp. Med.* **132**:775.

Daniels, C. A., Borsos, T., Rapp, H. J., Snyderman, R., and Notkins, A. L., 1970, Neutralization of sensitized virus by purified components of complement, *Proc. Nat. Acad. Sci.* **65**:528.

Davis, S. D., Janetta, A., and Wedgewood, R. J., 1972, Bactericidal reactions in serum, in: *Biological Activities of Complement* (D. G. Ingram, ed.), p. 43, Karger, Basel.

Donaldson, V. H., and Evans, R. R., 1963, A biochemical abnormality in hereditary angioneurotic edema: absence of serum inhibitor of C1 esterase, *Amer. J. Med.* **35**:37.

Donaldson, V. H., Merler, E., Rosen, F. S., Kretschmer, K. W., and Lepow, I. H., 1970, A polypeptide kinin in hereditary angioneurotic edema plasma: role of complement in its formation, *J. Lab. Clin. Med.* **76**:986.

Fischer, H., 1965, Lysophosphatide und Komplementlyse, *Bull. Schweiz. Akad. Med. Wiss.* **21**:471.

Gigli, I., and Austen, K. F., 1969, Fluid phase destruction of C2^{hu} by C1^{hu}. I. Its enhancement and inhibition by homologous and heterologous C4, *J. exp. Med.* **129**:679.

Gigli, I., Ruddy, S., and Austen, K. F., 1968, The stoichiometric measurement of the serum inhibitor of the first component of complement by the inhibition of immune hemolysis, *J. Immunol.* **100**:1154.

Gigli, I., Kaplan, A., and Austen, K. F., 1971, Alteration in complement component utilization following the interaction of C1^{hu} with kallikrein fragment, *J. Immunol.* **107**:311.

Green, H., Barrow, P., and Goldberg, B., 1959, Effect of antibody and complement on permeability control in ascites tumor cells and erythrocytes, *J. Exp. Med.* **110**:699.

Henson, P. M., 1972, Complement dependent adherence of cells to antigen and antibody mechanism and consequences, in: *Biologic Activities of Complement,* Guelph, 1970 (D. G. Ingram, ed.), pp. 173–210, Karger, Basel.

Hoffman, E. M., 1969a, Inhibition of complement by a substance isolated from human erythrocytes. I. Extraction from human erythrocyte stromata, *Immunochemistry* **6**:391.

Hoffman, E. M., 1969b, Inhibition of complement by a substance isolated from human erythrocytes. II. Studies on the site and mechanism of action, *Immunochemistry* **6**:405.

Hoffmann, L. G., 1960, Purification of the first and fourth component of guinea pig complement and studies on their mechanisms and action, Thesis, School of Hygiene and Public Health, Johns Hopkins University, Baltimore.

Humphrey, J. H., and Dourmashkin, R. R., 1969, The lesions in cell membranes caused by complement, *Adv. Immunol.* **11**:75.

Humphrey, J. H., Dourmashkin, R. R., and Payne, S. N., 1968, The nature of lesions in cell membranes produced by action of complement and antibodies, *The Fifth International Immunopathology Symposium* (P. A. Miescher and P. Grabar, eds.), pp. 209–220, Schwabe, Basel.

Iles, G. H., Seeman, P., Naylor, D., and Cinader, B., 1973, Membrane lesions in immune hemolysis. Surface rings, globule aggregates and transient openings, *J. Cell Biol.* **56**:528.

Ishizaka, T., Ishizaka, K., Borsos, T., and Rapp, H., 1966, C1 fixation by human isoagglutinin: fixation of C1 by γG and γM but not by γA antibody, *J. Immunol.* **97**:716.

Ishizaka, T., Ishizaka, K., Salomon, S., and Fudenberg, H., 1967, Biologic activities of aggregated γ-globulin: VIII. Aggregated immunoglobulins of different classes, *J. Immunol.* **99**:82.

Ishizaka, K., Ishizaka, T., and Lee, J. M., 1970, Biological function of the Fc-fragments of E-myeloma protein, *Immunochemistry* **7**:687.

Kaplan, A. D., and Vogt, W., 1974, Relation of complement with other plasma enzyme systems, in: *Progress in Immunology II,* Vol. I (L. Brent and J. Holborow, eds.), p. 305, North Holland Publishing Comp., Amsterdam and Oxford.

Kehoe, J. M., and Fougereau, M., 1969, Immunoglobulin peptide with complement fixing activity, *Nature* **224**:1212.

Klemperer, M. R., Rosen, F. S., and Donaldson, V. H., 1969, A polypeptide derived from the second component of human complement (c2) which increases vascular permeability, *J. Clin. Invest.* **48**:44a.

Koethe, S. M., Austen, K. F., and Gigli, I., 1973, Blocking of the hemolytic expression of the classical complement sequence by products of complement activation via the alternate pathway. Materials responsible for the blocking phenomenon and their proposed mechanism of action, *J. Immunol.* **110**:390.

Kolb, W. P., and Müller-Eberhard, H. J., 1973, The membrane attack mechanism of complement. Verification of the stable C5–9 complex in free solution, *J. Exp. Med.* **138**:438.

Lachmann, P. J., and Müller-Eberhard, H. J., 1968, The demonstration in human serum of "conglutinogen activating factor" and its effect on the third component of complement, *J. Immunol.* **100**:691.

Lachmann, P. J., and Thompson, R. A., 1970, Reactive lysis: the complement-mediated lysis of unsensitized cells. II. The characterization of activated reactor as C5b and the participation of C8 and C9, *J. Exp. Med.* **131**:643.

Leon, M. A., 1965, Complement: inactivation of second component by *p*-hydroxymercuribenzoate, *Science* **147**:1034.

Lepow, I. H., 1971, Biologically active fragments of complement, *Prog. Immunol.* **1**:579.

Lepow, I. H., Ratnoff, O. J., Rosen, F. S., and Pillemer, L., 1956a, Observation on a proesterase associated with partially purified first component of human complement, *Proc. Soc. Exp. Biol. Med.* **92**:32.

Lepow, I. H., Ratnoff, O. J., and Pillemer, L., 1956b, Elution of an esterase from antigen–antibody aggregates treated with human complement, *Proc. Soc. Exp. Biol. Med.* **92**:111.

Lepow, J. H., Naff, G. B., Todd, E., Pensky, J., and Hinz, Jr., C. F., 1963, Chromatographic resolution of the first component of human complement into three activities, *J. Exp. Med.* **117**:983.

Levy, L., and Lepow, I. H., 1959, Assay and properties of serum inhibitor of C1-esterase, *Proc. Soc. Exp. Biol. Med.* **101**:608.

Loos, M., Wolf, H. U., and Opferkuch, W., 1972, The C1-inactivation from guinea pig serum. III. Characterization and kinetic data of the reaction between the inactivator and EAC1 and EAC14, *Immunochemistry* **9**:451.

Loos, M., Borsos, T., and Rapp, H. J., 1973, The first component of complement in serum: evidence for a hitherto unrecognized factor in C1 necessary for internal activation, *J. Immunol.* **110**:205.

Manni, J., and Müller-Eberhard, H. J., 1969, The eighth component of human complement (C8): isolation, characterization, and hemolytic efficiency, *J. Exp. Med.* **130**:1145.

Mayer, M. M., 1960, *Development of the One-Hit Theory of Immune Hemolysis, Immunochemical Approaches to Problems in Microbiology,* Rutgers University Press, New Brunswick, New Jersey.

Mayer, M. M., 1964, Complement and complement fixation, in: *Experimental Immunochemistry* (Kabat, E. A. and Mayer, M. M., eds.), pp. 133–240, Charles Thomas, Springfield.

Mayer, M. M., 1972, Mechanism of cytolysis by complement, *Proc. Nat. Acad. Sci.* **69**:2954.

Mayer, M. M., 1973, The complement system: a foreign cell in the body is identified by antibody, but the cell is destroyed by other agents. Among them is "complement," an intricately linked set of enzymes, *Sci. Amer.* **229**:54.

Mayer, M. M., Levine, L., Rapp, H. J., and Marucci, A. A., 1954, Kinetic studies on immune hemolysis. VII. Decay of EAC1, 4, 2 fixation of C3 and other factors influencing the hemolytic action of complement, *J. Immunol.* **73**:443.

Mayer, M. M., Shin, S., and Miller, J. A., 1967, Fragmentation of guinea pig complement components C2 and C3c, *Prot. Biol. Fluids* **15**:411.

Miyakawa, Y., Sekine, T., Shimada, K., and Nishioka, K., 1969, High efficiency of SAC142 conversion to S* with EDTA-treated rat serum, *J. Immunol.* **103**:374.

Molenaar, J. L., Müller, M. A. R., Engelfriet, C. P., and Pondman, K. W., 1974, Changes in antigenic properties of human C3 upon activation and conversion by trypsin, *J. Immunol.* **112**:1444.

Muschel, L. H., 1965, Immune bactericidal and bacteriolytic reactions, in: *Wolstenholme and Knight Complement,* Ciba Foundation symposium, pp. 155–168, Little, Brown, and Co., Boston.

Müller, F., Feddersen, H., and Segerling, M., 1973, Studies on the action of lysozyme in immune immobilization of *Treponema pallidum* (Nichols strain), *Immunol.* 24:711.

Müller-Eberhard, H. J., 1974, Serum complement system, in: *Textbook of Immunopathology* 2nd Ed., (P. A. Miescher and H. J. Müller-Eberhard, eds.), p. 33, Gruner and Stratton, New York.

Müller-Eberhard, H. J., and Calcott, M. A., 1966, Interaction between C1q and gamma G-globulin, *Immunochemistry* 3:500.

Müller-Eberhard, H. J., Dalmasso, A. P., and Calcott, M. A., 1966, The reaction mechanism of β_1C-globulin in immune hemolysis, *J. Exp. Med.* 123:33.

Müller-Eberhard, H. J., Polley, M. J., and Calcott, M. A., 1967, Formation and functional significance of a molecular complex derived from the second and the fourth component of human complement, *J. Exp. Med.* 125:359.

Naff, G. B., and Ratnoff, O. D., 1968, The enzymatic nature of C1r. Conversion of C1s to C1 esterase and digestion of amino acid esters by C1r, *J. Exp. Med.* 128:571.

Nelson, R. A., 1962, Immune adherence, in: *IInd International Symposium on Immunopathology,* Brook Lodge, Michigan, p. 245, Schwabe, Basel.

Nelson, R. A., 1974, The complement system, in: *The Inflammatory Process,* 2nd Ed., Vol. 3, (B. W. Zweifach, R. T. Mc. Cluskey, and H. L. Gernat, eds.) Academic Press, New York.

Nilsson, U. R., and Mapes, J., 1973, Polyacrylamide gel electrophoresis (PAGE) of reduced and dissociated C3 and C5: studies of the polypeptide chain (PPC) subunits and their modifications by trypsin (TRY) and C$\overline{42}$—C$\overline{423}$, *J. Immunol.* 111:293.

Nilsson, U. R., Mandle, R. J., Jr., and McConnel-Mapes, J. A., 1975, Human C3 and C5: subunit structure and modifications by trypsin and C$\overline{42}$ and C$\overline{423}$, *J. Immunol.* 114:815.

Opferkuch, W., 1967, Physical and functional properties of guinea pig C1, *Prot. Biol. Fluids* 15:459.

Opferkuch, W., Loos, M., and Borsos, T., 1971a, Isolation and characterization of a factor from human and guinea pig serum that accelerates the decay of SAC$\overline{142}$, *J. Immunol.* 107:313.

Opferkuch, W., Rapp, H. J., Colten, H. R., and Borsos, T., 1971b, Immune hemolysis and the functional properties of the second (C2) and the fourth (C4) components of complement. II. Clustering of effective C$\overline{4,2}$ complexes at individual hemolytic sites, *J. Immunol.* 106:407.

Opferkuch, W., Rapp, H. J., Colten, H. R., and Borsos, T., 1971c, The hemolytic properties of the fourth component of complement. III. The efficiency of human and guinea pig C4 and C2 estimated with rat C′EDTA, *J. Immunol.* 106:927.

Patrick, R. A., Taubman, S. B., and Lepow, I. H., 1970, Cleavage of the fourth component of human complement (C4) by activated C1s, *Immunochemistry* 7:217.

Pepys, M. B., 1974, Role of complement in induction of antibody production in vivo. Effect of cobra factor and other C3-reactive agents on thymus dependent and thymus independent antibody response, *J. Exp. Med.* 140:126.

Perlmann, P., and Holm, G., 1969, Cytotoxic effects of lymphoid cells in vitro, *Adv. Immunol.* 11:117.

Perlmann, P., Perlmann, H., Müller-Eberhard, H. J., and Manni, H. A., 1969, Cytotoxic effects of leukocytes triggered by complement bound to target cells, *Science* 163:937.

Pillemer, L., Seifter, J., San Clemente, C. L., and Ecker, E. E., 1943, Immunochemical studies on human serum. III. The preparation and physico-chemical characterization of C1 of human complement, *J. Immunol.* 47:205.

Pillemer, L., Blum, L., Lepow, I. H., Ross, O. A., Todd, E. W., and Wardlaw, A. C., 1954, The properdin system and immunity. I. Demonstration and isolation of a new serum protein, properdin, and its role in immune phenomena, *Science* 120:279.

Polley, M. J., and Müller-Eberhard, H. J., 1966, Chemistry and mechanism of action of complement, *Prog. Hematol.* 5:1.

Polley, M. J., and Müller-Eberhard, H. J., 1967, Enhancement of the hemolytic activity of the second component of human complement by oxidation, *J. Exp. Med.* 126:1013.

Polley, M. J., and Müller-Eberhard, H. J., 1968, The second component of human complement: its isolation, fragmentation by C1-esterase and incorporation into C3 convertase, *J. Exp. Med.* 128:533.

Pondman, K. W., and Rother, K. O., 1972, Biochemistry and biology of the third component of complement. European Complement Workshop, Amsterdam, 1972.

Rapp, H. J., and Borsos, T., 1970, *Molecular Basis of Complement Action,* Appleton-Century-Crofts, New York.

Ratnoff, O. D., Pensky, J., Ogston, D., and Naff, G. B., 1969, The inhibition of plasmin, plasma

16

kallikrein, plasma permeability factor, and the C1r subcomponent of the first component of complement by serum C1 esterase inhibitor, *J. Exp. Med.* **129**:315.

Rother, K. (ed.), 1974, *Komplement: Biochemie und Pathologie,* Dr. D. Steinkopff-Verlag, Darmstadt.

Rother, U., Hausch, G., Menzel, J., and Rother, K., 1974, Deviated lysis: transfer of complement lytic activity to unsensitized cells. I. Generation of the transferable activity on the surface of complement resistant bacteria, *Z. Immun. Forsch.* **148**:172.

Ruddy, S., and Austen, K. F., 1971, C3b inactivator in man. II. Fragments produced by C3b inactivator cleavage of cell-bound or fluid phase C3b, *J. Immunol.* **107**:742.

Sakai, K., and Stroud, R. M., 1973, Purification, molecular properties, and activation of C1 proesterase, C1s, *J. Immunol.* **110**:1010.

Schreiber, R. D., and Müller-Eberhard, H. J., 1974, Fourth component of human complement. Description of a three polypeptide chain structure, *J. Exp. Med.* **140**:1324.

Segerling, M., Ohanian, S. H., and Borsos, T., 1975, Chemotherapeutic drugs increase killing of tumor cells by antibody and complement, *Science* **188**:55.

Shelton, E., Yonemasu, K., and Stroud, R. M., 1972, Ultrastructure of the human complement component, C1q, *Proc. Nat. Acad. Sci. U.S.A.* **69**:65.

Shin, H. S., and Mayer, M. M., 1968, The third component of guinea pig complement. II. Kinetic study of the reaction of EAC 42a with guinea pig C3. Enzymatic nature of C3 consumption, multiphasic character of fixation, and hemolytic titration of C3, *Biochemistry* **7**:2997.

Shin, H. S., Snyderman, R., Friedman, E., Mellors, A., and Mayer, M. M., 1968, Chemotactic and anaphylatoxic fragment cleaved from the fifth component of guinea pig complement, *Science* **162**:361.

Sitomer, G., Stroud, R. M., and Mayer, M. M., 1966, Reversible adsorption of C2 by EAC4: role of Mg^{2+}, enumeration of competent SAC4, two-step nature of C2a fixation and estimation of its efficiency, *Immunochemistry* **3**:57.

Stolfi, R. L., 1968, Immune lytic transformation: a state of irreversible damage generated as a result of the reaction of the eighth component in the guinea pig complement system, *J. Immunol.* **100**:46.

Stroud, R. M., Mayer, M. M., Miller, J. A., and McKenzie, A. T., 1966, C2a^d, an inactive derivative of C2 released during decay of EAC4, 2a, *Immunochemistry* **3**:163.

Tamura, N., and Nelson, R. A., 1967, Three naturally occurring inhibitors of components of complement in guinea pig and rabbit serum, *J. Immunol.* **99**:582.

Valentine, R. C., and Green, N. M., 1967, Electron microscopy of an antibody hapten complex, *J. Mol. Biol.* **27**:615.

Valet, G., and Cooper, N. R., 1974a, Isolation and characterization of the proenzyme form of C1s subunits of the first complement component, *J. Immunol.* **112**:339.

Valet, G., and Cooper, N. R., 1974b, Isolation and characterization of the proenzyme form of the C1r subunit of the first complement component, *J. Immunol.* **112**:1667.

Valet, G., and Opferkuch, W., 1975, Mechanism of complement induced cell lysis: demonstration of a three step mechanism of EAC1-8 lysis by C9 and of a nonosmotic swelling of the erythrocytes, *J. Immunol.* **115**:1028.

Vogt, W., 1974, Activation, activities and pharmacologically active products of complement, *Pharm. Rev.* **26**:125.

Wellek, B., and Opferkuch, W., 1975, A case of deficiency of the seventh component of complement in man. Biological properties of a C7-deficient serum and description of an C7 inactivating principle, *J. Clin. Exp. Immunol.* **19**:223.

Wellek, B., Hahn, H. H., and Opferkuch, W., 1975, Evidence for macrophage C3d-receptor active in phagocytosis, *J. Immunol.* **114**:1643.

Zimmermann, T. S., Arroyave, C. M., and Müller-Eberhard, H. J., 1971, A blood coagulation abnormality in rabbits, deficient in the sixth component of complement (C6) and its correction by purified C6, *J. Exp. Med.* **134**:1591.

2

Alternative Modes and Pathways of Complement Activation

HENRY GEWURZ and THOMAS F. LINT

1. Introduction

Complement (C) originally was detected by its ability to bring about cytolysis of antibody-sensitized bacteria and erythrocytes. Its name is derived from this ability to complement certain reactivities initiated by antibody. At least eleven C proteins, acting sequentially, are involved in mediating the usual antibody-initiated hemolysis. These proteins comprise the *classical,* or *primary,* C pathway, which is initiated upon interaction of erythrocyte (E) membrane antigens with receptors on the Fab portion of certain immunoglobulins (Ig), resulting in activation or exposure of a site on the immunoglobulin Fc portion which, in turn, binds with the C1q subcomponent to set the C interactions into motion. This pathway has been divided into recognition (C1q, C1r, C1s), activation (C4, C2, C3), and attack (C5, C6, C7, C8, C9) portions with respect to its function in cytolysis (Müller-Eberhard, 1972), and these interactions have recently been reviewed here (Opferkuch and Segerling, 1976) and elsewhere (Müller-Eberhard, 1975; Mayer, 1973; Ruddy *et al.,* 1972).

It is now clear that the C system mediates many reactivities that contribute to inflammation and host defense in addition to cytolysis and that the sequence can be initiated in multiple ways in addition to antigen–antibody reactions. The existence of a second pathway, alternative to but sharing with C1, C4, and C2 the ability to activate the C system at the level of C3, has recently been appreciated and has excited intense interest. It involves C3 (and C3b) itself, along with at least four or five additional interacting proteins, termed *Factor* D, *Factor* B, *properdin* (P), and *initiating factor* (IF) and/or *nephritic factor* (NF), and has been designated the

---

HENRY GEWURZ and **THOMAS F. LINT** • Department of Immunology, Rush Medical College, Chicago, Illinois

17

HENRY GEWURZ AND
THOMAS F. LINT

properdin, or *alternative, pathway.* Certain properties of the properdin system proteins are shown in Table 1. Several additional pathways to activation of the terminal C components that involve the proteins of the properdin system have been presented; one involves interaction of C1 with still undefined properdin-system factors and another involves a new enzyme termed *properdin convertase.* These considerations, some of which have recently been reviewed (Müller-Eberhard, 1975; Medicus *et al.,* 1976a), are elaborated below.

However, it should be noted that there are numerous means, alternative to both pathways just cited, by which components of C can be activated. These include the direct and indirect activation of C1s, C3 and C5 by bacterial or mammalian enzymes, and the nonenzymatic activation of C1 involving C1q by substances other than antigen–antibody complexes, including nonspecifically precipitated and coprecipitated Ig, certain polyanions and/or polyanion–polycation complexes, certain viruses, and C-reactive protein (CRP). The ubiquitous nature of these "nonimmune" activators suggests that initiation of C interactions by these means has real biologic importance. In this light, C has a role not only as a "complement" to antibody in the immune response, but also as a system that initiates and supports inflammatory and associated reactions of host defense in response to a variety of disturbances of body homeostasis. Finally, the C sequence can also be activated by heterotopically activated C components, i.e., C components activated at a site different from the one at or near which the reaction is completed.

We review herein these alternative modes and pathways of C activation, drawing in large part on recently published reviews by ourselves (Gewurz, 1972) and others. These are considered in three sections: (1) activation by agents that are not components of C, nor acting as antigens, at defined points of the primary C pathway; (2) activation involving factors of the properdin pathway; and (3) activation by heterotopically activated C components. Certain of these considerations and some of the multiple modes of initiating the C sequence at various entry points are shown in Figure 1.

It should be emphasized that we review here an area of most intense current investigation, with many of the major fundamental issues yet to be resolved. The material selected for presentation, admittedly, is influenced by the current interests and biases of the authors.

TABLE 1. Properties of the Alternative Pathway Components[a]

Protein	Molecular weight	Electrophoretic mobility	Serum concentration ($\mu g/ml$)
IF/NF	150,000	β/γ_1	trace
P	184,000	γ_2	25
B	93,000	β	200
D	24,000	α	trace
C3	180,000	β_2	1600
C3b	171,000	α_2	—
C3b-INA	100,000	β_2	25

[a]Data mainly from Müller-Eberhard (1975).

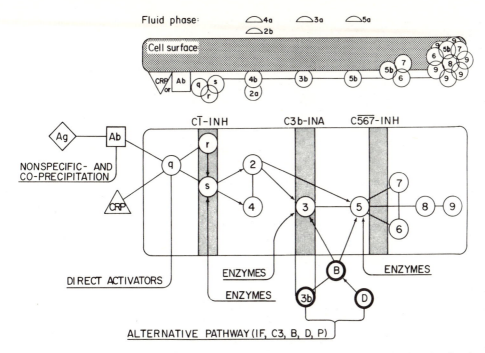

Figure 1. Diagrammatic representation of the primary C pathway (enclosed in rectangle), showing the alternative (properdin) pathway and additional modes of C activation. Enzymatic cleavages are represented by arrows; inhibitory activities, by shading. Above the pathways are shown the interactions of C components at the cell surface (stippled) and cleavage products released into the fluid phase. An important additional inhibitory factor, the C3b-INA accelerator (A·C3b-INA or β1H), has recently been described (Whaley and Ruddy, 1976).

2. Activation by Agents Not Components of C Nor Acting as Antigens

Agents that are not presently considered to be components of C nor to be acting as antigens are known to activate C via Ig and at least four other sites in the primary pathway: C1q, C1s, C3, and C5 (Figure 1). There is evidence that this also occurs at C1r and C4 and/or C2. Certain agents lead to marked consumption of only single components, while others initiate activation of the entire sequence with relative efficiency. When C is so activated at the erythrocyte surface, e.g., by CRP, hemolysis may readily ensue. However, in the fluid phase, these forms of C activation, like fluid-phase C activation generally, are relatively inefficient in bringing about the attachment and continuation of the sequence at surfaces of unsensitized bystander erythrocytes. Little information is available concerning these reactions on cells other than the erythrocyte. Twelve groups of activating agents, arranged according to their mode of entry into the primary C pathway, will be discussed.

2.1. Activation of the C Sequence by Nonspecific Aggregation of Gamma Globulins

Gamma globulins from many vertebrate species aggregated by such diverse nonimmune means as heating, ultrasonification, chemical coupling, and reaction with reduced insulin initiate sequential interaction and vigorous consumption of the classical C components with characteristics similar to C activation by immune complexes (Christian, 1960; Ishizaka and Ishizaka, 1959; Ishizaka *et al.,* 1961; Cantrell *et al.,* 1972). These interactions can result in deposition of C components and continuation of the C sequence on bystander membrane surfaces, particularly in the optimal milieu of high concentrations of acidified serum (Yachnin and Ruthenberg, 1965). However, efficient initiation or continuation of the C sequence on an unsensitized erythrocyte membrane also seems to require steps that promote the binding of the gamma globulin and/or activated C components to the target membrane surface. Thus, several agents (e.g., carbowax and tannic acid) which seem to appropriately modify both the erythrocyte membrane and gamma globulins or other serum proteins (Peck and Thomas, 1949; Cowan, 1954; Dalmasso and Müller-Eberhard, 1964; Leddy and Vaughan, 1964) induce passive lysis of unsensitized erythrocytes in the presence of fresh serum with such effectiveness that they have been offered as substitutes for antibody in assays of hemolytic C. Superimposed enzymic modification of the erythrocyte surface further facilitates attachment of C components (Dalmasso and Müller-Eberhard, 1964).

Interaction of C components with unsensitized erythrocytes also occurs at subphysiologic ionic strengths in the presence of sucrose (Rapp and Borsos, 1963) and has been interpreted to occur by a similar sequence of aggregation of gamma globulin with C activation and deposition (Mollison and Polley, 1964). Such mechanisms may be the basis for certain Coombs-positive erythrocyte disorders in which gamma globulins are not detected on the erythrocyte surface (Mollison and Polley, 1964).

Certain quantitative, if not qualitative, contrasts with immune complex-induced consumption of C seem to exist when C is activated in the fluid phase by aggregated human gamma globulin (AHGG) in the absence of membrane surfaces. AHGG seems to induce minimal if any consumption of C components C5–9 (Gewurz *et al.,* 1968c), generation of chemotactic factor from C5 (Snyderman *et al.,* 1968), or activation of C$\overline{56}$ as detected by reactive lysis (Thompson and Rowe, 1968). Whether these differences are absolute and whether they relate to the mode of antibody modification, the participation of antigen or membrane receptors, or to still other factors is not yet known.

2.2. Activation of the C Sequence by Interaction of a Staphylococcal Membrane Protein (Protein A) with the Fc Portion of the Immunoglobulin Molecule

A cell-wall protein of *Staphylococcus aureus,* termed *protein A,* can precipitate most of the normal human serum gamma globulins and myeloma proteins. It acts at the Fc portion of the molecule rather than at the antigen-combining site (Forsgren and Sjoquist, 1966). Precipitates prepared with protein A induce potent Arthus reactions when inoculated into rabbits (Gustafsen *et al.,* 1967) as well as marked depletion of hemolytic C activity when preincubated in normal serum (Sjoquist and Stalenheim, 1969); the latter involves extensive consumption of each of the primary pathway components (Kronvall and Gewurz, 1970; Stalenheim *et al.,* 1973). Accordingly, erythrocytes passively coated with protein A are lysed upon addition of fresh normal human or guinea pig serum (Stalenheim *et al.,* 1973).

2.3. Activation of the C Sequence by Direct Interaction of Polyanions with C1q

Multiple polyanions activate the primary C pathway by direct interaction with C1q. The first polyanion appreciated to do so was polyinosinic acid, which, in contrast to related polynucleotides, activates C1 and later-acting C components (Yachnin *et al.*, 1964) and brings about C-mediated hemolysis of unsensitized bystander erythrocytes (Yachnin and Ruthenberg, 1965). Only C1q of the C1 subcomponents loses its hemolytic function during preincubations with polyinosinic acid, and experiments in which this agent neither aggregated Ig nor acted as an antigen indicated that it initiates the C sequence by direct activation of C1q (Yachnin *et al.*, 1964). Similarly, DNA precipitates C1q from chelated human serum (Agnello *et al.*, 1970) and depletes hemolytic C activity (Agnello *et al.*, 1969); indeed, it has a greater affinity for C1q than has aggregated human gamma globulin (Volanakis and Stroud, 1973).

Certain other polyanions, including heparin (reviewed by Rent *et al.*, 1975), dextran sulfate (Loos *et al.*, 1974), polyvinyl sulfonate (Loos *et al.*, 1974), polyanethol sulfonate (liquid) (Loos *et al.*, 1974), carrageenin (Borsos *et al.*, 1965), cellulose sulfate (Eisen and Loveday, 1970), and SP 54 (Walb *et al.*, 1971; Loos *et al.*, 1972) also interact with C1 directly, probably at the level of C1q (Borsos *et al.*, 1965; Loos *et al.*, 1974), to bring about depletion of hemolytic C activity. Thus the ability to react with C1q and to deplete C1 seems to be a property shared by many highly polyanionic substances.

2.4. Activation of the C Sequence at the Level of C1q by Polyanion–Polycation Interactions

The interaction of certain polyanions with polycations, like the interaction of antibody with antigen, leads to a particularly marked activation of the first component of C. Heparin and protamine, in amounts far below those required for complement depletion by either agent alone, induce a virtually complete depletion of total hemolytic complement activity in fresh human serum with a predominant effect on C1. Under appropriate reaction conditions, C4 and C2 are depleted as well (Rent *et al.*, 1975). This consumption seems to occur via transient reactivity with C1 at the level of C1q; immunoglobulins are not required (Fiedel *et al.*, 1976). It seems to be limited by the ability to free heparin to potentiate the activity of CĪ-INH (Fiedel *et al.*, 1976) and perhaps also by the direct effect of heparin on the early-acting C components (Loos *et al.*, 1976).

Leonard and Thorne (1961) and Willoughby *et al.* (1973) observed that interactions of DNA and lysozyme deplete C activity in guinea pig serum; the latter investigators showed that this occurs via an activation of the classical C pathway, involves depletion of all the classical C component activities, and results in the generation of anaphylatoxin. Similarly, McCall *et al.* (1974) found that interaction between the counterions heparin and nitroblue tetrazolium results in activation of the primary C pathway and depletion of the classical C components. Therefore, it is not unlikely that C consumption initiated by interaction of polyanions and polycations is a commonly occurring phenomenon, which has a role in the initiation of certain inflammatory reactions.

Interestingly, this C activation is markedly potentiated in the presence of CRP, a trace serum factor that is also reactive with C1q and that elevates markedly in concentration (up to a thousandfold) during the acute inflammatory response. In recent experiments, amounts of heparin and protamine that together in the absence of CRP, or singly in the presence of CRP, had no effect on C1 or total C hemolytic activity, led to extensive activation of C1 and the classical C pathway when small amounts of CRP were present. Similar results were obtained when DNA, chondroitin sulfate, hyaluronic acid, or dextran sulfate were used as the model polyanion or when poly-L-lysine (4000 daltons) was used as the polycation. It therefore seems that the polyanion–polycation interaction can lead to even more extensive C activation than was first appreciated, and this is most evident when these reactions are performed under conditions approaching those present during the acute inflammatory response (Claus *et al.*, 1977).

2.5. Activation of the C Sequence at C1q by Direct Interaction with Viruses

Recently, it was found that a number of RNA viruses are inactivated upon interaction with fresh human serum by a process requiring C4 and C2 but not immunoglobulins (Welsh *et al.*, 1975). Incubation of the Moloney leukemia virus with fresh human serum was found to result in consumption of C1, C4, C2, C3, C5, and C9 as well as absorption of C1q and later-acting components of the classical C pathway to the viral surface, even in the absence of antibody (Cooper *et al.*, 1976). Similar results were obtained when vesicular stomatitis virus was used (Mills *et al.*, 1976). It was concluded that C1q in human serum interacts directly with these viruses in the apparent absence of antibody with resulting activation of the classical C pathway, deposition of C components on the viral surface, and viral lysis, and suggested that this natural resistance mechanism may limit oncornavirus infection in man.

2.6. Activation of the C Sequence by C-Reactive Protein at the Level of C1q

C-reactive protein (CRP) has now been shown to effectively activate the primary pathway at the level of C1q. CRP was described by Tillett and Francis (1930), and has long been known to appear in the sera of individuals during reactions of inflammation and tissue destruction. It has an average molecular weight of 120,000 to 140,000 daltons (Gotschlich and Edelman, 1965; Kushner and Somerville, 1970) and consists of six probably identical, noncovalently bound subunits (Gotschlich and Edelman, 1965). It differs from immunoglobulin in antigenicity (MacLeod and Avery, 1941), tertiary structure (Gotschlich and Edelman, 1965), homogeneity (Gotschlich and Edelman, 1965), stimuli required for formation and release (reviewed in Good, 1952), and binding specificities that, for at least certain reactivities of CRP, require calcium (Abernethy and Avery, 1941), and seem to be directed to phosphate esters and polycations generally (Gotschlich and Edelman, 1967; Volanakis and Kaplan, 1971; Siegel *et al.*, 1975). However, numerous functional similarities between CRP and immunoglobulins have been appreciated, including the ability to initiate reactions of precipitation (Tillett and Francis, 1930), agglutination (Gal and Miltenyi, 1955; Osmand *et al.*, 1975), capsular swelling

(Löfström. 1944), and enhancement of phagocytosis (Hokama *et al.,* 1962; Kind-mark, 1971). More recently, CRP has been found to bind selectively to T (but not B) lymphocytes and to platelets and to inhibit certain of their functions (Mortensen *et al.,* 1975; Fiedel and Gewurz, 1976).

The functional similarities between CRP and Ig were found to extend to the ability to activate the C sequence. Kaplan and Volanakis (1974) showed that interactions of CRP with C-polysaccharide (CPS) or the choline phosphatides sphingomyelin or lecithin in human serum resulted in consumption of C1, C4, and C2, with electrophoretic conversion of C3, and in an accompanying study, Volanakis and Kaplan (1974) showed that this occurred at the level of C1q. Siegel *et al.* (1974, 1975) observed that protamine and certain other polycations, including polymers of poly-L-lysine, histones, myelin basic proteins, and leukocyte cationic proteins, also activated the C system via CRP and, along with reactions between CRP and CPS, led to extensive consumption of C1–5. CRP was found to react with cell-bound CPS to initiate the C-dependent reactions of adherence, phagocytosis (for which the presence of CRP was required), and cytolysis (Osmand *et al.,* 1975; Mortensen *et al.,* 1976).

CRP, like IgG, could bind to purified C1 in the fluid phase, and this binding was markedly enhanced when CRP was aggregated or reacted with CPS. Similarly, C1 was found to bind to and transfer from CRP which had been reacted with its cell-bound substrates. Direct binding studies involving radiolabeled CRP and C1q, respectively, C1q-mediated hemagglutination and C1q inhibition of C1 binding, each confirmed that the CRP–C1 interaction involved the participation of C1q (Siegel *et al.,* 1976). Thus, CRP is remarkably similar to immunoglobulins in its ability to react with and activate the C system, and has been so represented in Figure 1.

It is of interest that, as a naturally occurring host factor with a widely distributed binding specificity(ies) and the capacity to activate the C system to its full biological potential, CRP fits well into the philosophical framework drawn by Pillemer *et al.* (1954) for properdin at the time of its discovery.

2.7. Activation of the Primary C Pathway at the Level of C1r

The C1r subcomponent of C1 has been postulated to be both a bridge between C1q and C1s and the protease responsible for the enzymatic activation of C1s (Naff and Ratnoff, 1968; de Bracco and Stroud, 1971; Ziccardi and Cooper, 1976). Recently, Assimeh and Painter (1975) have presented evidence that C1r may serve as a second point in C1 for attachment to immunoglobulin, involving a site on the Fc portion of IgG distinct from the C1q-specific site. Evidence has also been presented, using DNP-polylysine haptens, that the lysine portion of the hapten–antibody complex interacts directly with C1r and, to a lesser extent, with C1s to activate C1 (Goers *et al.,* 1976). Thus it would seem that C1r must also be considered as an additional site by which the C system can be activated.

2.8. Direct Activation of the Classical C Pathway at the Level of C1s

One of the first alternative pathways to activation of C is now known to involve direct activation of the C1s portion of the C1 macromolecule. Earlier observations that plasmin (directly) and streptokinase (via activation of plasmin) activate C1 under conditions that exclude an underlying antigen–antibody interaction (Pillemer *et al.*, 1953c; Lepow *et al.*, 1954) were extended to show that both plasmin and trypsin activate the isolated C1s proesterase to full esterase activity on C4, C2, and synthetic amino ester substrates (Ratnoff and Naff, 1967). Substantial consumption of hemolytic C1, C4, and C2 activities, with only modest reduction of C3–9 were observed (Pillemer *et al.*, 1953c; Lepow *et al.*, 1954), and under the optimal condition of concentrated acidified serum, C-dependent lysis of unsensitized erythrocytes could ensue (Yachnin and Ruthenberg, 1965). Kallikrein has also been shown to activate C1s (Donaldson, 1968). Therefore components of at least two other major blood enzyme cascades can activate C by direct interaction with C1s. It has been suggested that such a reaction sequence may be operative in hereditary angioedema.

2.9. Possible Direct Activation of the Primary C Pathway at the Level of C4 and C2

Few reports demonstrating direct activation of C4 and C2 have appeared. A euglobulin separated from the serum of the nurse shark, upon activation by such procedures as incubation at 37°C, leads to selective inactivation of C4 hemolytic activity *in vitro* and *in vivo* (Jensen, 1969). A substance in the venom of the cottonmouth moccasin (Zarco *et al.*, 1967), as well as factors from several additional snake venoms (Birdsey *et al.*, 1971), seem to deplete C4, C2, and C3–9 without the depletion or requirement of C1. Similarly, factors have been separated from the exotoxin of *Clostridium histolyticum* (Goldlust *et al.*, 1968) and from the venom of the snake *Lachesis muta* (Birdsey *et al.*, 1971) that lead to the selective inactivation of hemolytic C2 and C3–9. Whether these interactions are associated with the generation of biological activities remains to be seen.

2.10. Direct Activation of C3 (Excluding the Properdin Pathway)

Pathways to direct activation of C3 include cleavage by plasmin, by which chemotactic activity was first observed to be released from C3 (Ward, 1967); trypsin, which induces the release of both an anaphylatoxin and a neutrophil chemotactic factor (Bokisch *et al.*, 1969); tissue proteases, which also release chemotactic activity (Hill and Ward, 1969); and thrombin (Bokisch *et al.*, 1969). The capacity of enzymes generated during hemostasis and tissue damage to release biological activities from C3 emphasizes the potential importance of this C component in nonimmune as well as immune inflammation.

2.11. Direct Activation of C5 (Excluding the Properdin Pathway)

Trypsin and lysosomal enzymes derived from peripheral leukocytes cleave C5 with the release of an anaphylatoxin and a neutrophil chemotactic factor (Jensen, 1967; Ward and Hill, 1970; Taubman *et al.*, 1970; Snyderman *et al.*, 1972; Arroyave and Müller-Eberhard, 1973; Goldstein and Weissmann, 1974). A substance in the venom of the brown recluse spider, *Loxoceles reclusa,* is reported to induce cleavage of C5 via still unidentified serum factors (Kniker and Morgan, 1967). It has been emphasized that agents in this category frequently have been among those stated to generate anaphylatoxin by extra-immune-reaction mechanisms (Vogt and Schmidt, 1966); the hypothesis that C5 represents an anaphylatoxinogen that is accessible to pathways of activation that are alternate to immune complexes interacting with early-acting C components brought these observations into perspective (Jensen, 1967). Possible direct activation of C5 by membrane constituents of normal or altered cells is discussed in the next section.

2.12. Possible Direct Activation of C Components at the Cell Membrane

Silicic acid (Landsteiner, 1901), tannic acid (Peck and Thomas, 1949; Leddy and Vaughan, 1964), and polyethylene glycol or Carbowax 4000 (Cowan, 1954; Dalmasso and Müller-Eberhard, 1964) induce the attachment of C components to unsensitized erythrocytes in the presence and/or upon the addition of autologous or absorbed serum. In the presence of favorable reaction conditions, the C cascade can continue to hemolysis. This has suggested that these agents expose or activate a membrane substrate that reacts directly with components of C at the early stages of the sequence (Peck and Thomas, 1949; Cowan, 1954). That these agents also modify and/or favor adsorption of certain other serum proteins, including gamma globulins, has already been noted.

Similarly, in experiments inspired by the peculiar susceptibility of paroxysmal nocturnal hemoglobinuria cells to C-mediated hemolysis, pretreatment of unsensitized normal erythrocytes with any of several enzymes (trypsin, papain, ficin, or neuraminidase) was found to render them lysable by purified components of C corresponding to C5–C9 (Yachnin et al., 1961; Yachnin, 1965, 1966). This suggested that a membrane substrate which could directly activate the C system, in this case at a later step (C5) in the sequence, was exposed or generated. It has been generally found that cells treated in these ways are much more susceptible to C-mediated hemolysis than are untreated normal erythrocytes and that the enzyme modifications favor the binding of C components (Yachnin, 1965; Rosse and Dacie, 1966; Logue et al., 1973). However, the degree to which this corresponds to direct activation of the C system by membrane constituents as opposed to enhanced binding of and/or reactivity with C components activated in other ways (e.g., by conventional immune reactions in the fluid phase or on the membrane surface or during purification) is not yet clear.

Platts-Mills and Ishizaka (1974) have shown that rabbit erythrocytes undergo C-dependent lysis in human serum by an antibody-independent mechanism involving components of the properdin system, and Zimmerman and Kolb (1976) have shown that platelet–serum interactions result in the assembly and attachment of the C attack mechanism in autologous sera. The factors involved in the initiation of these reactions, and their relationship and implications to direct activation of the primary C pathway, is yet to be elaborated.

Direct activation of the C cascade by certain bacteria (Sterzl, 1963; Miler et al., 1964) and bacterial surface structures (Skarnes, 1965) has been reported, but the question of involvement of natural antibody has persisted. C activation by interaction of virus surface constituents with C1q has recently been shown and was discussed in Section 2.5.

HENRY GEWURZ AND
THOMAS F. LINT

3. The Alternative or Properdin Pathway of C Activation

3.1. Introduction

In 1954, driven by an interest in natural defense mechanisms and perhaps prepared by his then-recent finding of antibody-independent activation of C1 by plasmin, Pillemer and his colleagues described an antibody-independent pathway to C activation that involved a new serum protein termed *properdin*. In the ensuing years, this was widely accepted and investigated, but later it was successively challenged, doubted, and ridiculed. By 1961, virtually no papers concerning properdin were appearing from the major laboratories investigating the C system. The recent rediscovery of this alternative pathway has again brought these earlier studies to attention. They are reviewed here in some detail, not only because they provide the basis for the terminology currently in use, but because they also have provided concepts and methodology that were integral in the more recent investigations establishing the existence and features of this pathway.

3.2. Historic Aspects

Yeast cells (Coca, 1914) and the insoluble yeast extracts zymin (Whitehead *et al.,* 1925) and zymosan (Pillemer and Ecker, 1941) originally prepared for this purpose, bring about depletion of classical C3 hemolytic activity with relatively little apparent loss of C1, C4, and C2 when preincubated with relatively undiluted serum at 37°C (Pillemer *et al.,* 1942; Pillemer, 1943). Hypothesizing absorption of C3 as the underlying mechanism, Pillemer *et al.* (1953a,b) sought to purify human C3 by absorption to and elution from zymosan, but the reaction was found to be much more complex: Other serum factors were required for zymosan to fix C3 and when so fixed, its biological activity could not be recovered even by a variety of procedures. Attention thus was shifted to the reaction(s) that lead to C3 consumption by zymosan and, after initial reservations (Pillemer, 1953a,b), led to the announcement of an alternative pathway to C activation (Pillemer *et al.,* 1954, 1955, 1956). It was thought to be initiated by a newly discovered serum protein termed *properdin* ("destructive substance") rather than by antibody; to require the participation of serum factors similar to or identical with C1, C4, and C2 as well as Mg^{2+}; and, under reaction conditions similar to those optimal for classical C hemolysis, to lead to the preferential consumption and binding of C3 (Pillemer *et al.,* 1954). In addition, the ability of zymosan to fix C3 was found to be shared by many other high-molecular-weight polysaccharides, polysaccharide complexes, and bacterial cell walls (Pillemer *et al.,* 1955), and these reactivities were thought to have a fundamental role in host defense (Pillemer *et al.,* 1954; Pillemer *et al.,* 1956). Certain of the issues raised by these investigations and the consequent supporting and challenging studies of others have been reviewed (Lepow, 1961; Mayer, 1961; Muschel, 1961; Osler, 1961; Austen and Cohn, 1963) and will be summarized briefly.

3.2.1. Antibody

It was emphasized initially that antibody is not required for properdin-mediated activities (Pillemer *et al.,* 1954). Properdin was thought to interact directly with various foreign substances and had many features, including lack of serologic specificity, distinguishing it from known natural antibodies. However, natural antibodies to zymosan were found in normal sera (Nelson, 1958), and specific antibodies were found to initiate bactericidal reactions attributed to properdin (Muschel, 1961). Subsequently, a serum factor absorbed by zymosan at 0°C and required for zymosan to interact with properdin and C was found. This 0°C factor further displayed serologic specificity in reacting with various polysaccharide and bacterial cell-wall antigens (Blum *et al.,* 1959a; Blum, 1964). The failure to recognize this feature of properdin previously was considered an "error of omission" (Lepow, 1961). The 0°C factor was considered to be a natural antibody separable from naturally occurring antizymosan agglutinins (Lepow, 1961; Blum, 1964; Lepow, 1965) but was not classified in modern terminology. Major questions concerning the nature of natural antibodies and recognition factors have been discussed (Franek *et al.,* 1961; Boyden, 1966; Landy and Weidenz, 1964).

3.2.2. Properdin

Properdin was defined as a serum factor that is removed by absorption with zymosan at 17°C and required for zymosan to consume C3 at 37°C (in the presence of optimal amounts of 0°C factor).

3.2.3. Complement-like Factors

It was appreciated that early-acting C components or remarkably similar factors were required for zymosan to deplete C3, because this reaction did not occur in sera depleted of C1, C4, or C2 ('R1, R4, R2') heated serum or serum pretreated with immune complexes at 37°C (Pillemer *et al.,* 1953a,b). However, some contrasts to C were observed, most notably an inability of streptokinase-activated plasmin, which depletes the hemolytic activity of the early-acting C components, to deplete the serum factors mediating the C3 consuming activity of zymosan. At first it was interpreted that the properdin-utilizing and hemolytic C activities probably resided in the same chemical structure (Pillemer *et al.,* 1953a,b), but further experimentation indicated that properdin reacted with two new serum factors alternate to C1, C4, and C2 in order to consume C3. These were termed as follows:

Factor A (Hydrazine-Sensitive Factor). Like C4, this was sensitive to hydrazine, but less sensitive in serum than is C4 to addition of streptokinase at 37°C or of immune precipitates and C1 at 0°C; it was more depleted than C4 in R1 and R3 (Pensky *et al.,* 1959).

Factor B (Heat-Labile Factor). Like C2, this was labile at 56°C for $\frac{1}{2}$ hr, but less sensitive in serum than is C2 to addition of streptokinase at 37°C or of immune precipitates at 0°C; it was more depleted in R2, but more sensitive to heat and to zymosan (Blum *et al.,* 1959b).

A role for C1 was not included in this modified scheme.

3.2.4. Zymosan–C Complexes

An intermediate was formed between zymosan and the reactive serum factors (P–Z complex) that, in its ability to consume C3 in serum-EDTA, displayed many similarities to the lysis of $EAC\overline{142}$ by C3 in serum-EDTA (Leon, 1956, 1957, 1958, 1960).

3.2.5. Preferential Reactivity with C3

HENRY GEWURZ AND
THOMAS F. LINT

Zymosan added to normal human serum was found to deplete C3 with minimal reduction of C1, C4, and C2. By contrast, immune complexes induced substantial depletion of C1, C4, and C2 with minimal reduction of C3. Therefore, zymosan was interpreted to bring about a preferential consumption of C3 (Pillemer *et al.,* 1942; Pillemer *et al.,* 1954). Later, it was cautioned that this could represent an artifact of the assay systems then extant. Both zymosan and small amounts of immune complexes, used in intended analogy to complexes formed with natural antibody, were shown to consume equal numbers of units of both C1, C4 (C1 and C4 assayed in tandem), and C3, but since there was less C3 activity available, C3 showed a much greater percentage of depletion (Nelson, 1958).

In summary, the properdin system was eventuallly presented by its proponents as an alternate pathway to the activation of the terminal C components, which was activated by certain predominantly polysaccharide antigens. It was stated to consist of a naturally occurring specific antibody (0°C factor), properdin, and at least two additional proteins, Factors A and B, which are similar to C4 and C2, respectively, although having properties somewhat different from these complement components. Their interaction, during which an intermediate capable of consuming C3 was formed, resulted in a preferential depletion of the terminal C components.

3.3. Rediscovery of the Properdin System

The work of many investigators, particularly Nelson (1958) and Muschel (1961), emphasized that the properdin system indeed operated with a specificity that was dependent on factors indistinguishable from antibody and that the apparent preferential reactivity with C3 was a mathematical artifact. This refutation was generally accepted. With these special features of the properdin system effectively (and emotionally) challenged, the importance, if not the existence, of properdin, Factor A, and Factor B was questioned, and these were considered by many to be manifestations of antibody and/or known C components. Despite a continuing advance in the physicochemical definition of properdin as a distinct protein (Pensky *et al.,* 1968), there remained a distinct negative stigma associated with the investigations that had advanced the existence and the importance of this system, clearly reflected in the review articles of the early 1960s.

It was approximately 10 years later that the activity and existence of this pathway began to be reappreciated. As seen by the present authors, it was again brought to attention by studies of the interactions between endotoxic lipopolysaccharides (LPS) and the C system, which clearly established that certain substances (e.g., LPS and zymosan), indeed, could induce preferential consumption of C3–C9 with relative sparing of the early-acting C components (Bladen *et al.,* 1967), a pattern that contrasted markedly with that seen upon C activation by classical immune complexes or aggregated human gamma globulin. This finding was fortified when it was found that *each* of the six terminal C components was consumed in the process (Gewurz *et al.,* 1968c), with generation of anaphylatoxins (Lichtenstein *et al.,* 1969) and neutrophil chemotactic factors (Snyderman *et al.,* 1968, 1969). These reactions were further described (Gewurz *et al.,* 1968a; Mergenhagen *et al.,* 1968; Day *et al.,* 1970; Gewurz, 1971; reviewed in Gewurz *et al.,* 1969b; Gewurz, 1971b,

1972; Mergenhagen *et al.*, 1969) and found to occur in a variety of immunoglobulin-deficient sera (Gewurz *et al.*, 1970b), emphasizing the possibility that an alternative pathway analogous to that proposed by Pillemer *et al.* was involved (e.g., Gewurz *et al.*, 1968b, 1969a).

This possibility was reinforced upon investigation of C-component depletion patterns (profiles) in patients with renal diseases: the early- and late-acting portions of the C sequence were depleted in patients with systemic lupus erythematosus and serum sickness nephritis, whereas only the late-acting components were depleted in acute glomerulonephritis and hypocomplementemic chronic glomerulonephritis (Gewurz *et al.*, 1968b, 1970a). These contrasting depletion patterns were interpreted to reflect two distinctly different modes of C activation dependent either on different antibodies or other serum factors. These contrasts and interpretations, along with the then-recent purification and characterization of properdin (Pensky *et al.*, 1968), led to an investigation of serum properdin titers in the renal diseases just mentioned. Properdin levels were indeed found to be decreased selectively in the two diseases associated with preferential depletion of C3–C9 (Gewurz *et al.*, 1969a), and this finding clearly refocused the issues raised by Pillemer in the clinical as well as the experimental perspectives. Shortly thereafter, in extension of this latter investigation, properdin was found deposited on the renal tissues of patients with acute glomerulonephritis and hypocomplementemic chronic glomerulonephritis (Westberg *et al.*, 1971).

Appreciation of an alternative pathway of C activation also derived from studies of a C-consuming activity found in the venoms of a variety of species of cobra (CVF) (Flexner and Noguchi, 1903; Nelson, 1966; Müller-Eberhard *et al.*, 1966; Müller-Eberhard and Fjellström, 1971; Birdsey *et al.*, 1971). Cobra venom, long known to preferentially deplete C3 in whole serum via a heat-labile factor(s) (reviewed in Gewurz, 1972), was first thought to inhibit C3 selectively, but later it was found to generate anaphylatoxin from C3 (Cochrane and Müller-Eberhard, 1968), to generate neutrophil chemotactic activity from C5 or later-acting C components (Shin *et al.*, 1969), to deplete *each* of the C3–9 component activities (Shin *et al.*, 1969), and to induce C-mediated lysis of bystander erythrocytes (Pickering *et al.*, 1969; Ballow and Cochrane, 1969). This indicated that CVF was activating the entire terminal C-component sequence rather than inhibiting a single C component. Studies were directed to the 5 S serum beta globulin through which it operated (Müller-Eberhard *et al.*, 1966; Gewurz *et al.*, 1971a), and the possibility that the CVF cofactor might be involved in endotoxin-induced C depletion was proposed (Gewurz *et al.*, 1969b). CVF emerged as perhaps the critical tool that allowed the establishment of the existence of the alternative pathway.

At this point multiple lines of evidence rapidly accumulated to establish the existence of the properdin pathway and to initiate its definitive characterization. First, certain guinea pig immunoglobulins and, later, F(ab′)₂ fragments, were shown to induce preferential consumption of the six terminal C components selectively in a manner similar to that seen when LPS and zymosan were used (Osler *et al.*, 1969; Sandberg *et al.*, 1971a,b). This clarified earlier observations of the peculiar C consumption induced by F(ab′)₂ fragments (Schur and Becker, 1963; Cerrotini and Fitch, 1968), later shown to be independent of C1q (Isliker *et al.*, 1967; Reid, 1971) and, for the first time, defined a host factor capable of initiating this pattern of C depletion. These incisive investigations were later extended to show directly the relationship of this type of C activation to the alternative C pathway (Sandberg *et al.*, 1971a). Second, earlier collaborative studies, which showed that a C3-consuming intermediate was formed during the LPS-C interaction, were extended to show that the activity of this intermediate could *not* be inhibited by amounts of anti-C2 antiserum which readily inhibited the ability of EAC$\overline{142}$ to react with C3, implying the existence of a "new" C3-converting enzyme on LPS distinct from the known (C4b2a) C3-convertase (Marcus *et al.*, 1971). Third, the elegant detection and definition of guinea pigs lacking C4, establishment of a colony of such animals, and elucidation of the range of LPS-induced reactivities in such animals and their sera (including the demonstration of extensive consumption of C3) clearly displayed the presence of an alternative means of activating the terminal C components (Ellman *et al.*, 1970; Frank *et al.*, 1971). Finally, the definitive classic investigations of Götze and Müller-Eberhard (1971) isolating the serum factor reactive with CVF and identifying it as Factor B of the properdin system, as well as studies by Goodkofsky and Lepow (1971) and Alper *et al.* (1973), placed the various previous indications of an alternative pathway in a sharp new molecular perspective, established the existence of the properdin pathway and provided the framework for future studies, as reviewed in the next section.

3.4. Current Understanding of the Properdin System

3.4.1. Chemistry of the Alternative Pathway Factors

Details of the properties of the known alternative pathway components have recently been reviewed (Müller-Eberhard, 1975), and some are shown in Table 1.

Factor B (B). This factor is a heat-labile beta pseudoglobulin with a molecular weight of 93,000 daltons. It is also known as C3 proactivator (C3PA) and glycine-rich beta globulin (GBG) (Alper *et al.*, 1973). The activated form of Factor B ($\overline{B}$) possesses C3-convertase enzymatic activity (Götze and Müller-Eberhard, 1971). Factor B is split into two fragments by $\overline{D}$ (see below), one of which migrates as a gamma globulin and possesses the enzymatic activity. This fragment has variously been called Bb, C3 activator (C3A), β_2-glycoprotein II, or glycine-rich gamma globulin (GGG). The nonactive fragment has alpha electrophoretic mobility and has been called Ba or glycine-rich alpha globulin (GAG). While cleavage of B is associated with the appearance of C3-convertase activity and is often used as an indicator of alternative pathway activation, it is now clear that the molecule need not be cleaved to be activated (Schreiber *et al.*, 1975; Fearon and Austen, 1975a).

Factor D (D). This factor, also known as C3PA-convertase, acts enzymatically to activate and cleave B (Müller-Eberhard and Götze, 1972; Hunsicker *et al.*, 1973). It is an alpha euglobulin of 24,000 daltons and has serine esterase activity, since it is inactivated by diisopropylfluorophosphate (DFP) (Fearon *et al.*, 1974). It also exists in serum as a DFP-insensitive precursor, designated D. The nature of the conversion of D to $\overline{D}$ in serum is poorly understood at present, though in isolated systems trypsin has been used to induce this activation (Fearon *et al.*, 1974).

Properdin (P). This factor is a euglobulin of 184,000 daltons, which is composed of 4 subunits of about 46,000 daltons (Müller-Eberhard, 1975). In nearly all studies of properdin performed to date, it has been isolated in an active form, designated $\overline{P}$, which reacts directly with C3 (Stitzel and Spitzer, 1974; Schreiber *et al.*, 1975;

Fearon and Austen, 1975a) and C3b (Schreiber *et al.*, 1975; Fearon and Austen, 1975a,b), and may initiate or enhance the formation of C3- and C5-convertases as a result of these reactions, but the mechanism by which P becomes activated in serum is unclear. One report suggests that conversion of P to $\overline{P}$ is due to the action of an enzyme, properdin convertase (Stitzel and Spitzer, 1974). It has been reported that $\overline{P}$ reacts with C3b, while native P reacts only with $\overline{C3bB}$ (Medicus *et al.*, 1976a).

Nephritic Factor (NF). This factor is a 150,000-dalton gamma globulin that is difficult to separate from IgG, but that has been clearly shown to be a distinct protein (Vallota *et al.*, 1974). It is found in an activated form in sera of patients with hypocomplementemic nephritis (Spitzer *et al.*, 1969) and causes C3 activation by a pathway requiring B and $\overline{D}$ (Schreiber *et al.*, 1975). An analogue of NF has been found in normal sera using anti-NF antiserum (Vallota *et al.*, 1974) and may represent a precursor form of NF, termed *initiating factor* (IF).

C3. This factor is a 180,000-dalton beta-2 globulin that seems to be both a component and a substrate of the initial alternative pathway convertase (Schreiber *et al.*, 1975; Fearon and Austen, 1975b; Medicus *et al.*, 1976a). It is identical to Factor A, the hydrazine-sensitive factor of the alternative pathway described by Pillemer and his colleagues (Müller-Eberhard and Götze, 1972).

C3b. This factor, the major cleavage product of C3, is a 171,000-dalton alpha-2 globulin possessing numerous biological activities and can form a C3-convertase in the presence of B, $\overline{D}$, and Mg^{2+} (Müller-Eberhard and Götze, 1972).

C3b Inactivator (C3b-INA). This factor, also known as *conglutinin activating factor* (KAF), exerts an essential control on alternative-pathway activation. It is a 100,000-dalton beta globulin, which cleaves and inactivates C3b (Lachmann and Müller-Eberhard, 1968; Ruddy *et al.*, 1972b; Gitlin *et al.*, 1975), and probably is identical to the properdin-receptor-destroying enzyme (Medicus *et al.*, 1976a,b).

3.4.2. Enzymes of the Alternative Pathway

It is now clear that there are two major early-acting enzymes in the properdin pathway and, surprisingly, both are C3-convertases. They act sequentially; the first requires native C3, while the second requires C3b. The reaction mechanisms of the C3b-dependent convertase are generally agreed upon and are shown diagrammatically in Figure 1. The same components also generate a C5-convertase, and its assembly is described later.

The C3-Dependent C3-Convertase. This enzyme, which involves B, D, and other serum factors, is the first enzyme formed and seems to be required for activation of the alternative pathway by such substances as zymosan or inulin. There are, at this writing, two views concerning the nature of this initial convertase. One suggests that the nephritic factor analogue (IF) interacts with C3, B, $\overline{D}$, and Mg^{2+}, in the absence of properdin, to form an enzyme capable of cleaving C3 to C3b. In this view, properdin is not required in the initial enzyme, but IF is (Medicus *et al.*, 1976a). The other hypothesis suggests that C3, B, $\overline{D}$, and Mg^{2+} alone form this C3-convertase, and $\overline{P}$ stabilizes this enzyme; no role for IF is postulated at this stage of the sequence (Fearon and Austen, 1975a,b). There is essential agreement as to the events subsequent to the formation of the initial convertase. The C3b generated by this convertase, in turn, initiates the formation of the second C3-convertase.

HENRY GEWURZ AND
THOMAS F. LINT

The C3b-Dependent C3-Convertase. This enzyme was shown by two separate lines of evidence. The first followed the purification of the appropriate components when it was found that the addition of $\overline{D}$ to B and Mg^{2+} did not cause conversion of purified C3 unless C3b was also present (Müller-Eberhard and Götze, 1972). Thus, C3b was shown to initiate the assembly of a labile C3-convertase ($C\overline{3bB}$), which was later shown to be stabilized by the binding of properdin or NF (Daha *et al.*, 1976a; Medicus *et al.*, 1976b; Schreiber *et al.*, 1976). This enzyme acts on native C3 to produce additional C3b and thus to function as part of a positive feedback loop. Such a mechanism would necessarily require control to prevent the complete utilization of C3 whenever C3b is formed. This limiting role is performed by the C3b inactivator, a protein found in all normal human sera. Studies on its activity have contributed the second line of evidence for the existence of the C3b-dependent C3-convertase. When C3b-INA is immunochemically removed from serum (Lachmann *et al.*, 1973), or when it is congenitally deficient (Alper *et al.*, 1972), spontaneous activation of the alternative pathway occurs, resulting in the generation of C3b, which in turn initiates the virtually total cleavage of the available C3. Normal C3 turnover is restored upon readdition of C3b-INA both *in vitro* (Lachmann *et al.*, 1973) and *in vivo* (Ziegler *et al.*, 1975).

Cobra venom factor (CVF) has been useful in delineating the molecular interactions of the C3b-dependent C3-convertase. Like C3b, CVF reacts with Mg^{2+}, B, and $\overline{D}$ to form a C3-convertase (Cooper, 1973). CVF binds to purified B in the presence of Mg^{2+} to generate minimal but distinct C3-converting activity; the binding is reversible, and B is not cleaved. However, B is cleaved when $\overline{D}$ is present; the binding between $\overline{B}$ and CVF is much more stable, and full C3-converting activity is realized (Cooper, 1973). This reaction is analogous to C3b-initiated generation of the C3-convertase and may be explained by the finding (Alper and Balavitch, 1976) that CVF is cobra C3b.

The C5-Convertase. This enzyme seems to acquire full activity upon the addition of a second C3b molecule to the $C\overline{3bB}$ enzyme (Medicus *et al.*, 1976a,b; Daha *et al.*, 1976b). The $C\overline{3bB}$ enzyme is analogous to $C\overline{4b2a}$ of the classical pathway; formation of both enzymes requires Mg^{2+} and a serine esterase ($\overline{D}$ or $C\overline{1s}$, respectively), and both are labile, decaying with loss of $\overline{B}$ and C2a, respectively. When the convertases cleave C3 and bind C3b, the enzymes $C\overline{3bB3b}$ or $C\overline{4b2a3b}$ are formed; both are C5-convertases and susceptible to decay or the action of the C3b inactivator. The enzymatic activity for both substrates, C3 and C5, seems to reside on the decayable fragments, $\overline{B}$ or C2a (Figure 1). No analogue of $\overline{P}$ has been found to stabilize the classical pathway enzymes.

3.4.3. Role of P and NF

It is now clear that both $\overline{P}$ and NF stabilize the $C\overline{3bB}$ enzyme, which decays by the loss of $\overline{B}$ or through the action of C3b-INA (Schreiber *et al.*, 1975; Fearon and Austen, 1975a; Daha *et al.*, 1976a,b; Medicus *et al.*, 1976a,b). In this role, P and NF act analogously. However, an additional role for properdin has been suggested by one group in the stabilization of the *initial* C3-dependent C3-convertase (Fearon and Austen, 1975b), while another group has proposed that the NF analogue (IF) plays the essential role in the formation of this initial enzyme (Medicus *et al.*, 1976a). Whether P and NF act in an analogous fashion in stabilizing the C3-

dependent convertase, as they do in stabilizing the C3b-dependent enzyme, would seem to be a critical issue.

3.4.4. Regulation of the Properdin Pathway

The C3b-INA plays a critical role in the control of the alternative pathway. In addition to its ability to limit the availability of C3b as an initiator of the feedback loop, it has been shown to inactivate the properdin- or NF-stabilized C3- and C5-convertases (Medicus *et al.*, 1976a,b; Daha *et al.*, 1976b). Thus, C3b-INA acts to prevent the formation of these enzymes as well as to dissociate them once they are formed. An important additional inhibitory factor, the C3b-INA accelerator (A·C3b-INA or β1H), has recently been described (Whaley and Ruddy, 1976). Other regulatory mechanisms may also exist. Thus, fluid-phase C3b has been postulated to cause dissembly of the C3b-dependent convertase (Schreiber *et al.*, 1975; Medicus *et al.*, 1976a). Longer ago, an alpha-2 globulin inhibitor to a zymosan-bound convertase was reported in certain human sera (Willers *et al.*, 1959), but to our knowledge its characterization was not pursued.

3.4.5. Other Pathways

Additional alternative pathways to C3 activation have been proposed, requiring some of the factors just described. Using C4-deficient guinea pig serum or C2-deficient human serum, May and Frank (1973a,b) found that heavily sensitized erythrocytes could be lysed by a mechanism apparently involving C1 and components of the properdin pathway. Indeed, it has been suggested that C1s plays an essential role in the activation of the alternative pathway (Volanakis *et al.*, 1976).

A novel enzyme, properdin convertase, has been described that can cleave properdin, which in turn was reported to activate C3 and C5 directly (Stitzel and Spitzer, 1974; Spitzer *et al.*, 1976). Its place in the alternative-pathway-reaction sequence remains to be established.

Direct enzymatic cleavage of alternative pathway components provide an additional means of activating this pathway. Trypsin, plasmin, or pronase can replace $\overline{D}$ in the activation of B (Brade *et al.*, 1974) and, also, the conversion of D to $\overline{D}$ has been accomplished with trypsin (Fearon *et al.*, 1974). Leukocyte lysosomal enzymes have been shown to cause direct activation of the alternative pathway, but their site of action has not been defined (Goldstein and Weissmann, 1974).

3.4.6. Unsolved Questions

A number of questions concerning the activation and reaction mechanisms of the alternative pathway seem particularly urgent. For example, what is the initiating factor(s) and how is it activated? What is the role of immunoglobulin and of C1 in the activation of the alternative pathway? How is Factor D activated physiologically, and what are the identities and/or roles of any additional factors involved in the activation, interactions, and control of this system? Answers to these and related questions should help pave the way to an understanding of the role of the alternative pathway in health and disease and ways in which it can be interpreted and manipulated to diagnostic and therapeutic benefit.

4. Initiation of the C Sequence by Heterotopically Activated Complement Components

A third category of C activation involves a C sequence initiated at one site and completed at another (even distant) site, independent of the initiating event. Such continuation or transfer of the C cascade can occur at an unsensitized membrane in at least five groups of ways.

4.1. Classical Passive Hemolysis by Antigens Adsorbed to the Erythrocyte Surface

Antigens passively adsorbed or chemically coupled to the erythrocyte surface can initiate cell lysis in the presence of the homologous antibody and complement, even though the immune reaction is initiated by a nonerythrocytic antigen (Adler, 1950; Mayer, 1961).

4.2. Chemical Coupling of Activated C Components to Erythrocytes

It has been found that functionally active C1 can initiate lysis of an unsensitized erythrocyte to which it has been coupled by chemical bonds when components C2–C9 are provided (Inai et al., 1968; Linscott et al., 1969).

4.3. Activation in the Fluid Phase by Previously Activated C Components

Large amounts of certain purified C components, however activated, can initiate C deposition onto bystanding unsensitized erythrocytes, albeit with low orders of efficiency, and the continuation of the C sequence to bystander hemolysis. Thus, fluid-phase $\overline{C1}$ can induce binding of C4 and $\overline{C42}$ (Müller-Eberhard and Lepow, 1965); $\overline{C4^{oxy}23}$ can induce binding of C5 (Götze and Müller-Eberhard, 1970) and $\overline{C1}$, plus C2–7 (Müller-Eberhard, 1968) can induce formation of sites that are capable of reacting with C8. As mentioned, binding is favored on certain enzyme-modified membranes. Attachment to the cell surface when the C sequence is activated in the fluid phase via the properdin system is also markedly enhanced when C3b is present on the bysander cell (Fearon et al., 1973) or if a cell with a C3 receptor is the target (Theofilopoulos et al., 1974).

4.4. Transfer of Free or Antibody-Bound Activated C Components

Activated $\overline{C1}$ (Borsos and Rapp, 1963) and $\overline{C5b}$ (Shin et al., 1971a; Shin et al., 1971b) have been observed to transfer from their site of activation to receptors in the states EA and EAC4, and $EAC\overline{423}$, respectively, such that the subsequent steps of the C sequence can be continued at the new site. Similarly, complexes of antibody and early-acting C components, e.g., $AC\overline{42}$, have been shown to transfer to appropriate unsensitized cells and in the presence of C3–9 (C-EDTA) to initiate their hemolysis (Willoughby and Mayer, 1965).

4.5. Reactive Lysis

35

ALTERNATIVE
MODES AND
PATHWAYS OF
COMPLEMENT
ACTIVATION

This phenomenon represents a distinct, if related, mechanism for inducing lysis of unsensitized cells initiated by a stable $\overline{C56}$ intermediate generated by C activation at a distance (Thompson and Rowe, 1968; Lachmann and Thompson, 1970; Thompson and Lachmann, 1970; Götze and Müller-Eberhard, 1970). An activated complex of C5 and C6 ($\overline{C56}$) can be formed in certain acute phase sera during C activation by certain antigens, such as zymosan. When an additional source of C7 is provided, $\overline{C567}$ is formed, which for a short time can attach to an unsensitized bystander erythrocyte to result in a cellular intermediate, which is lysable by C8 and C9.

An activity in serum recognized by its ability to inhibit the attachment of $\overline{C567}$ to bystanding cells during the short time it is capable of doing so has been described (McLeod *et al.*, 1974a). The serum components responsible have been termed $\overline{C567}$ *inhibitor* ($\overline{C567}$-INH) (McLeod *et al.*, 1974b) and represent a heterogeneous group of heat-stable alpha-migrating pseudoglobulins (McLeod *et al.*, 1975a), which include lipoproteins (Lint and Behrends, 1976). Polycations such as poly-L-lysine enhance reactive lysis by counteracting $\overline{C567}$-INH, while polyanions such as dextran sulfate share $\overline{C567}$-INH activity (McLeod *et al.*, 1975b; Baker *et al.*, 1975).

Lysis mediated via $\overline{C567}$ is greatly enhanced when the bystander cells have C3b on their surfaces (Hammer *et al.*, 1976). However, it readily occurs upon the addition of cobra venom factor— and zymosan—serum complexes to normal unsensitized erythrocytes in C-EDTA or upon addition of zymosan, endotoxin, immune complexes, or AHGG to mixtures of similar erythrocytes in serum under appropriate conditions, which include high cell concentrations and the presence of agents to neutralize $\overline{C567}$-INH (McLeod *et al.*, 1975c; Behrends *et al.*, 1975; Lint *et al.*, 1976).

Thus, it is likely that $\overline{C567}$ is generated when C5 is activated in solution, either by earlier-acting C components or other means, but inhibited by $\overline{C567}$-INH from binding to bystander cells. Synthetic polycations neutralize this inhibitor to allow $\overline{C567}$-mediated bystander hemolysis to occur in whole serum; naturally occurring polycations, such as the cationic proteins of leukocytes, also have this activity (Baker *et al.*, 1976). Perhaps any C activator or, indeed, any enzyme that leads to activation of C5 has the potential to initiate membrane damage via formation of fluid phase $\overline{C567}$ under appropriate conditions, which include those that favor either increased formation, binding efficiency, or stability of $\overline{C567}$, or involve neutralization of $\overline{C567}$-INH. This mechanism thus may well participate in "nonspecific" tissue damage as C is activated during inflammatory reactions.

Cobra venom factor–induced hemolysis (Pickering *et al.*, 1969; Ballow and Cochrane, 1969) has been postulated to occur, at least in part, via this "reactive lysis" mechanism (Fearon *et al.*, 1973; McLeod *et al.*, 1975c).

4.6. Deviated Lysis

Rother and his colleagues (1974) described a novel form of lysis that they termed *deviated lysis*. This involves a lytic activity detectable in the supernatant upon incubation of C-resistant *Salmonella* strain C5 organisms with complement. It was dependent on the C5–9 complement components both for its formation and for its activity, was active for more than 30 min, and effectively lysed unsensitized chicken erythrocytes in EDTA in the absence of additional serum factors. Its relationship to other complexes of the C attack mechanism was not reported.

5. Summary

The C system was long perceived as a single pathway, activated only by antigen–antibody reactions. The realization of a second major activation pathway eventually evolved, despite extensive resistance at times. Today, many activating agents and points of entry into both the classical and properdin pathways are appreciated. The intertwining of C with other blood enzyme systems and cells associated with inflammation and host defense is now tenet, and C is known not only as a "complement" to antibody in the immune response, but also as a system that initiates and supports inflammatory and associated reactions of host defense in response to a variety of disturbances of body equilibrium. Perhaps these extensive achievements are still only a beginning of an appreciation of the seemingly diverse limbs of the C system and the various real functions that its components, acting singly or as a group, can and do perform. Such understanding should help not only to definitively interpret its enormous power, but also to help lead to a pharmacology geared to its control.

References

Abernethy, T. J., and Avery, O. T., 1941, The occurrence during acute infections of a protein not normally present in the blood. I. Distribution of the reactive protein in patients' sera and the effect of calcium on the flocculation reaction with C polysaccharide of pneumococcus, *J. Exp. Med.* **73**:173–182.

Adler, F. L., 1950, On hemolysis mediated by non-erythrocytic antigens, their homologous antibodies and complement, *Proc. Soc. Exp. Biol. Med.* **74**:561–565.

Agnello, V., Carr, R. I., Koffler, D., and Kunkel, H. G., 1969, Gel diffusion reactions of C1q with aggregated globulin, DNA, and other anionic substances, *Fed. Proc. Fed. Amer. Soc. Exp. Biol.* **28**:696 (abstract).

Agnello, V., Winchester, R., and Kunkel, K., 1970, Precipitin reactions of the C1q component of complement with aggregated γ-globulin and immune complexes in gel diffusion, *Immunology* **19**:909–919.

Alper, C. A., and Balavitch, D., 1976, Cobra venom factor: evidence for its being altered cobra C3 (the third component of complement), *Science* **191**:1275–1276.

Alper, C. A., Rosen, F. S., and Lachmann, P. J., 1972, Inactivator of the third component of complement as an inhibitor in the properdin pathway, *Proc. Nat. Acad. Sci. U.S.A.* **69**:2910–2913.

Alper, C. A., Goodkofsky, I., and Lepow, I. H., 1973, The relationship of glycine-rich β-glycoprotein to factor B in the properdin system and to the cobra factor-binding protein of human serum, *J. Exp. Med.* **137**:424–437.

Arroyave, C. M., and Müller-Eberhard, H. J., 1973, Interactions between human C5, C6, and C7, and their functional significance in complement-dependent cytolysis, *J. Immunol.* **111**:536–545.

Assimeh, S. N., and Painter, R. H., 1975, The macromolecular structure of the first component of complement, *J. Immunol.* **115**:488–494.

Austen, K. F., and Cohn, Z. A., 1963, Contribution of serum and cellular factors in host defense reactions, *N. Engl. J. Med.* **268**:994–1000.

Baker, P. J., Lint, T. F., McLeod, B. C., Behrends, C., and Gewurz, H., 1975, Studies on the inhibition of C56-induced lysis (reactive lysis). VI. Modulation of C5̄6̄-induced lysis by polyanions and polycations, *J. Immunol.* **114**:554–558.

Baker, P. J., Lint, T. F., Siegel, J., Kies, M. W., and Gewurz, H., 1976, Potentiation of C56-initiated lysis by leukocyte cationic proteins, myelin basic proteins, and lysine rich histones, *Immunology* **30**:467–473.

Ballow, M., and Cochrane, C. G., 1969, Two anticomplementary factors in cobra venom. Hemolysis of guinea pig erythrocytes by one of them, *J. Immunol.* **103**:944–952.

Behrends, C. L., Lint, T. F., Baker, P. J., McLeod, B. C., and Gewurz, H., 1975, Zymosan (Z)-induced hemolysis via the alternative complement (C) pathway: control by C567-INH and polycations, *Fed. Proc. Fed. Amer. Soc. Exp. Biol.* **34**:854 (abstract).

Birdsey, V., Lindhoffer, J., and Gewurz, H., 1971, Interactions of toxic venoms with the complement system, *Immunology* **21**:299–310.

Bladen, H. A., Gewurz, H., and Mergenhagen, S. E., 1967, Interactions of the complement system with the surface and endotoxic lipopolysaccharide of *Veillonella alcalescens*, *J. Exp. Med.* **125**:767–786.

Blum, L., 1964, Evidence for immunological specificity of the properdin system: demonstration, isolation and properties of a serum factor which interacts with zymosan and other polysaccharides at 0°C, *J. Immunol.* **92**:61–72.

Blum, L., Pillemer, L., and Lepow, I. H., 1959a, The properdin system and immunity. XI. Studies on the interaction of zymosan with the properdin system, *Z. Immunitätsforsch.* **118**:313–328.

Blum, L., Pillemer, L., and Lepow, I. H., 1959b, The properdin system and immunity. XIII. Assay and properties of a heat labile serum factor (factor B) in the properdin system, *Z. Immunitätsforsch.* **118**:349–357.

Bokisch, V. A., Müller-Eberhard, H. J., and Cochrane, C. G., 1969, Isolation of a fragment (C3a) of the third component of human complement containing anaphylatoxin and chemotactic activity and description of an anaphylatoxin inactivator of human serum, *J. Exp. Med.* **129**:1109–1130.

Borsos, T., and Rapp, H. J., 1963, Chromatographic separation of the first component of complement and its assay on a molecular basis, *J. Immunol.* **91**:851–858.

Borsos, T., Rapp, H. J., and Crisler, C., 1965, The interaction between carrageenan and the first component of complement, *J. Immunol.* **94**:662–666.

Boyden, S. V., 1966, Natural antibodies and the immune response, *Adv. Immunol.* **5**:1–28.

de Bracco, M. M. E., and Stroud, R. M., 1971, C1r, subunit of the first complement component: purification, properties, and assay based on its linking role, *J. Clin. Invest.* **50**:838–848.

Brade, V., Nicholson, A., Bitter-Seurmann, D., and Hadding, U., 1974, Formation of the C3-cleaving properdin enzyme on zymosan. Demonstration that factor D is replaceable by proteolytic enzymes, *J. Immunol.* **113**:1735–1743.

Cantrell, J. W., Stroud, R. M., and Pruitt, K. M., 1972, Insulin and IgG complexes: an immunologic bypass for complement activation, *Diabetes* **21**:872–880.

Cerottini, J. C., and Fitch, F., 1968, Complement-fixing ability and antibody activity of rabbit F(ab′)₂ antibody, *Int. Arch, Allergy Appl. Immunol.* **34**:188–200.

Christian, C. L., 1960, Studies of aggregated gamma globulin. I. Sedimentation, electrophoretic and anticomplementary properties, *J. Immunol.* **84**:112–116.

Claus, D. R., Siegel, J., Petras, K., Skor, D., Osmand, A. P., and Gewurz, H., 1977, Complement activation by interaction of polyanions and polycations. III. Complement activation by interaction of multiple polyanions and polycations in the presence of C-reactive protein, *J. Immunol.*, in press.

Coca, A. F., 1914, A study of the anticomplementary action of yeast, of certain bacteria, and of cobra venom, *Z. Immunitätsforschung* **21**:604–622.

Cochrane, C. G., and Müller-Eberhard, H. J., 1968, The derivation of two distinct anaphylatoxin activities from the third and fifth components of human complement, *J. Exp. Med.* **127**:371–386.

Cooper, N. R., 1973, Formation and function of a complex of the C3 proactivator with a protein from cobra venom, *J. Exp. Med.* **137**:451–460.

Cooper, N. R., Jensen, F. C., Welsh, R. M., and Oldstone, M. B. A., 1976, Lysis of RNA tumor viruses by human serum: direct antibody-independent triggering of the classical complement pathway, *J. Exp. Med.* **144**:970–984.

Cowan, K., 1954, Lysis of sheep erythrocytes by a long-chain polymer, polyethylene glycol, and complement, Dissertation, School of Hygiene and Public Health, Johns Hopkins University, Baltimore.

Daha, M. R., Fearon, D. T., and Austen, K. F., 1976a, C3 nephritic factor (C3NeF): stabilization of fluid phase and cell bound alternative pathway convertase, *J. Immunol.* **116**:1–7.

Daha, M. R., Fearon, D. T., and Austen, K. F., 1976b, Additional C3 requirement for alternative pathway C5 convertase, *Fed. Proc. Fed. Amer. Soc. Exp. Biol.* **35**:654 (abstract).

Dalmasso, A. P., and Müller-Eberhard, H. J., 1964, Interaction of autologous complement with red cells in the absence of antibody, *Proc. Soc. Exp. Biol. Med.* **117**:643–650.

Day, N. K., Good, R. A., Finstad, J., Johannsen, R., Pickering, R. J., and Gewurz, H., 1970, Interactions between endotoxic lipopolysaccharides and the complement system in the sera of lower vertebrates, *Proc. Soc. Exp. Biol. Med.* **133**:1397–1401.

Donaldson, V. H., 1968, Mechanisms of activation of C′1 esterase in hereditary angio-neurotic edema plasma in vitro, *J. Exp. Med.* **127**:411–429.

Eisen, V., and Loveday, C., 1970, Effect of cellulose sulphate on serum complement, *Br. J. Pharmacol.* **39**:831–833.

Ellman, L., Green, I., and Frank, M. M., 1970, Genetically controlled total deficiency of the fourth component of complement in the guinea pig, *Science* **170**:74, 75.

Fearon, D. T., and Austen, K. F., 1975a, Properdin: binding to C3b and stabilization of the C3b-dependent C3 convertase, *J. Exp. Med.* **142**:856–863.

Fearon, D. T., and Austen, K. F., 1975b, Properdin: initiation of alternative complement pathway, *Proc. Nat. Acad. Sci. U.S.A.* **72**:3220–3224.

Fearon, D. T., Austen, K. F., and Ruddy, S., 1973, Formation of a hemolytically active cellular intermediate by the interaction between properdin factors B and D and the activated third component of complement, *J. Exp. Med.* **138**:1305–1313.

Fearon, D. T., Austen, K. F., and Ruddy, S., 1974, Properdin factor D: characterization of its active site and isolation of the precursor form, *J. Exp. Med.* **139**:355–366.

Fiedel, B. A., and Gewurz, H., 1976, Effects of C-reactive protein on platelet function. I. Inhibition of platelet aggregation and release reactions, *J. Immunol.* **116**:1289–1294.

Fiedel, B. A., Rent, R., Myhrman, R., and Gewurz, H., 1976, Complement activation by interaction of polyanions and polycations. II. Precipitation and role of IgG, C1q, and C1-INH during heparin-protamine-induced consumption of complement, *Immunology* **30**:161–169.

Flexner, S., and Noguchi, H., 1903, Snake venom in relation to hemolysis, bacteriolysis and toxicity, *J. Exp. Med.* **6**:277–301.

Forsgren, A., and Sjoquist, J., 1966, 'Protein A' from *S. aureus.* I. Pseudoimmune reaction with human γ-globulin, *J. Immunol.* **97**:822–827.

Franek, F., Riha, I., and Sterzl, J., 1961, Characteristics of γ-globulin lacking antibody properties in newborn pigs, *Nature, Lond.* **189**:1020–1022.

Frank, M. M., May, J. E., Gaither, T., and Ellman, L., 1971, In vitro studies of complement function in sera of C4-deficient guinea pigs, *J. Exp. Med.* **134**:176–187.

Gal, K., and Miltenyi, M., 1955, Hemagglutination test for the demonstration of CRP, *Acta Microbiol. Acad. Sci. Hung.* **3**:41–46.

Gewurz, H., 1971, Interactions between endotoxic lipopolysaccharides and the complement system. Solubilization of complement-consuming substances during brief absorptions at 0°C, *Proc. Soc. Exp. Biol. Med.* **136**:561–564.

Gewurz, H., 1972, Alternate pathways to activation of the complement system, in: *Biological Activities of Complement,* Fifth International Symposium of the Canadian Society of Immunology, Guelph, August 27–29, 1970 (D. G. Ingram, ed.), pp. 56–88, Karger, Basel.

Gewurz, H., Mergenhagen, S. E., Nowotny, A., and Phillips, J. K., 1968a, Interactions of the complement system with native and chemically modified endotoxins, *J. Bacteriol.* **95**:397–445.

Gewurz, H., Pickering, R. J., Mergenhagen, S. E., and Good, R. A., 1968b, The complement profile in acute glomerulonephritis, systemic lupus erythematosus and hypocomplementemic chronic glomerulonephritis. Contrasts and experimental correlations, *Int. Arch. Allergy Appl. Immunol.* **34**:556–570.

Gewurz, H., Shin, H. S., and Mergenhagen, S. E., 1968c, Interactions of the complement system with endotoxic lipopolysaccharide. Consumption of each of the six terminal complement components, *J. Exp. Med.* **128**:1049–1057.

Gewurz, H., Pickering, R. J., Naff, G., Snyderman, R., Mergenhagen, S. E., and Good, R. A., 1969a, Decreased properdin activity in acute glomerulonephritis, *Int. Arch. Allergy Appl. Immunol.* **36**:592–598.

Gewurz, H., Shin, H. S., Pickering, R. J., Snyderman, R., Lichtenstein, L., Good, R. A., and Mergenhagen, S. E., 1969b, Interactions of the complement system with endotoxic lipopolysaccharides: complement-membrane interactions and endotoxin-induced inflammation, in: *Cellular Recognition* (Smith and Good, eds.), pp. 305–315, Appleton-Century-Crofts, New York.

Gewurz, H., Pickering, R. J., Moberg, A., Simmons, R. L., Good, R. A., and Najarin, J. S., 1970a, Reactivities to horse anti-lymphocyte globulin. II. Serum sickness nephritis with complement alterations in man, *Int. Arch, Allergy Appl. Immunol.* **39**:210–220.

Gewurz, H., Pickering, R. J., Synderman, R., Lichtenstein, L. M., Good, R. A., and Mergenhagen, S. E., 1970b, Interactions of the complement system with endotoxic lipopolysaccharides in immuno-globulin-deficient sera, *J. Exp. Med.* **131**:817–831.

Gewurz, H., Pickering, R., Day, N., and Good, R., 1971a, Cobra venom factor–induced activation of the complement system: developmental, experimental and clinical considerations of an alternate pathway of complement activation, *Int. Arch. Allergy Appl. Immunol.* **40**:47–58.

Gewurz, H., Snyderman, R., Mergenhagen, S. E., and Shin, H. S., 1971b, Effects of endotoxic lipopolysaccharides on the complement system, in: *Microbial Toxins* Vol. 5 (S. J. Ajl, G. Weinbaum, and S. Kodis, eds.), pp. 127–149, Academic Press, New York.

Gitlin, J. D., Rosen, F. S., and Lachmann, P. J., 1975, The mechanism of action of the C3b inactivator (conglutinogen-activating factor) on its naturally occurring substrate, the major fragment of the third component of complement (C3b), *J. Exp. Med.* **141**:1221–1226.

Goers, J., Ziccardi, B., Glovsky, M., and Schumaker, V., 1976, Studies on the activation of C1 by a univalent hapten-antibody complex, *J. Immunol.* **116**:1734, 1935 (abstract).

Goldlust, M. B., Luzzati, A., and Levine, L., 1968, Complement-inactivating proteinase(s) from *Clostridium histolyticum, J. Bacteriol.* **96**: 1961–1968.

Goldstein, I. M., and Weissmann, G., 1974, Generation of C5-derived lysosomal enzyme-releasing activity (C5a) by lysates of leukocyte lysosomes, *J. Immunol.* **113**:1583–1588.

Good, R. A., 1952, Acute phase reactions in rheumatic fever, in: *Rheumatic Fever* (L. Thomas, ed.), p. 115, University of Minnesota Press, Minneapolis.

Goodkofsky, I., and Lepow, I. H., 1971, Functional relationship of factor B in the properdin system to C3 proactivator of human serum, *J. Immunol.* **107**:1200–1204.

Gotschlich, E. C., and Edelman, G. M., 1965, C-reactive protein: a molecule composed of subunits, *Proc. Nat. Acad. Sci. U.S.A.* **54**:558–566.

Gotschlich, E. C., and Edelman, G. M., 1967, Binding properties and specificity of C-reactive protein, *Proc. Nat. Acad. Sci. U.S.A.* **57**:706–712.

Götze, O., and Müller-Eberhard, H. J., 1970, Lysis of erythrocytes by antibody in the absence of antibody, *J. Exp. Med.* **132**:898–915.

Götze, O., and Müller-Eberhard, H. J., 1971, The C3 activator system: an alternate pathway of complement activation, *J. Exp. Med.* **134**:90s–108s.

Götze, O., and Müller-Eberhard, H. J., 1974, The role of properdin in the alternate pathway of complement activation, *J. Exp. Med.* **139**:44–57.

Gustafsen, G. T., Sjoquist, J., and Stalenheim, G., 1967, "Protein A" from *Staphylococcus aureus.* II. Arthus-like reaction produced in rabbits by interaction of protein A and human γ-globulin, *J. Immunol.* **98**:1178–1181.

Hammer, C. H., Abramovitz, A. S., and Mayer, M. M., 1976, A new activity of complement component C3: cell bound C3b potentiates lysis of erythrocytes by C5b, 6 and terminal components *J. Immunol.* **117**:830–834.

Hill, J. H., and Ward, P. A., 1969, C3 leukotactic factors produced by a tissue protease, *J. Exp. Med.* **130**:505–518.

Hokama, Y., Coleman, M. K., and Riley, R. F., 1962, *In vitro* effects of C-reactive protein on phagocytosis, *J. Bacteriol.* **83**:1017–1024.

Hunsicker, L. G., Ruddy, S., and Austen, K. F., 1973, Alternate complement pathway: factors involved in cobra venom factor (CoVF) activation of the third component of complement (C3), *J. Immunol.* **110**:128–138.

Inai, S., Tsuyuguchi, I., and Hiramatsu, S., 1968, Hemolysis of sheep erythrocytes by complement without participation of antibody, *J. Immunol.* **102**:1336–1337.

Ishizaka, T., and Ishizaka, K., 1959, Biological activities of aggregated γ-globulin. I. Skin reactive and complement-fixing properties of heat-denatured γ-globulin, *Proc. Soc. Exp. Biol. Med.* **101**:845–850.

Ishizaka, T., Ishizaka, K., and Borsos, T., 1961, Biological activities of aggregated γ-globulin. IV. Mechanism of complement fixation, *J. Immunol.* **87**:433–438.

Isliker, H., Jocot-Guillarmod, H., Waldesbühl, M., von Fellenberg, R., and Cerottini, J. C., 1967, Complement fixation by different IgG preparations and fragments, in: *Fifth International Sympo-*

HENRY GEWURZ AND
THOMAS F. LINT

sium on Immunopathology. Mechanisms of Inflammation Induced by Immune Injury (Meischer and Grabar, eds.), pp. 197–206, Schwabe, Basel.

Jensen, J., 1967, Anaphylatoxin and its relation to the complement system, *Science* **155**:1122–1123.

Jensen, J. A., 1969, A specific inactivator of mammalian C′4 isolated from nurse shark *(Ginglymostoma cirratum)* serum, *J. Exp. Med.* **130**:217–241.

Kaplan, M. H., and Volanakis, J. E., 1974, Interactions of C-reactive protein complexes with the complement system. I. Consumption of human complement associated with the reaction of C-reactive protein with pneumococcal C-polysaccharide and with the choline phosphatides, lecithin and sphingomyelin, *J. Immunol.* **112**:2135–2147.

Kindmark, C.-O., 1971, Stimulating effect of C-reactive protein on phagocytosis of various species of pathogenic bacteria, *Clin. Exp. Immunol.* **8**:941–948.

Kniker, W. T., and Morgan, P. N., 1967, An inactivator in spider venom of the fifth component of complement, *Fed. Proc.* **26**:362 (abstract).

Kronvall, G., and Gewurz, H., 1970, Activation and inhibition of IgG mediated complement fixation by staphylococcal protein A, *Clin. Exp. Immunol.* **7**:211–220.

Kushner, I., and Somerville, J. A., 1970, Estimation of the molecular size of C-reactive protein and Cx-reactive protein in serum, *Biochim. Biophys. Acta* **207**:105–114.

Lachmann, P. J., and Müller-Eberhard, H. J., 1968, The demonstration in human serum of conglutino-gen-activating factor and its effect on the third component of complement, *J. Immunol.* **100**:691–698.

Lachmann, P. J., and Thompson, R. A., 1970, Reactive lysis: the complement-mediated lysis of unsensitized cells. II. The characterization of activated reactor as C56 and the participation of C8 and C9, *J. Exp. Med.* **131**:643–657.

Lachmann, P. J., Nicol, P., and Aston, W. P., 1973, Further studies on the C3b inactivator or conglutinogen activating factor (KAF), *Immunochemistry* **10**:695–700.

Landsteiner, K., 1901, Reprinted in: *The Specificity of Serological Reactions,* Oxford University Press, London, 1945.

Landy, M., and Weidenz, W. P., 1964, Natural antibodies against gram-negative bacteria, in: *Bacterial Endotoxins* (Landy and Braun, eds.), pp. 275–290, Rutgers University Press, New Brunswick, New Jersey.

Leddy, J. P., and Vaughan, J. H., 1964, Auto-sensitization of trypsin-treated human red cells by complement, *Proc. Soc. Exp. Biol. N. Y.* **117**:734–738.

Leon, M. A., 1956, Quantitative studies on the properdin-complement system, *J. Exp. Med.* **103**:285–293.

Leon, M. A., 1957, Quantitative studies on the properdin-complement system. II. Kinetics of the reaction between properdin and zymosan, *J. Exp. Med.* **105**:403–415.

Leon, M. A., 1958, Quantitative studies on the properdin-complement system. III. Kinetics of the reaction between C′3 and the properdin-zymosan complex, *J. Immunol.* **81**:23–28.

Leon, M. A., 1960, The reactions between dextrans and the properdin-complement system. I. Inhibition by excess dextran, *J. Immunol.* **85**:190–196.

Leonard, C. G., and Thorne, C. B., 1961, Studies on the nonspecific precipitation of basic serum proteins with γ-glutamyl polypeptides, *J. Immunol.* **87**:175–188.

Lepow, I. H., 1961, The properdin system: a review of current concepts, in: *Immunochemical Approaches to Problems in Microbiology* (Heidelberger and Plescia, eds.), pp. 280–294, Rutgers University Press, New Brunswick, New Jersey.

Lepow, I. H., 1965, Serum complement and properdin, in: *Immunological Diseases* (Samter and Alexander, eds.), pp. 188–210, Churchill, London.

Lepow, I. H., Wurz, L., Ratnoff, O. D., and Pillemer, L., 1954, Studies on the mechanism of inactivation of human complement by plasmin and by antigen–antibody aggregates. I. The requirement for a factor resembling C′1 and the role of Ca++, *J. Immunol.* **73**:146–185.

Lichtenstein, L., Gewurz, H., Adkinson, N. F., Shin, H. S., and Mergenhagen, S. E., 1969, Interactions of the complement system with endotoxic lipopolysaccharide: the generation of an anaphylatoxin, *Immunology* **16**:327–336.

Linscott, W. D., Faulk, W. P., and Perucca, P. J., 1969, Complement: chemical coupling of a functionally active component to erythrocytes in the absence of antibody, *J. Immunol.* **103**:474–479.

Lint, T. F., and Behrends, C. L., 1976, Control of the complement (C) attack mechanism by serum lipoproteins, *Fed. Proc. Fed. Amer. Soc. Exp. Biol.* **35**:493 (abstract).

Lint, T. F., Behrends, C. L., Baker, P. J., and Gewurz, H., 1976, Activation of the complement attack mechanism in the fluid phase and its control by $C\overline{567}$-INH: lysis of normal erythrocytes initiated by zymosan, endotoxin, and immune complexes, *J. Immunol.,* in press.

Löfström, G., 1944, Comparison between the reactions of acute phase serum with pneumococcus C-polysaccharide and with pneumococcus type 27, *Br. J. Exp. Pathol.* **25**:21–26.

Logue, G. L., Rosse, W. F., and Adams, J. P., 1973, Mechanisms of immune lysis of red blood cells in vitro. I. Paroxysmal nocturnal hemoglobinuria cells, *J. Clin. Invest.* **52**:1129–1137.

Loos, M., Borsos, T., and Rapp, H. J., 1972, Activation of the first component of complement. Evidence for an internal activation step. *J. Immunol.* **108**:683–688.

Loos, M., Raepple, E., Hadding, U., and Bitter-Suermann, D., 1974, Interaction of polyanions with the first and third component of complement, *Fed. Proc. Fed. Amer. Soc. Exp. Biol.* **33**:775 (abstract).

Loos, M., Volanakis, J. E., and Stroud, R. M., 1976, Mode of interaction of different polyanions with the first (C1, $C\overline{1}$) the second (C2) and the fourth (C4) component of complement. II. Effect of polyanions on the binding of C2 to EAC4b, *Immunochemistry* **13**:257–261.

MacLeod, C. M., and Avery, O. T., 1941, The occurrence during acute infections of a protein not normally present in the blood. III. Immunological properties of the C-reactive protein and its differentiation from normal blood proteins, *J. Exp. Med.* **73**:191–200.

McCall, C. E., DeChatelet, L. R., Butler, R., and Brown, D. 1974, Enhanced phagocytic capacity: the biologic basis for the elevated histochemical nitroblue tetrazolium reaction, *J. Clin. Invest.* **54**:1227–1234.

McLeod, B., Baker, P., and Gewurz, H., 1974a, Studies on the inhibition of $C\overline{56}$-initiated lysis (reactive lysis). I. Description of the phenomenon and methods of assay, *Immunology* **26**:1145–1157.

McLeod, B. C., Baker, P., and Gewurz, H., 1974b, studies on the inhibition of $C\overline{56}$-initiated lysis (reactive lysis). II. $C\overline{567}$-INH—an inhibitor of the $C\overline{567}$ trimolecular complex of complement, *Int. Arch. Allergy Appl. Immunol.* **47**:623–632.

McLeod, B. C., Baker, P., and Gewurz, H., 1975a, Studies on the inhibition of $C\overline{56}$-initiated lysis (reactive lysis). III. Characterization of the inhibitory activity $C\overline{567}$-INH and its mode of action, *Immunology* **28**:133–149.

McLeod, B. C., Baker, P., Behrends, C., and Gewurz, H., 1975b, Studies on the inhibition of $C\overline{56}$-initiated lysis (reactive lysis). IV. Antagonism of the inhibitory activity $C\overline{567}$-INH by poly-L-lysine, *Immunology* **28**:379–390.

McLeod, B. C., Lint, T. F., Baker, P., Behrends, C., and Gewurz, H., 1975c, Studies on the inhibition of $C\overline{56}$-initiated lysis (reactive lysis). V. The role of $C\overline{567}$-INH in the regulation of complement-dependent hemolysis initiated by cobra venom factor, *Immunology* **28**:741–754.

Marcus, R. L., Shin, H. S., and Mayer, M. M., 1971, An alternate complement pathway: C3 cleaving activity, not due to C4, 2a, on endotoxic lipopolysaccharide after treatment with guinea pig serum: relation to properdin, *Proc. Nat. Acad. Sci. U.S.A.* **68**:1351–1354.

May, J. E., and Frank, M. M., 1973a, Hemolysis of sheep erythrocytes in guinea pig serum deficient in the fourth component of complement. I. Antibody and serum requirements, *J. Immunol.* **111**:1661–1667.

May, J. E., and Frank, M. M., 1973b, Hemolysis of sheep erythrocytes in guinea pig serum deficient in the fourth component of complement. II. Evidence for involvement of C1 and components of the alternate complement pathway, *J. Immunol.* **111**:1668–1676.

Mayer, M. M., 1961, Complement and complement fixation, in: *Experimental Immunochemistry* (Kabat and Mayer, eds.), pp. 133–240, Charles C Thomas, Springfield.

Mayer, M. M., 1973, The complement system, *Sci. Amer.* **229**:54–66.

Medicus, R. G., Schreiber, R. D., Götze, O., and Müller-Eberhard, H. J., 1976a, A molecular concept of the properdin pathway, *Proc. Nat. Acad. Sci. U.S.A.* **73**:612–616.

Medicus, R. G., Götze, O., and Müller-Eberhard, H. J., 1976b, C3b inactivator: the properdin receptor destroying enzyme, *Fed. Proc. Fed. Amer. Soc. Exp. Biol.* **35**:654 (abstract).

Mergenhagen, S. E., Gewurz, H., Bladen, H. A., Nowotny, A., Kasai, N., and Lüderitz, O., 1968, Interactions of the complement system with endoxtoxins from a *Salmonella minnesota* mutant deficient in O-polysaccharide and heptose, *J. Immunol.* **100**:227–229.

Mergenhagen, S. E., Snyderman, R., Gewurz, H., and Shin, H. S., 1969, Significance of complement to the mechanism of action of endotoxin, *Curr. Top. Microbiol. Immunol.* **50**:37–77.

Miler, I., Sterzl, H., Kostka, J., and Lanc, A., 1964, Effect of antigens of the intestinal flora on the development of specific and nonspecific reactions in newborns of different species, in: *Bacterial*

Endotoxins (Landy and Braun, eds.), pp. 291–305, Rutgers University Press, Rahway, New Jersey.

Mills, B. J., Oldstone, M. B. A., and Cooper, N. R., 1976, Complement dependent lysis of vesicular somatitis virus, *Fed. Proc. Fed. Amer. Soc. Exp. Biol.* **35**:494 (abstract).

Mollison, P. L., and Polley, M. J., 1964, Uptake of γ-globulin and complement by red cells exposed to serum at low ionic strength, *Nature London* **203**:535, 536.

Mortensen, R. F., Osmand, A. P., and Gewurz, H., 1975, Effects of C-reactive protein on the lymphoid system. I. Binding to thymus-dependent lymphocytes and alteration of their functions, *J. Exp. Med.* **141**:821–839.

Mortensen, R. F., Osmand, A. P., Lint, T. F., and Gewurz, H., 1976, Interaction of C-reactive protein with lymphocytes and monocytes. Complement-dependent adherence and phagocytosis, *J. Immunol.* **117**:774–781.

Müller-Eberhard, H. J., Nilsson, U. R., Dalmasso, A. P., Polley, M. J., and Calcott, M. A., 1966, A molecular concept of immune cytolysis, *Arch. Pathol.* **82**:205–217.

Müller-Eberhard, H. J., 1968, Chemistry and reaction mechanisms of complement, *Adv. Immunol.* **8**:1–80.

Müller-Eberhard, H. J., 1972, The molecular basis of the biological activities of complement, in: *The Harvey Lectures* (1970–1971), pp. 75–104, Academic Press, New York.

Müller-Eberhard, H. J., 1975, Complement, *Annu. Rev. Biochem.* **44**:697–724.

Müller-Eberhard, H. J., and Fjellström, K. E., 1971, Isolation of the anticomplementary protein from cobra venom and its mode of action on C3, *J. Immunol.* **107**:1666–1672.

Müller-Eberhard, H. J., and Götze, O., 1972, C3 proactivator convertase and its mode of action, *J. Exp. Med.* **135**:1003–1008.

Nelson, R. A., 1958, An alternative mechanism for the properdin system, *J. Exp. Med.* **108**:515–535.

Nelson, R. A., 1966, A new concept of immunosuppression in hypersensitivity reactions and in transplantation immunity, *Surv. Ophthalmol.* **11**:498–505.

Opferkuch, W., and Segerling, M., 1976, Biochemistry and biology of complement activation, this volume.

Osler, A. G., 1961, Functions of the complement system, *Adv. Immunol.* **1**:131–210.

Osler, A. G., Oliveira, B., Shin, H. S., and Sandberg, A. L., 1969, The fixation of guinea pig complement by γ_1 and γ_2 immunoglobulins, *J. Immunol.* **102**:269–271.

Osmand, A. P., Mortensen, R. F., Siegel, J., and Gewurz, H., 1975, Interactions of C-reactive protein with the complement system. III. Complement-dependent passive hemolysis initiated by CRP, *J. Exp. Med.* **142**:1065–1077.

Peck, J. L., and Thomas, L., 1949, Studies in the hemolysis of human erythrocytes by homologous complement in the presence of tannic acid, *Bull. Johns Hopkins Hosp.* **84**:216–237.

Pensky, J., Wurz, L., Pillemer, L., and Lepow, I. H., 1959, The properdin system and immunity, XIII. Assay, properties, and partial purification of a hydrazine-sensitive serum factor (factor A) in the properdin system, *Z. Immunitätsforch.* **118**:329–348.

Pensky, J., Hinz, C. F., Todd, E. W., Wedgwood, R. J., Boyer, J. T., and Lepow, I. H., 1968, Properties of highly purified human properdin, *J. Immunol.* **100**:142–158.

Pickering, R. J., Wolfson, M. R., Good, R. A., and Gewurz, H., 1969, Passive hemolysis by serum and cobra venom factor. A new mechanism inducing membrane damage by complement, *Proc. Nat. Acad. Sci. U.S.A.* **62**:521–527.

Pillemer, L., 1943, Recent advances in the chemistry of complement, *Chem. Rev.* **33**:1–26.

Pillemer, L., Blum, L., Lepow, I. H., Ross, O. A., Todd, E. W., and Wardlaw, A. C., 1954, The properdin system and immunity. I. Demonstration and isolation of a new serum protein, properdin, and its role in immune phenomena, *Science* **120**:279–285.

Pillemer, L., Blum, L., Lepow, I. H., Wurz, L., and Todd, E. W., 1956, The properdin system and immunity. III. The zymosan assay of properdin, *J. Exp. Med.* **103**:1–13.

Pillemer, L., and Ecker, E. E., 1941, Anticomplementary factor in yeast, *J. Biol. Chem.* **137**:139–142.

Pillemer, L., Seifter, S., and Ecker, E. E., 1942, The role of the components of complement in specific immune fixation, *J. Exp. Med.* **75**:421–435.

Pillemer, L., Blum, L., Pensky, J., and Lepow, I. H., 1953a, The requirement for magnesium ions in the inactivation of the third component of human complement (C′3) by insoluble residues of yeast cells (zymosan), *J. Immunol.* **71**:331–338.

Pillemer, L., Lepow, I. H., and Blum, L., 1953b, The requirement for a hydrazine-sensitive serum factor and heat-labile serum factors in the inactivation of human C'3 by zymosan, *J. Immunol.* **71**:339–345.

Pillemer, L., Ratnoff, O. D., Blum, L., and Lepow, I. H., 1953c, The inactivation of complement and its components by plasmin, *J. Exp. Med.* **97**:573–589.

Pillemer, L., Schoenberg, M. D., Blum, L., and Wurz, L., 1955, Properdin system and immunity. II. Interaction of the properdin system with polysaccharides, *Science* **122**:545–549.

Platts-Mills, T. A. E., and Ishizaka, K., 1974, Activation of the alternate pathway of human complement by rabbit cells, *J. Immunol.* **113**:348–358.

Rapp, H. J., and Borsos, T., 1963, Effects of low ionic strength on immune hemolysis, *J. Immunol.* **91**:826–832.

Ratnoff, O. D., and Naff, G. B., 1967, The conversion of C'1s to C'1-esterase by plasmin and trypsin, *J. Exp. Med.* **125**:337–358.

Reid, K. B. M., 1971, Complement fixation by the F(ab')$_2$-fragment of pepsin treated rabbit antibody, *Immunology* **20**:649–658.

Rent, R., Ertel, N., Eisenstein, R., and Gewurz, H., 1975, Complement activation by interaction of polyanions and polycations. I. Heparin-protamine induced consumption of complement, *J. Immunol.* **114**:120–124.

Rosse, W. F., and Dacie, J. V., 1966, Immune lysis of normal human and paroxysmal nocturnal hemoglobinuria (PNH) red blood cells, II. The role of complement components in the increased sensitivity of PNH red cells to immune lysis, *J. Clin. Invest.* **45**:749–757.

Rother, U., Hänsch, G., Menzel, J., and Rother, K., 1974, Deviated lysis: transfer of complement lytic activity to unsensitized cells. I. Generation of the transferable activity on the surface of complement resistant bacteria, *Z. Immunitätsforsch.* **148**:172–186.

Ruddy, S., Gigli, I., and Austen, K. F., 1972a, The complement system of man, *N. Engl. J. Med.* **287**:489–495; 545–549; 592–596; 642–646.

Ruddy, S., Hunsicker, L. G., and Austen, K. F., 1972b, C3b inactivator in man. III. Further purification and production of antibody to C3b INA, *J. Immunol.* **108**:657–664.

Sandberg, A. L., Götze, O., Müller-Eberhard, H. J., and Osler, A. G., 1971a, Complement utilization by guinea pig γ_1 and γ_2 immunoglobulins through the C3 activator system, *J. Immunol.* **107**:920–923. 923.

Sandberg, A. L., Oliveira, B., and Osler, A. G., 1971b, Two complement interaction sites in guinea pig immunoglobulins, *J. Immunol.* **106**:282–285.

Schreiber, R. D., Medicus, R. G., Götze, O., and Müller-Eberhard, H. J., 1975, Properdin- and nephritic factor-dependent C3 convertases: requirement of native C3 for enzyme formation and the function of bound C3b as properdin receptor, *J. Exp. Med.* **142**:760–772.

Schreiber, R. D., Götze, O., and Müller-Eberhard, H. J., 1976, Nephritic factor and initiating factor C3/C5 convertases, *Fed. Proc. Fed. Amer. Soc. Exp. Biol.* **35**:253 (abstract).

Schur, P. H., and Becker, E. L., 1963, Pepsin digestion of rabbit and sheep antibodies. The effect on complement fixation, *J. Exp. Med.* **118**:891–904.

Shin, H. S., Gewurz, H., and Snyderman, R., 1969, Reaction of a cobra venom factor with guinea pig complement and generation of an activity chemotactic for polymorphonuclear leukocytes, *Proc. Soc. Exp. Biol. Med.* **131**:203–207.

Shin, H. S., Pickering, R. J., and Mayer, M. M., 1971a, The fifth component of the guinea pig complement system. II. Mechanism of SAC$\overline{1}$, $\overline{423}$, 5b formation and C5 consumption by EAC$\overline{1}$, $\overline{423}$, *J. Immunol.* **106**:473–479.

Shin, H. S., Pickering, R. J., and Mayer, M. M., 1971b, The fifth component of the guinea pig complement system. III. Dissociation and transfer of C5b, and the probable site of C5b fixation, *J. Immunol.* **106**:480–493.

Siegel, J., Rent, R., and Gewurz, H., 1974, Interactions of C-reactive protein with the complement system. I. Protamine-induced consumption of complement in acute phase sera, *J. Exp. Med.* **140**:631–647.

Siegel, J., Osmand, A. P., Wilson, J. F., and Gewurz, H., 1975, Interactions of C-reactive protein with the complement system. II C-reactive protein mediated consumption of complement by poly-L-lysine polymers and other polycations, *J. Exp. Med.* **142**:709–721.

Siegel, J., Claus, D., and Petras, K., 1976, Interactions of C-reactive protein (CRP) and C1, *Fed. Proc. Fed. Amer. Soc. Exp. Biol.* **35**:493 (abstract).

Sjoquist, J., and Stalenheim, G., 1969, Protein A from *Staphylococcus aureus*. IX. Complement-fixing activity of protein A–IgG complexes, *J. Immunol.* **103**:467–473.

Skarnes, R. C., 1965, Nonspecific hemolysis of erythrocytes modified with bacterial endotoxins, *Ann. Inst. Pasteur* **109**:66–79.

Snyderman, R., Gewurz, H., and Mergenhagen, S. E., 1968, Interactions of the complement system with endotoxic lipopolysaccharide. Generation of a factor chemotactic for polymorphonuclear leukocytes, *J. Exp. Med.* **128**:259–275.

Snyderman, R., Shin, H. S., Phillips, J. K., Gewurz, H., and Mergenhagen, S. E., 1969, A neutrophil chemotactic factor derived from C′5 upon interaction of guinea pig serum with endotoxin, *J. Immunol.* **103**:413–422.

Snyderman, R., Shin, H. S., and Dannenberg, A. M., Jr., 1972, Macrophage proteinase and inflammation: the production of chemotactic activity from the fifth component of complement by macrophage proteinases, *J. Immunol.* **109**:896–898.

Spitzer, R. E., Vallota, E. H., Forristal, J., Sudora, E., Stitzel, A., Davis, N. C., and West, C. D., 1969, Serum C3 lytic system in patients with glomerulonephritis, *Science* **164**:436, 437.

Spitzer, R. E., Stitzel, A. E., and Urmson, J., 1976, Interaction of properdin convertase and properdin in the alternative pathway of complement activation, *Immunochemistry* **13**:15–20.

Stalenheim, G., Götze, O., Cooper, N. R., Sjöquist, J., and Müler-Eberhard, H. J., 1973, Consumption of human complement components by complexes of IgG with protein A of *Staphylococcus aureus, Immunochemistry* **10**:501–507.

Sterzl, J., 1963, The opsonic activity of complement in sera without antibody, *Folia Microbiol. Prague.* **8**:240–244.

Stitzel, A. E., and Spitzer, R. E., 1974, The utilization of properdin in the alternate pathway of complement activation: isolation of properdin convertase, *J. Immunol.* **112**:56–62.

Taubman, S. B., Goldschmidt, P. R., and Lepow, I. H., 1970, Effects of lysosomal enzymes from human leukocytes on human complement components, *Fed. Proc. Fed. Amer. Soc. Exp. Biol.* **29**:434.

Theofilopoulos, A. N., Bokisch, V. A., and Dixon, F. J., 1974, Receptor for soluble C3 and C3b on human lymphoblastoid (Raji) cells: properties and biological significance, *J. Exp. Med.* **139**:696–711.

Thompson, R. A., and Lachmann, P. J., 1970, Reactive lysis: the complement-mediated lysis of unsensitized cells. I. The characterization of the indicator factor and its identification as C7, *J. Exp. Med.* **131**:629–641.

Thompson, R. A., and Rowe, D. S., 1968, Reactive hemolysis. A distinctive form of red cell lysis, *Immunology London* **14**:745–762.

Tillett, W. S., and Francis, T., Jr., 1930, Serological reactions in pneumonia with a non-protein somatic fraction of pneumococcus, *J. Exp. Med.* **52**:561–571.

Vallota, E. H., Götze, O., Spiegelberg, H. L., Forristal, J., West, C. F., and Müller-Eberhard, H. J., 1974, A serum factor in chronic hypocomplementemic nephritis distinct from immunoglobulins and activating the alternative pathway of complement, *J. Exp. Med.* **139**:1249–1261.

Vogt, W., and Schmidt, G., 1966, Formation of an anaphylatoxin in rat plasma, a specific enzymic process, *Biochem. Pharmacol.* **15**:905–914.

Volanakis, J. E., and Kaplan, M. H., 1971, Specificity of C-reactive protein for choline phosphate residues of pneumococcal C-polysaccharide, *Proc. Soc. Exp. Biol. Med.* **136**:612–614.

Volanakis, J. E., and Kaplan, M. H., 1974, Interaction of C-reactive protein complexes with the complement system. II. Consumption of guinea pig complement by CRP complexes: requirement for human C1q, *J. Immunol.* **113**:9–17.

Volanakis, J. E., and Stroud, R. M., 1973, Properties of radiolabeled C1q, *J. Immunol.* **111**:313–314 (abstract).

Volanakis, J. E., Schultz, D. R., and Stroud, R. M., 1976, Evidence that C1̄s participates in the alternative complement pathway, *Int. Arch. Allergy Appl. Immunol.* **50**:68–80.

Walb, D., Loos, M., and Hadding, U., 1971, *In vitro* Untersuchungen über Angriffspunkt und Wirkungsunterschiede zum Heparin. Antikomplementäre Wirkung eines semisynthetischen Pentosan-polysulfo-esters, *Z. Naturforsch. (B)* **26**:403–408.

Ward, P. A., 1967, A plasmin-split fragment of C′3 as a new chemotactic factor, *J. Exp. Med.* **126**:189–206.

Ward, P. A., and Hill. J. H., 1970, C5 chemotactic fragments produced by an enzyme in lysosomal granules of neutrophils, *J. Immunol.* **104**:535–543.

Welsh, R. M., Cooper, N. R., Jensen, F. C., and Oldstone, M. B. A., 1975, Human serum lyses RNA tumor viruses, *Nature* **257**:612–614.

Westberg, N. D., Naff, G. B., Boyer, J. T., and Michael, A. F., 1971, Glomerular deposition of properdin in acute and chronic glomerulonephritis with hypocomplementemia, *J. Clin. Invest.* **50**:642–649.

Whaley, K., and Ruddy, S., 1976, Modulation of C3b hemolytic activity by a plasma protein distinct from C3b inactivator, *Science* **193**:1011–1013.

Whitehead, H. R., Gordon, J., and Wormall, A., 1925, XCII. The "third component" or heat-stable factor of complement, *Biochem. J.* **19**:618–625.

Willers, J. M. N., Pondman, K. W., and Winkler, K. C., 1959, An improved properdin titration, based on the elimination of an inhibitor, *Vox Sang.* **4**:21–32.

Willoughby, W. F., and Mayer, M. M., 1965, Antibody–complement complexes, *Science* **150**:907, 908.

Willoughby, W. F., Ford, R. T., and Shin, H. S., 1973, Complement activation by lysozyme-DNA compleses, *J. Immunol.* **111**:296 (abstract).

Yachnin, S., 1965, The hemolysis of red cells from patients with paroxysmal nocturnal hemoglobinuria by partially purified subcomponents of the third complement component, *J. Clin. Invest.* **44**:1534–1546.

Yachnin, S., 1966, Further studies on the hemolysis of human red cells by late acting complement components, *Immunochemistry* **3**:505 (abstract).

Yachnin, S., and Ruthenberg, J. M., 1965, The initiation and enhancement of human red cell lysis by activation of the first component of complement and by first component esterase. Studies using normal red cells and red cells from patients with paroxysmal nocturnal hemoglobinuria, *J. Clin. Invest.* **44**:518–534.

Yachnin, S., Laforet, M. T., and Gardner, F. H., 1961, pH-Dependent hemolytic systems. I. Their relationship to paroxysmal nocturnal hemoglobinuria, *Blood* **17**:83–96.

Yachnin, S., Rosenblum, D., and Chatman, D., 1964, Biological properties of polynucleotides. V. Studies on the inhibition of the first component of complement by polyinosinic acid; the interaction with C′1q, *J. Immunol.* **93**:542–548.

Zarco, R. M., Schultz, D., and Vroon, D. D., 1967, Inactivation of guinea pig complement and Agkistrodon piscivorus (cottonmouth moccasin) venom, *Fed. Proc.* **26**:362 (abstract).

Ziccardi, R. J., and Cooper, N. R., 1976, Activation of C1r by proteolytic cleavage, *J. Immunol.* **116**:504–509.

Ziegler, J. B., Alper, C. A., Rosen, F. S., Lachmann, P. J., and Sherington, L., 1975, Restoration by purified C3b inactivator of complement-mediated function *in vivo* in a patient with C3b inactivator deficiency, *J. Clin. Invest.* **55**:668–672.

Zimmerman, T. S., and Kolb, W. P., 1976, Human platelet-initiated formation and uptake of the C5-9 complex of human complement, *J. Clin. Invest.* **57**:203–211.

3

Complement Synthesis

HARVEY R. COLTEN

1. Introduction

In the past two decades, considerable progress has been made in the study of complement biosynthesis, following the isolation and characterization of the individual components of complement, the design of suitable immunochemical and functional assays for complement proteins, and improvements in tissue- and organ-culture techniques. These advances have made it possible to identify the sites of synthesis of most of the complement proteins and, more recently with these methods, an approcah to questions of more general biological interest has been possible. Genetic variants of complement proteins have been recognized and well-defined deficiencies of complement have been described in humans and experimental animals, providing excellent models for studies of genetic control of protein synthesis. In addition, changes in serum complement resulting from the *acute phase response* or in specific autoimmune diseases have raised important general questions about the control of plasma protein metabolism, which can be approached with current methods. One purpose of this chapter is to emphasize these actual and potential applications of studies of complement biosynthesis.

2. Methods for Studies of Complement Synthesis

2.1. Tissue Culture Conditions: Media and Cells

The development of suitable tissue-culture techniques for studies of protein synthesis by eukaryotic cells *in vitro* have progressed largely on a trial-and-error basis. Outside of requirements for nutritionally balanced media with optimal concentrations of ionic species and adequate buffering capacity, there are few data that would permit a rational choice of the best medium for any specific experiment. In addition, several supplements (e.g., calf serum, hormones, and vitamins) are often used to improve longevity of cells and tissues in culture, frequently without

HARVEY R. COLTEN • Division of Allergy, Department of Medicine, Children's Hospital Medical Center and Department of Pediatrics, Harvard Medical School, Boston, Massachusetts.

complete understanding of the specific effects of these constituents. Additional considerations must be taken into account in the choice of medium, particularly if functional assay systems are used to monitor protein synthesis; e.g., the protein must be stable under the conditions of culture. In studies of synthesis of the early-acting complement components C4 and C2, complex media supplemented with fetal calf serum have been used successfully (Colten, 1972a). For detection of biologically active C1, C3, and C5–C9, two media may be substituted for M199 or MEM in short-term (72 hr) experiments (Colten, 1973). One is a commercially available preparation, Neuman and Tytell's serumless medium (Grand Island Biological Co.); the other is a special minimal medium designed for studies of biosynthesis of the late-acting complement components (Colten, 1973).

Studies of primary cell cultures or organ cultures require considerable preliminary preparation, since all tissues contain large quantities of preformed complement components. In order to demonstrate synthesis of relatively small amounts of complement *in vitro,* baseline levels must be achieved without damaging the tissues. Established cell lines have also been used in many studies of complement synthesis. Use of permanent cell lines have many advantages in that large cell numbers are easily obtained and, aside from problems of genetic drift, are identical from time to time (i.e., reproducibility of conditions is maximized). However, interpretation of results of studies in which these cells are used requires caution, since the cell lines, generally, must be maintained in media supplemented with serum, and the cells may be capable of adsorbing or ingesting proteins from the media. Release of these proteins must be distinguished from *de novo* synthesis of protein. Furthermore, one cannot draw conclusions regarding the normal site of synthesis from the origin of the tissue or cell giving rise to permanent cell lines, although these cells may be particularly valuable for investigations of the regulation of inducible and noninducible cell functions.

Identification of the specific cellular sites of complement biosynthesis has been approached with two methods: fluorescent antibody staining of individual cells with anti-complement-component antibodies and a modification of the hemolysis in gel technique, used successfully in studies of antibody synthesis. Fluorescent antibody techniques have the principal advantage of simplicity but are limited for biosynthetic studies by the fact that the technique is qualitative. Even with appropriate controls, it is difficult or impossible to establish that the cell in question is actively synthesizing the specific protein; and the number or types of cells synthesizing the protein may be grossly underestimated, since there is evidence to suggest that under normal conditions, plasma proteins are rapidly secreted following synthesis and assembly (Colten, 1974b). A method for detection of antibody production by single cells was introduced by Jerne and Nordin (1963) and Ingraham and Bussard (1964). Plaquelike zones of hemolysis surrounding the antibody-forming cells are easily detectable. At the Ciba Symposium on Complement, Lepow (1965) suggested that a modification of this method permits studies of complement synthesis by individual cells. Lepow's suggestion has been picked up by several investigators and has been particularly useful in studies of synthesis of the early-acting complement components, C1, C4, and C2 (Colten *et al.,* 1968b; Littleton *et al.,* 1970; Wyatt *et al.,* 1972).

Although many technical problems still remain, recent studies of the cell-free biosynthesis of C3 and C4 indicate that fundamental problems in molecular biology may yield to this approach (Hall and Colten, unpublished data; Hall *et al.*, unpublished data). This is particularly significant when one considers that, in preliminary experiments, it has been possible not only to detect synthesis of immunochemically identifiable C3 and C4 polypeptides, but also the production of biologically active C4 in cell-free systems. Basically, methods in use at this time consist of preparation of polysomes from liver, spleen, or peritoneal cells, priming with initiation factors from wheat germ or rabbit reticulocyte lysates, and monitoring of synthesis with immunochemical and functional assays for the individual complement proteins. The size of newly synthesized protein is estimated on polyacrylamide gels, and the presence of uniform incorporation of radiolabeled amino acids is detected with radioautography of peptide maps. Problems inherent in this approach are magnified by the relatively small amounts of specific complement proteins synthesized in relation to total protein synthesis. This stands in contradistinction to the relatively large proportion of hemoglobin or immunoglobulin to total protein synthesized by polysomes prepared from reticulocytes and myeloma plasma cells, respectively.

2.2. Assay Systems

Ideally, one would wish to monitor production of complement *in vitro* by organs, cells, or subcellular components with a detection system that is sensitive, specific, reproducible, capable of detecting active and inactive complement proteins, and able to distinguish newly synthesized from preformed protein. No single method satisfies all these criteria, but it is possible to approach the ideal condition with the use of several methods in combination. As noted earlier, the hemolytic assays for individual complement components are extremely sensitive and specific (Rapp and Borsos, 1970). Nanogram quantities of the biologically active component can be detected in complex mixtures, which is a decided advantage for measurements of complement in tissue-culture media. Because of the specificity of these measurements, the biologically active complement components can be detected in complex mixtures of proteins without fractionating or concentrating the sample. More detail on the theoretical and practical aspects of these assays can be found in Rapp and Borsos (1970).

The hemolytic assays for individual components vary in their efficiency of detection. Therefore, even discounting other potential problems of stability of the component in various tissue-culture media and efficiency of uptake of the components on the indicator cells, certain components are more easily detected with this method. Direct comparison of rates of synthesis of the individual components must take these differences into account. Moreover, these measurements, of course, do not detect hemolytically inactive complement proteins, nor do they permit a distinction between preformed and newly synthesized protein. Other biological activities of complement components, such as immune adherence and chemotactic activity, may be used for quantitation of biosynthesis, but these have had only limited use in synthesis studies because of a lack of specificity or sensitivity or both.

Biosynthesis of complement components *in vitro* was first detected by means of immunoprecipitation of specific proteins by Hochwald *et al.* (1961). Using this method, the incorporation of radiolabeled amino acids into specific proteins may be estimated by a variety of techniques, including scintillation counting and radioautography of immunoprecipitation bands in gels. Although considerably less sensitive than the functional assay described above, if proper controls are included, the immunochemical method is capable of differentiating newly synthesized from preformed protein. Generally, because of the extremely small amount of labeled protein produced in short-term experiments, carrier, unlabeled protein must be added to detect immunoprecipitation of radiolabeled protein. The effect of inhibitors of protein synthesis on incorporation and suitable controls for nonspecific binding must be included. In spite of these controls, the limitations of this method are considerable, particularly if it represents the only evidence of complement synthesis, since an unlabeled component may be bound to a radiolabeled antigen–antibody complex. Additional controls to test for incorporation of radiolabel into complement protein can be performed by taking advantage of the specificity of interaction of a component with a suitable erythrocyte intermediate. For example, in studies of the biosynthesis of C2 by guinea pig tissues *in vitro* (Rubin *et al.,* 1971), it was shown that immunoprecipitable radiolabeled C2 was removed by adsorption with EAC4 but not by EA, and that adsorption of the labeled protein was associated with the uptake of hemolytically active C2, since the EAC4 could then be lysed by addition of C1, C3, and C5–9. In several studies (Rommel *et al.,* 1970; Strunk *et al.,* 1975; Bing *et al.,* 1975), it has also been possible to show, using a variety of physicochemical and immunoabsorbent column methods, that radiolabel was incorporated into authentic complement proteins. That is, the physicochemical characteristics of the newly formed proteins corresponded to those of the native proteins in whole serum. It is obvious from the foregoing that several methods must be employed in a given set of studies of synthesis *in vitro* in order to offset the limitations of each one.

2.3. Biosynthesis *in Vivo*

While many questions regarding biosynthesis can be tested with *in vitro* methods, it is apparent that control of plasma protein concentration *in vivo* is dependent not only on synthesis rates, but also on immune and nonimmune catabolic rates. Moreover, the possibility that synthesis rates are affected by circulating factors, produced at sites remote from the primary site of synthesis, cannot be studied *in vitro* without prior evidence obtained from metabolic studies in the intact organism. Some of the first investigations of sites of complement biosynthesis were performed in experimental animals, but these required destruction or ablation of organ systems. More sophisticated techniques permit a study of metabolism of several of the complement components using trace-labeled purified components. From the rate of disappearance of radiolabeled protein in plasma, one can calculate the catabolic rate as a percentage of the plasma pool, the synthesis rate, and the extravascular-to-plasma-pool ratio, using the analytic method of Mathews (1957). The validity of this analysis depends on two critical assumptions: first, that catabolism occurs in a pool in equilibrium with the plasma pool; i.e., sequestration of labeled protein in an inaccessible pool does not occur; and, second, that a steady-state condition for the protein under study is obtained throughout the period of observation. These conditions have been satisfied in most of the published accounts of complement metabolism in man. Two additional approaches to investigations of complement synthesis *in vivo* have been applied to both clinical conditions and studies in experimental animals. First, advantage has been taken of organ transplantation to determine sites of synthesis of human plasma proteins (Merrill *et al.*, 1964; Kashiwagi *et al.*, 1968), including specific complement components (Alper *et al.*, 1969). Similar studies have been performed in experimental animals (Phillips and Thorbecke, 1965; Phillips *et al.*, 1969). Second, the availability of genetically determined deficiencies of complement proteins (reviewed by Alper and Rosen, 1971; Stroud and Donaldson, 1974) has made it possible to study fetal synthesis of complement and to test for transplacental transfer of complement in humans and experimental animals. The results of these studies will be described at length in subsequent sections.

3. Sites of Synthesis of Complement Components

3.1. Biosynthesis of the First Component

In 1966, a series of experiments designed to identify the site of synthesis of biologically active C1 indicated that, in the guinea pig (Colten *et al.*, 1966) and in man (Colten *et al.*, 1968a), macromolecular C1 was synthesized primarily, if not exclusively, in the small and large intestines. This conclusion was based on observations that isolated segments of intestine, in short-term organ culture, were the only tissues capable of producing hemolytically active C1. Production of C1 *in vitro* was temperature-dependent, reversibly inhibited by actinomycin D and puromycin, and accompanied by incorporation of ^{14}C-labeled amino acids into a molecule functionally similar to C1. In subsequent studies (Colten *et al.*, 1968b), with a modification of the Jerne plaque technique, which is capable of detecting production of hemolytically active C1 by individual cells, evidence was presented that, in the guinea pig, columnar epithelial cells were the site of C1 synthesis.

At about the same time, Thorbecke *et al.* (Stecher and Thorbecke, 1967a; Stecher *et al.*, 1967) reported production of C1q *in vitro* by human and monkey liver, spleen, bone marrow, and lung, as well as by isolated macrophages from peritoneal exudates and lung washings. Their conclusions were based solely on detection of radiolabeled C1q precipitin lines developed with an anti-C1q antiserum in the presence of carrier serum or euglobulin. In a study of the ontogenetic development of C1q in the piglet, Day *et al.* (1970) failed to find hemolytic C1 in any of the embryonic tissues examined. Accordingly, they used a modification of Thorbecke's method for the detection of incorporation of labeled amino acids into C1q protein. Portions of the fore, mid, and hind gut were the first tissues to synthesize C1q protein as estimated by this technique. This was detectable in the earliest tissue examined. Lymph node, spleen, liver, and lung cultures obtained from fetuses later in gestation also contained labeled C1q. Labeling was significantly reduced in cultures incubated in medium containing chloramphenicol. Although the cellular site of C1q synthesis was not identified, these workers suggested that since nonintestinal tissues, particularly those rich in lymphoid cells, also produced C1q, a mesenchymal cell, not an epithelial cell, was the site of synthesis. Several clinical observations, indicating independent control of C1q, C1r, and C1s concentrations in sera of some patients with severe combined immunodeficiency (O'Connel *et al.*, 1967; Gewurz *et al.*, 1968; Stroud *et al.*, 1970) and in a patient with selective deficiency of C1r (Pickering *et al.*, 1970) suggested the possibility that the known subcomponents of C1 might be synthesized in different cell lines, with assembly of the macromolecule in one of the cell types. Moreover, bone marrow transplantation for severe, combined immunodeficiency resulted in an apparent reconstitution of C1q (Ballow *et al.*, 1973; Yount *et al.*, 1974). From these and other studies (Kohler and Müller-Eberhard, 1969), it was postulated that the synthesis of C1q and IgG were linked. Two observations make this an untenable hypothesis at the present time. Metabolic studies of trace-labeled C1q in patients with agammaglobulinemia revealed accelerated catabolism, not depressed synthesis (Kohler and Müller-Eberhard, 1972), and serum levels of C1q and IgG vary coincidentally with exogenous gamma globulin administration in patients with agammaglobulinemia (Pickering, unpublished, cited in Gabrielson *et al.*, 1974).

Renewed interest in epithelial cells as a site of C1 synthesis has been generated by a series of elegant experiments by Bing *et al.* (1975). They demonstrated synthesis of macromolecular C1 and C1s in long-term primary suspension cultures of normal human colon, adenocarcinoma of the colon, and transitional epithelial cells of bladder, urethra, and reneal pelvis but not in cultures of prostate, renal cell carcinoma, or fibroblasts. It is believed that the epithelial cells of the urogenital tract and the colon may have a common (endodermal) origin, since early in embryonic life, the hindgut and mesonephric duct are continuous with the cloaca. Synthesis of biologically active C1 was inhibited by cycloheximide and was accompanied by incorporation of radiolabeled amino acids into macromolecular C1 and its subcomponent of C1s. Moreover, the newly formed protein was isolated from the tissue-culture medium by means of specific-affinity column chromatography. Subcloning experiments, now in progress, should establish finally whether, as it appears, all the subcomponents of C1 are synthesized in a single cell type. Wyatt (1974) has also provided preliminary evidence that the HEK (human embryonic kidney) and MA177 (human embryonic intestine) cell lines produce C1 *in vitro,* but the precise cells of origin and homogeneity of these lines are not known. A report (van Zaipel, 1970) has appeared of synthesis of a C1-like molecule by HeLa cells (derived from a cervical carcinoma), but examination of at least two other HeLa lines has failed to reveal synthesis of either C1q (Stecher and Thorbecke, 1967c; Colten and Wyatt, 1972), C1s, or intact C1 (Colten, 1972b). These contradictory findings can probably be accounted for by extensive genetic drift during many years in culture and the resulting heterogeneity of HeLa cell lines.

3.2. Biosynthesis of the Second Component

Several authors, using a variety of methods, have concluded that the macrophage is the site of C2 biosynthesis. Early studies of C2 biosynthesis (Siboo and Vas, 1965; Rubin *et al.*, 1971; Colten, 1972a) indicated that production of hemolytically active C2 could be detected in many organs, including lung, bone marrow, spleen, and, in some species, liver. In several of these studies, it was shown that C2 production was, in fact, due to *de novo* synthesis, inasmuch as the appearance of C2 in culture was reversibly inhibited by cycloheximide and was accompanied by incorporation of radiolabeled amino acids into a protein that is immunochemically and functionally identical with C2. Subsequently, using a modification of the Jerne plaque technique to detect guinea pig C2 synthesis (Wyatt *et al.*, 1972) and isopyknic density-gradient centrifugation of fetal liver cells to partially purify cells that synthesize human C2 (Colten, 1972a), it was shown in each case that C2 was produced by large mononuclear cells, probably macrophages.

Recently, a significant advance in methodology, permitting maintenance of human peripheral blood monocytes in primary culture for prolonged periods (10–12 wk), has made it possible to demonstrate C2 synthesis by circulating cells of the monocyte/macrophage series (Einstein *et al.*, 1976). These cells maintain the capacity to synthesize C2 and lysozyme, to phagocytize large latex particles, to kill *Listeria monocytogenes,* and to rosette with IgG-sensitized erythrocytes. Within the limits of the methods employed, these appear to be pure monocyte cultures.

A cell line developed by Wyatt (1974) should also be useful for long-term studies of C2 synthesis *in vitro*. This cell, obtained from a peritoneal exudate induced in strain 2 guinea pigs, has a mean generation time of 40 hr, an epitheloid appearance, and adheres firmly to surfaces, resisting attempts to dislodge them from plastic tissue-culture dishes with EDTA-trypsin. C2 production by this cell line has continued through more than 22 passages over a 15-month period. Several reports of C2 synthesis by hepatoma cell lines have appeared (Levisohn and Thompson, 1973; Strunk *et al.,* 1975). Some of these cells are highly differentiated and have retained many functions that are characteristic of hepatic parenchymal cells. In spite of these findings, since in primary culture only monocytes or macrophages synthesize C2, it is likely that in the liver, the Kupffer cell, not a parenchymal cell, is the site of C2 production.

3.3. Biosynthesis of the Fourth Component

Several independent lines of evidence indicate that the macrophage is a site of C4 biosynthesis. Interest in the liver as a primary site of C4 synthesis initially depended on experiments showing marked depression of serum C4 levels in animals exposed to hepatotoxins or following hepatectomy (Dick, 1913; Gordon, 1955). Jensen *et al.* (1971), in the first study of synthesis of functional C4 *in vitro,* demonstrated synthesis by liver and concluded that the parenchymal cell was the likely site of C4 production. On the other hand, Thorbecke and her colleagues (Thorbecke *et al.,* 1965; Stecher and Thorbecke, 1967a) suggested that the macrophage was the principal site of C4 synthesis, but these studies were incomplete, since no studies of biologically active C4 were performed. Indirect evidence that macrophages produce biologically active C4 was also obtained by others (Chan, 1970; Füst and Surján, 1971; Chan and Cebra, 1966). Work by at least two groups (Littleton *et al.,* 1970; Wyatt *et al.,* 1972) has confirmed these observations and extended the initial experiments to include direct measurements of production of biologically active C4. The adherent cells in guinea pig peritoneal exudates, spleen cells (Ilgen and Burkholder, 1974), and cells from upper fractions of discontinuous density-gradient ultracentrifugation of human fetal (Colten, 1972a) or guinea pig liver (Ilgen and Burkholder, 1974) are capable of synthesizing biologically active C4 in short-term tissue culture. Moreover, it has been demonstrated that at least some of the cells capable of synthesizing C4 also synthesize C2 (Wyatt *et al.,* 1972). At least two sources of mononuclear phagocytes, human peripheral blood and lung macrophages, yield cells that synthesize C2 but produce no hemolytically active C4.

[14]C-labeled amino acids are apparently incorporated into C4 protein, but attempts to detect the appearance of active C4 in these cultures have thus far been unsuccessful (Einstein *et al.*, 1976; Laguarda, unpublished data). Studies underway should indicate whether this finding represents heterogeneity of macrophages, production of a fragment of C4, or, least likely, a technical problem in the detection system.

Biosynthesis of C4 by established cell lines has also been demonstrated (Stecher and Thorbecke, 1967c; Wyatt, 1974; Strunk *et al.*, 1975) using both functional and immunochemical methods. Several lines derived from normal rat liver or hepatomas produce significant quantities of C4 in culture. One of these lines has been subcloned and has many characteristics of liver parenchymal cells.

3.4. Biosynthesis of the Third Component

The first studies of C3 biosynthesis *in vitro* suggested that this component was synthesized by many tissues and cell types. Claims were made by Thorbecke *et al.* (1965) that lymph nodes, spleen, liver, lung, bone marrow, adult thymus, and the fibria of the fallopian tube were sites of synthesis of C3. This conclusion was based solely on detection of radiolabeled C3 precipitin arcs on immunoelectrophoresis of culture media. One group (Glade and Chessin, 1968) has suggested that the lymphocyte was the cellular site of C3 synthesis, but several authors (Stecher *et al.*, 1967; Lepow, 1965) have provided both direct and indirect evidence that this is not the case. Others (Stecher and Thorbecke, 1967a; Lai A Fat and van Furth, 1975) have indicated that macrophages synthesize C3 but again with one possible exception (Colten, 1974b), this was based on immunochemical detection of ^{14}C-labeled amino acid incorporation into B_1C protein.

Alper *et al.* (1969) performed an interesting experiment, making use of the technique of prolonged agarose electrophoresis to detect polymorphic forms of C3, and showed that the liver was the principal, if not the only, site of C3 synthesis. In this study, a patient with a hepatoma received a liver transplant following total hepatectomy. The recipient had a rare C3 type ($FS_{0.6}$). The donor was C3 type SS. Within 20 hr following transplantation, the C3 type changed almost completely from that of the recipient to the donor type, and by 6 weeks postoperatively, no C3F or $S_{0.6}$ type could be detected. A concomitant change in haptoglobin type (another protein synthesized by the liver) was also noted, confirming the observations of Merrill *et al.* (1964) and Kashiwagi *et al.* (1968). Additional evidence that the liver is the major site of C3 synthesis was obtained in experiments (Johnson *et al.*, 1971b) showing staining of hepatic parenchymal cells with fluorescent-labeled anti-C3 antiserum. In addition, production of hemolytically active C3 has been detected *in vitro* in cultures of human fetal and postnatal liver (Colten, 1972a). Extrahepatic production of hemolytically active C3 has been detected in synovial tissues from patients with rheumatoid arthritis but not from patients with traumatic or degenerative joint disease (Ruddy and Colten, 1974). This study and other studies would indicate the necessity to study C3 synthesis under a variety of conditions before excluding the possibility that a given cell type is not a site of C3 synthesis. As with many of the other complement proteins, production of C3 by long-term, established cell lines has been reported (Stecher and Thorbecke, 1967c; Strunk *et al.*, 1975).

55

COMPLEMENT
SYNTHESIS

These cell lines have been particularly useful in studies of the microenvironmental control of complement synthesis.

3.5. Biosynthesis of C5 and C6

In early studies of C5 biosynthesis, Phillips *et al.* (1969) made use of the observation that several mouse strains were known to be deficient in C5 or MuB1 (the immunochemically defined C5 protein) (Rosenberg and Tachibana, 1962; Terry *et al.*, 1964; Cinader and Dubiski, 1963). Bone marrow cells from allogeneic or apparent congenic strains were injected into C5 deficient X-irradiated recipients. Total complement activity was detected in sera of recipients of the marrow within 2–3 days and persisted for almost 3 weeks following the transplant, indicating production of biologically active C5 by bone marrow cells. Examination of sera of each of the recipient mice immunoelectrophoretically did not reveal MuB1 protein following transplantation. This discrepancy between the immunochemical and hemolytic data was no doubt due to differences in sensitivity of the assay systems. *In vitro* studies indicated that the C5-producing marrow cells were present in the recipient spleen since cultures of this organ prepared 3–4 weeks after establishment of chimerism showed labeling of MuB1 when incubated in the presence of ^{14}C-labeled amino acids.

Much later, Levy *et al.* (1973) demonstrated that the adherent cells from the spleen of B10D2 new line mice were the only cells of those examined, capable of synthesizing C5 as judged by the appearance of hemolytic C5 activity in media harvested from spleen cell cultures. Puromycin inhibited C5 production, indicating active synthesis. These experiments suggested that the macrophage was a site of C5 synthesis. This conclusion was not confirmed in studies of the adherent cell population isolated from guinea pig peritoneal exudates (Colten, 1974b). Although hemolytically active C5 was present in media harvested from peritoneal cell cultures, there was no net increase in C5 activity and no effect of temperature nor inhibitors of protein synthesis on the appearance of C5. This indicated that substantial quantities of preformed C5, either bound to or within the peritoneal cells, were released under the culture conditions. The reasons for this finding are not clear at the present time. In any case, it is likely that a widely distributed cell type is the site of C5 synthesis as evidenced by studies of biosynthesis of this component in man. Two studies of human C5 biosynthesis have been reported. In one of these (Colten, 1973), production of biologically active C5 was detected in the lung, liver, spleen, and fetal intestine. In the other study (Kohler, 1973), C5 production, as judged by incorporation of radiolabeled amino acids, was detected in the thymus, placenta, peritoneal cells, and bone marrow as well. Thus far, the specific cell type that synthesizes human C5 has not been identified.

Several clonal strains of rat hepatoma, including a strain that also synthesized C3, C9, C1 inhibitor, albumin, and tyrosine aminotransferase, synthesize biologically active C5 (Strunk *et al.*, 1975). As with other studies of protein synthesis by long-term cell lines, it would be imprudent to conclude on the basis of this study that hepatic parenchymal cells are a site of C5 synthesis. However, primary rat liver cell cultures, rich in parenchymal cells and relatively depleted of Kupffer cells, produce C5 in culture (Breslow *et al.*, unpublished data). A difference in species is an unlikely explanation to account for the different observations with respect to C5 synthesis by mouse and rat or guinea pig cell types. Final conclusions must, therefore, await additional studies.

The availability of rabbits deficient in C6 (Rother *et al.*, 1966) and a recent report of C6 deficiency in humans (Leddy *et al.*, 1974) suggest the need for more extensive studies of C6 synthesis. In the single report of C6 biosynthesis (Rother *et al.*, 1968), it appeared that the liver was the major site of C6 production, but synthesis of C6 by other tissues could not be excluded. The precise cellular site of synthesis was not defined. In fact, many technical problems encountered in that work have subsequently been resolved so that a reexamination of C6 synthesis *in vitro* might now be fruitful.

3.6. Biosynthesis of C7 and C8

The biosynthesis of C7 has not been studied, and only isolated reports of C8 synthesis are available. For example, Geiger *et al.* (1972) have investigated the ontogeny and synthesis of C8 by tissue obtained from fetal piglets. Significant C8 production was noted in the spleen, liver, lung, intestine, and kidney, but not in the lymph nodes, thymus, or bone marrow. In the lung, reversible inhibition of C8 production was noted in the presence of cycloheximide and actinomycin D, and production was temperature dependent in cultures of fetal kidney, spleen, liver, and lung.

3.7. Biosynthesis of C9

Synthesis of C9 by a long-term rat hepatoma cell strain was demonstrated several years ago (Rommell *et al.*, 1970). This line is highly differentiated, having many features characteristic of normal hepatic parenchymal cells. For example, it is capable of synthesizing albumin, C3, C1 inhibitor, and C6 but not C1, C4, or significant amounts of C2 (Strunk *et al.*, 1975). Moreover, in this cell, the glucuronide-conjugating system is intact. More recently, Breslow *et al.* (unpublished data) found that primary rat liver cell cultures, enriched in parenchymal cells, produced substantial amounts of hemolytically active C9 in culture; production was reversibly inhibited by cycloheximide. Based on these experiments, it is likely, but not yet firmly established, that C9 is synthesized by liver parenchymal cells.

3.8. Complement-Associated Proteins

The synthesis of C1 inhibitor by liver has been demonstrated in short-term cultures using both functional (Colten, 1972a) and immunochemical (Gitlin and Biassucci, 1969; Colten, 1972a) assays. Based on fluorescence, approximately 5–10% of normal human liver parenchymal cells produce C1 inhibitor (Johnson *et al.*, 1971a). Fluorescence of Kupffer or other liver cells was not noted. Synthesis of the C3b inactivator and the proteins of the properdin system have not yet been studied in any detail.

Genetically determined complement deficiencies in man and experimental animals (reviewed by Alper and Rosen, 1971, and Stroud and Donaldson, 1974) have provided material for several promising lines of investigation, using methods developed in modern studies of complement biosynthesis.

4.1. C4 Deficiency

Following the discovery and development of a strain of guinea pigs genetically deficient in C4 (Ellman *et al.,* 1970), Colten and Frank (1972) studied the biosynthesis of C2 and C4 by tissues and cells isolated from affected animals. The study of C2 biosynthesis by tissues from C4 deficient animals was of particular interest, since it had been shown that in some but not all homozygous C4-deficient animals, the C2 serum levels were approximately one-half normal (Frank *et al.,* 1971). Measurements of complement synthesis in short- and long-term cell cultures indicated that homozygous deficient animals produced no detectable C4 and that the rate of C2 synthesis was approximately 40% of normal. Tissues and cells from heterozygous deficient animals produced C4 at a rate that is intermediate between that of the normal and the homozygous deficient. In each case, the relative reduction in rates of *in vitro* C2 and C4 synthesis by heterozygous and homozygous deficient cells correlated well with the reduced serum levels of the corresponding component. In an attempt to define the genetic lesion responsible for C4 deficiency, peritoneal exudate cells from a homozygous C4-deficient guinea pig were fused *in vitro* with a cell line of human origin. The resulting hybrid cells derived from parental cells, each incapable of C4 biosynthesis by themselves (Stecher and Thorbecke, 1967c, and Colten and Frank, 1972), synthesized functionally active human C4 but no detectable guinea pig C4 (Colten and Parkman, 1972). Several explanations for these results were considered. Among these was the possibility that, in hybrid cells, a product of the C4 deficient genome was capable of derepressing the human C4 gene but that the defective guinea pig C4 gene could not respond to the signal. In order to test this possibility, attempts were made to identify the putative derepressor. Peritoneal cells isolated from C4 deficient guinea pigs, although incapable of synthesizing C4, produced a factor that specifically induced synthesis and secretion of functionally active C4 by HeLa cells (Colten, 1972b). Operationally, this substance has been designated a regulator factor, since the site of action of the factor in the indicator (HeLa) cells is not known. The factor from the C4-deficient cells was found to be heat-stable (at 56° for 1 hr), nondialyzable, and partially inactivated by RNAase and trypsin, but not by DNAase. Chromatography on Sephadex G-100 demonstrated that the activity eluted in a position corresponding to a 45,000-molecular-weight market (Colten, 1974a).

A few preliminary generalizations about the regulator are warranted at this time: (1) The regulator factor appears to initiate biosynthesis of a specific protein without affecting total protein synthesis in the responsive cell. (2) The effect of the regulator is reversible. (3) The regulator is not species specific; i.e., a human cell is capable of recognizing and responding to guinea pig regulator. (4) Synthesis of the regulator and the response to it are both sensitive to inhibition by relatively low concentrations of actinomycin D and other inhibitors of protein synthesis. (5) The amount of regulator recovered from genetically deficient peritoneal cells was about 5–10 times that recovered from primary cultures of normal peritoneal cells. This could be the result of increased synthesis or decreased degradation of the factor in genetically deficient cells. These observations suggest the possibility that in deficient cells the regulator of C4 gene function accumulates perhaps because an interruption in the normal C4 biosynthetic pathway prevents normal feedback control. It has been shown that, in hybrid cells, activation or expression of a specialized gene function may depend on gene dose (Davidson and Benda, 1970; Fougere *et al.*, 1972), and that it is possible to demonstrate cross-species induction of gene function in the hybrid cell when one of the parent cells has a greater than normal chromosome complement (Peterson and Weiss, 1972). The results of the experiment with C4-deficient cells suggest the possibility of a somewhat similar mechanism of ''activation'' of a silent gene. In hybrid cells, an increased gene dose may supply a regulator factor or a similar mediator in sufficient quantity to initiate synthesis of a specialized gene product, whereas, in genetically deficient cells, defective feedback control may lead to increased production or accumulation of a regulator. A search for other specific regulator factors seems warranted, particularly in those genetic lesions that result in total absence of gene product.

4.2. C5 Deficiency

In a similar study of the molecular basis of C5 deficiency, Levy and his co-workers (Levy and Ladda, 1971; Levy *et al.*, 1973) have also made use of the technique of somatic-cell hybridization *in vitro*. The two closely related mouse strains, B10D2 old (C5 deficient) and new (C5 sufficient) lines, were used as sources of parent cells for the hybridization studies. As mentioned in an earlier section of this review, splenic macrophages from new line mice were the only cells capable of synthesizing C5. Hybridization of B10D2 new-line kidney cells with B10D2 old-line splenic macrophages and between B10D2 old-line macrophages and adult chicken erythrocytes indicated that whereas none of the parent cells were capable of producing C5 by themselves, the hybrids produced C5 in tissue culture. Injection of the hybrid cells into old-line mice resulted in the appearance of hemolytic complement activity in their sera. This activity peaked between 3 and 6 days after injection, gradually declined, and was undetectable at 21 days following the injection, coincident with the appearance of anti-C5 antibody (Levy and Ladda, 1971). Appropriate controls ruled out a nonspecific effect of (1) Sendai virus (used to increase the frequency of fusion) and (2) fusion itself, with the use of cells that would not expect to provide adequate gene complementation. Several interpretations of these experiments were considered: (1) complementation of the structural gene derived from a kidney cell and the regulator from splenic macrophages (results with the mouse by chicken erythrocyte hybrids were inconsistent with this interpretation, since mouse C5 was produced.); (2) the possibility that subunits of C5 were supplied by the chicken and other subunits by the deficient mouse cells, but neither immunochemical nor structural data are available to rule this possibility in or out; and (3) lack of a derepressor or presence of an abnormal repressor in the C5 deficient mouse cells. The experiments argue against these possibilities, but do not rigorously exclude them.

Recently, it has been possible to extend this approach to a study of a complement deficiency in man. With the use of a method for prolonged culture of human peripheral blood monocytes, it was shown that monocytes from three homozygous C2 deficient individuals synthesized no detectable C2 *in vitro,* even after 8 weeks in culture, whereas normal and heterozygote deficient monocytes synthesized C2 throughout this period (Einstein *et al.,* 1975). Although monocytes from some heterozygous deficient individuals synthesized C2 at slower rates than monocytes from normals, there was no direct relationship between rates of C2 synthesis *in vitro* and the serum C2 concentrations. Perhaps this was due to stimulation of C2 synthesis in heterozygous deficient cells by *in vitro* factors (e.g., fetal calf serum, glass surfaces) to a proportionately greater extent than in normal monocytes. Alternatively, release of the cells from *in vivo* regulatory factors may have been sufficient to account for these findings. Of note is an earlier observation that C2 synthesis by peritoneal macrophages from homozygous C4 deficient guinea pigs was stimulated to a greater extent than was C2 synthesis by normal macrophages when both were exposed to heat-killed pneumococci (Colten and Frank, 1972).

Monocytes from normal and heterozygous deficient individuals incorporated radiolabeled amino acids into protein that was immunochemically dentified as C2; there was no labeled C2 in the medium harvested from homozygous deficient monocytes. Incorporation of radiolabel into total protein was similar in monocytes from homozygous and heterozygous deficient individuals and normals. Moreover, monocytes from the C2 deficient children could not be distinguished from the monocytes of other family members or the unrelated normal subject on the basis of morphology. They were equally capable of phagocytizing 5.7-μm diameter latex particles, forming rosettes with IgG or C3 coated erythrocytes, and killing *L. monocytogenes,* indicating that the defect was apparently specific for C2 synthesis.

Fusion between C2-deficient monocytes or normal monocytes and undifferentiated cells, with assays for C2 production and HLA cell-surface determinants should make it possible to define the genetic lesion in C2 deficiency and to test whether both functions (C2 production and HLA antigens) are invariably expressed coincidentally in hybrid cells. Hybrids between mouse macrophages and L cells express several macrophage-specific markers, including H-2 antigens (Gordon *et al.,* 1971). Unfortunately, C2 synthesis by these hybrids was not studied. Others have shown that, in hybrid cells, C2 synthesis may be expressed (Levisohn and Thompson, 1973) and persist for many months in culture (Parkman *et al.,* unpublished data). In one of these studies, some hybrids between human fetal liver and mouse 3T3 cells continued to synthesize and secrete human C2 up to 1 year after hybridization, although, as is characteristic of mouse–human hybrids, most of the human chromosomes had been lost. It appeared, based on examination of several clones, that persistence of a group C human chromosome correlated with the capacity to synthesize C2. This group C chromosome seemed to correspond to chromosome 6, but fluorescence banding techniques were not sufficiently refined to determine this with certainty. These data, however, are not incompatible with the localization of HL-A loci to chromosome 6 (van Someren *et al.,* 1974; Lamm *et al.,* 1974) and the close linkage between C2 deficiency and HL-A type (Fu *et al.,* 1974).

The mechanisms of other genetic diseases of the complement system may also yield to this type of analysis. The advantage of using complement as a model system for genetic studies is based primarily on the ease of detecting the gene product, the large number of well-characterized genetic abnormalities, and the availability of cell lines capable of synthesizing individual complement proteins.

5. Nongenetic Control of Complement Biosynthesis

The recognition of the importance of complement in host defenses has prompted many studies of complement levels in patients with a variety of diseases and particularly those with acute infections. Although all such studies were limited by the fact that a static measure of serum-complement concentration cannot reveal the dynamics of synthesis, catabolism, and distribution of a plasma protein, many interesting and provocative observations have resulted from this approach. In some fulminant infections, such as meningococcal meningitis (Ecker *et al.*, 1946) and dengue fever with shock (Bokisch *et al.*, 1973), levels were often reduced largely as a result of increased consumption but perhaps also due to depressed synthesis. On the other hand, it was found that during the course of most acute infections with pyogenic organisms, there is often a marked increase in complement levels (Dick, 1912; Ecker *et al.*, 1946). These clinical observations have been explored experimentally, but as yet no unifying control mechanisms have been uncovered. For example, staphylococcal bacteremia leads to a transient decline and then a marked increase in total complement activity in the sera of experimental animals (Baltch *et al.*, 1962) as well as a change in apparent synthesis rates (Williams *et al.*, 1963). Viable microorganisms are apparently not required for this effect, as shown by the experiments of Jungeblut and Berlot (1926) many years before, indicating a similar effect of India ink. Ample evidence exists for a stimulatory effect of endotoxin on synthesis of certain plasma proteins, including C-reactive protein and C3 (Hurlimann *et al.*, 1966; Thorbecke *et al.*, 1965; Stecher and Thorbecke, 1967b). Whether these effects are mediated by similar or distinct mechanisms is not known.

In view of a recent series of investigations, the possibility must be considered that phagocytosis or "activation" of cells of the reticuloendothelial system may account, in part, for the aforementioned findings. Studies in which normal guinea pig macrophages were exposed *in vitro* to heat-killed pneumococci revealed up to a tenfold increase in C2 and C4 production over baseline rates (Colten, 1974b). In these experiments, the cells were maintained in a serum-free medium because normal serum also contains a factor, or factors, that stimulate C2 and C4 biosynthesis *in vitro* (Stecher and Thorbecke, 1967b; Colten, 1974a,b). The mechanism by which serum or phagocytic activity affects the rates of complement biosynthesis is not clear at the present, but the effects are strikingly similar to those of identical stimuli on intracellular enzyme activities (Cohn and Benson, 1965). It is unlikely that the serum stimulatory factor is a complement component, inasmuch as serum from guinea pigs with a genetic deficiency of C4 was as effective as normal guinea pig serum in stimulating C4 synthesis by guinea pig peritoneal macrophages (Colten and Frank, 1972). The signal for a change in rate of complement synthesis and the details of the cellular response to this signal have, therefore, not been defined. However, in the case of a "phagocytic" stimulus, there was suggestive evidence that increased secretion of C2 by cells exposed to particles in suspension required new protein synthesis, not merely an accelerated release of preformed protein.

These experiments raised the possibility that control of local production of complement at a site of inflammation may be of importance in affecting the balance between host defenses and an invading microorganism. A similar finding, noted in studies of complement synthesis by synovial tissues (Ruddy and Colten, 1974) seems to confirm this hypothesis. Evidence has also been obtained that sterile inflammatory reactions *in vivo* may affect the capacity of mononuclear cells at remote sites to synthesize C2 and C4. For instance, when turpentine or complete Freund's adjuvant were injected intramuscularly to induce inflammatory reactions, preliminary results suggested than an inflammatory reaction at a remote site will lead to a five- to tenfold increase in C2 and C4 synthesis rates by peritoneal cells even when the cells are maintained in culture for 72–96 hr. These results are quite similar to those reported by Hartveit *et al.* (1973), who demonstrated in mice a stimulatory effect of an inflammatory response on C3 synthesis. In addition, they found that the extent of this response was genetically determined. Developmental changes also must be taken into account when one considers that, for example, adult mouse or rat liver failed to synthesize C3 *in vitro* except after stimulation of the animal with endotoxin (Thorbecke *et al.*, 1965), whereas C3 synthesis was easily demonstrated in liver from unstimulated juvenile animals. Perhaps the latter situation is analogous to the striking increase in plasma protein synthesis by liver, including C3 (Thorbecke *et al.*, 1965) and C4 (Füst *et al.*, 1972), several days following a partial hepatectomy. That is, the stimulus for proliferation of liver cells and control of protein synthesis in each case (normal development and post hepatectomy) may be similar. Both functions persist in short-term tissue culture, and therefore do not require a continuing external stimulus. Perhaps these factors, in addition to stimulation by microbial agents, account for the rapid rise in complement levels in the early months of postnatal life (Fireman *et al.*, 1969).

Several investigators have studied the metabolism of C1q (Kohler and Müller-Eberhard, 1972), C3 (Alper *et al.*, 1966), and C4 (Carpenter *et al.*, 1969) *in vivo* in normal subjects and in patients with acquired abnormalities of the complement system, using radiolabeled purified complement proteins. Metabolic studies of C3 in patients with membranoproliferative glomerulonephritis (MPGN) have suggested that decreased C3 biosynthesis often contributes to depressed serum levels of C3 (Alper *et al.*, 1966; Peters *et al.*, 1972). Other authors (Hunsicker *et al.*, 1972) have claimed that the decrease in serum C3 associated with MPGN is solely a consequence of increased C3 catabolism. As indicated above, recent work (Colten, 1972a) has confirmed that the liver is a principal site of C3 biosynthesis in that short-term cultures of liver produced biologically active C3, production of C3 was temperature-dependent and reversibly inhibited by cycloheximide, and [^{14}C]amino acids were incorporated into C3 protein. Liver biopsies were obtained from patients with MPGN, patients with other hypocomplementemic renal diseases, and controls (patients without renal diseases). In general, rates of biosynthesis of C3 by liver specimens *in vitro* corresponded to synthesis rates calculated from metabolic turnover studies (Colten *et al.*, 1973). Liver samples from two patients with MPGN failed to produce detectable C3 *in vitro*, although they were capable of synthesizing C2 and C5. Studies of the metabolic turnover of radiolabeled C3 in these two patients also indicated a depression of C3 biosynthesis. The rates of C3 synthesis did not correlate with the serum concentration of C3; i.e., some patients with low serum C3 levels had greater synthesis rates than those with higher serum C3 levels and vice versa. Preliminary data suggested two possible mechanisms for decreased C3 biosynthesis in MPGN: (1) a relative deficiency of a normal heat-stable serum factor that stimulates C3 biosynthesis. [A comparable effect of serum on C3 and transferrin synthesis by murine cells has also been observed (Stecher and Thorbecke, 1967b)]; and (2) perhaps an inability of the liver from patients with MPGN to respond to this C3 stimulating factor. In short, both increased catabolism and decreased synthesis account for depression of C3 levels in MPGN.

A similar finding was noted in studies of C3 metabolism in systemic lupus erythematosis (SLE), but results were somewhat more variable (Alper and Rosen, 1967; Hunsicker et al., 1972; Sliwinski and Zvaifler, 1972). For example, in one study, two of three patients with untreated SLE and low serum C3 levels had depressed synthesis rates, whereas the synthesis rate was normal in the third patient. C1q and C4 turnover were markedly increased and in another study C1q synthesis rates were found to be significantly increased as well (Kohler and Müller-Eberhard, 1972). Treatment with between 40–120 mg Prednisone per day resulted in an increase in the C3 synthesis rate in each of the patients and a variable effect on the C3 catabolic rate (Sliwinski and Zvaifler, 1972). Apparently, contradictory data were obtained in a study of C3 levels following administration of cortisone to experimental animals (Atkinson and Frank, 1973). Guinea pigs treated with cortisone acetate (5 mg/kg) demonstrated a 20% and a 51% elevation of CH50 and C1 titers, respectively. C4, C2, and C3–9 complex were all somewhat higher, but not statistically different from controls. At 20 mg/kg, C1 was 137% of control values and the other components were essentially unchanged. At 100 mg/kg, C1 and C9 were the only components not significantly depressed. Periorbital abscesses, secondary to bleeding procedures, abolished the depression of CH50, C4, and C3–9 complex, again emphasizing the effect of inflammation on complement levels. Direct experiments showed that in tissue culture the presence of hydrocortisone at a concentration of approximately 10^{-6} M stimulated synthesis of C3 and transferrin as judged by semiquantitative methods (Stecher and Thorbecke, 1967b). In experiments designed to quantitate the magnitude of this effect of cortisone, it was shown that incubation of a well-differentiated rat hepatoma in the presence of hydrocortisone succinate (4×10^{-7} M) increased rates of C3 production up to ninefold over baseline but had no effect on C5 synthesis (Strunk et al., 1975). The possibility that this effect was restricted to malignant cells was considered and ruled out by showing a comparable effect of hydrocortisone on C3 synthesis by primary cultures of normal rat liver (Breslow et al., unpublished data).

Suggestive evidence has been obtained that hormones other than cortisol may also affect complement synthesis, but these preliminary observations have not been pursued to any significant degree. For example, Urbach and Cinader (1966) first noted that the concentration of MuB1 (C5) protein in sera of normal male mice was approximately twice that of normal females. Churchill et al. (1967) found that late-acting complement components (C3–C9 complex) in sera from male mice were eight to ten times higher than the corresponding components in sera from female mice. Evidence was presented that this difference is due to the effect of androgens and estrogens on late-acting complement components, which were tentatively identified as C5 and C6. In humans, it is known that total complement activity (Ecker and Rees, 1922) and C3 (Propp and Alper, 1968) is significantly increased late in pregnancy. Studies of complement metabolism and of the effects of sex hormones on complement synthesis *in vitro* should elucidate the mechanisms responsible for these phenomena.

6. Conclusion

The sites of synthesis of most of the complement proteins have now been established. Preliminary probes of the molecular events controlling complement production have been of considerable interest and will no doubt stimulate additional work on this problem. Applications of studies of complement synthesis may therefore contribute to a more sophisticated understanding of fundamental problems in medicine, biology, and biochemical genetics.

ACKNOWLEDGMENT

I thank Ms. Barbara Caruso and Ms. Rita Callan for assistance in preparing this manuscript.

Dr. Colten is a recipient of USPHS Research Career Development Award 5 K04 HD70558.

References

Alper, C. A., and Rosen, F. S., 1967, Studies of the *in vivo* behavior of human C3 in normal subjects and patients, *J. Clin. Invest.* **46**:2021–2034.

Alper, C. A., and Rosen, F. S., 1971, Genetic aspects of the complement system, in: *Advances in Immunology* (H. G. Kunkel and F. J. Dixon, eds.), vol. 14, pp. 252–290, Academic Press, New York.

Alper, C. A., Levin, A. S., and Rosen, F. S., 1966, Beta-1C-globulin: metabolism in glomerulonephritis, *Science* **153**:180–183.

Alper, C. A., Johnson, A. M., Birtch, A. G., and Moore, F. D., 1969, Human C'3: evidence for the liver as the primary site of synthesis, *Science* **163**:286–288.

Atkinson, J. P., and Frank, M. M., 1973, Effect of cortisone therapy on serum complement components, *J. Immunol.* **111**:1061–1066.

Ballow, M., Day, N. K., Biggar, W. D., Park, B. H., Yount, W. J., and Good, R. A., 1973, Reconstitution of C1q after bone marrow transplantation in patients with severe combined immunodeficiency, *Clin. Immunol. Immunopathol.* **2**:28–35.

Baltch, A. L., Osborne, W., Canarile, L., Hassirdjian, A., and Bunn, P., 1962, Serum properdin complement and agglutinin changes in dogs with staphylococcal bacteremia, *J. Immunol.* **88**:361–368.

Bing, D. H., Spurlock, S. E., and Bern, M. M., 1975, Synthesis of the first component of complement by primary cultures of human tumors of the colon and urogenital tract and comparable normal tissue, *Clin. Immunol. Immunopath.* **4**:341–351.

Bokisch, V. A., Top, F. H., Russell, P. K., Dixon, F. J., and Müller-Eberhard, H. J., 1973, The potential pathogenic role of complement in dengue hemorrhagic shock syndrome, *New Eng. J. Med.* **289**:996–1000.

Carpenter, C. B., Ruddy, S., Shehadeh, I. H., Müller-Eberhard, H. J., Merrill, J. P. and Austen, K. F., 1969, Complement metabolism in man: hypercatabolism of the fourth (C4) and third (C3) components in patients with renal allograft rejection and hereditary angioedema (HAE), *J. Clin. Invest.* **48**:1495–1505.

Chan, P. C. Y., 1970, Detection of complement-producing cells with macrophage antisera, *Experientia* **26**:189.

Chan, P. C. Y., and Cebra, J. J., 1966, Studies of the fourth component of guinea pig serum, *Immunochemistry* **3**:496 (abstract).

Churchill, W. H., Weintraub, R. M., Borsos, T., and Rapp, H. J., 1967, Mouse complement: the effect of sex hormones and castration on two of the late acting components, *J. Exp. Med.* **125**:657–672.

Cinader, B., and Dubiski, S., 1963, An alpha-globulin allotype in the mouse (MuB1), *Nature London* **200**:781.

Cohn, Z. A., and Benson, B., 1965, The *in vitro* differentiation of mononuclear phagocytes. II. The influence of serum on granule formation hydrolase production and pinocytosis, *J. Exp. Med.* **121**:835–848.

Colten, H. R., 1972a, Ontogeny of the human complement system: *in vitro* biosynthesis of individual complement components by fetal tissues, *J. Clin. Invest.* **51**:725–730.

Colten, H. R., 1972b, *In vitro* synthesis of a regulator of mammalian gene expression, *Proc. Nat. Acad. Sci. U.S.A.* **69**:2233–2236.

Colten, H. R., 1973, Biosynthesis of the fifth component (C5) of human complement, *Clin. Immunol. Immunopath.* **1**:346–352.

Colten, H. R., 1974a, Deficiency of the fourth component of complement (C4): studies of the molecular basis of the genetic abnormality, in: *Somatic Cell Hybridization* (R. L. Davidson and F. F. de la Cruz, eds.), Raven Press, New York.

Colten, H. R., 1974b, Biosynthesis of serum complement, in: *Proceedings of the IInd International Congress of Immunology* (L. Brent and J. Holbrow, eds.), Vol. 1, pp. 183–190b, North Holland, Amsterdam.

Colten, H. R., and Frank, M. M., 1972, Biosynthesis of the second and fourth components of complement *in vitro* by tissues isolated from guinea pigs with genetically determined C4 deficiency, *Immunology* **22**:991–999.

Colten, H. R., and Parkman, R., 1972, Biosynthesis of the fourth component of complement (C4) by C4-deficient guinea pig-HeLa cell hybrids, *Science* **176**:1029–1031.

Colten, H. R., and Wyatt, H. V., 1972, Biosynthesis of serum complement, in: *Biological Activities of Complement*, (D. G. Ingram, ed.), pp. 244–255, Karger, Basel.

Colten, H. R., Borsos, T., and Rapp, H. J., 1966, *In vitro* synthesis of the first component of complement by guinea pig small intestine, *Proc. Nat. Acad. Sci. U.S.A.* **56**:1158–1163.

Colten, H. R., Gordon, J. M., Borsos, T., and Rapp, H. J., 1968a, Synthesis of the first component of human complement *in vitro*, *J. Exp. Med.* **128**:595–604.

Colten, H. R., Gordon, J. M., Rapp, H. J., and Borsos, T., 1968b, Synthesis of the first component of guinea pig complement by columnar epithelial cells of the small intestine, *J. Immunol.* **100**:788–792.

Colten, H. R., Levey, R. H., Rosen, F. S., and Alper, C. A., 1973, Decreased synthesis of C3 in membranoproliferative glomerulonephritis, *J. Clin. Invest.* **52**:20a (abstract).

Davidson, R. L., and Benda, P., 1970, Regulation of specific functions of glial cells in somatic hybrids. II. Control of inducability of glycerol-3-phosphate dehydrogenase, *Proc. Nat. Acad. Sci. U.S.A.* **67**:1870–1877.

Day, N. K., Gewurz, H., Pickering, R. J., and Good, R. A., 1970, Ontogenetic development of C1q synthesis in the piglet, *J. Immunol.* **104**:1316–1319.

Dick, G. F., 1912, On the development of proteolytic ferments in the blood during pneumonia, *J. Inf. Dis.* **10**:383–387.

Dick, G. F., 1913, On the origin and action of hemolytic complement, *J. Inf. Dis.* **12**:111–126.

Ecker, E. E., and Rees, H. M., 1922, Effect of hemorrhage on complement, *J. Infect. Dis.* **31**:361–367.

Ecker, E. E., Seifter, S., Dozois, T. F., and Barr, L., 1946, Complement in infectious disease in man, *J. Clin. Invest.* **25**:800–808.

Einstein, L. P., Alper, C. A., Bloch, K. H., Herrin, J. T., Rosen, F. S., David, J. R., and Colten, H. R., 1975, Biosynthetic defect in monocytes from human beings with genetic deficiency of the second component of complement (C2), *N. Engl. J. Med.* **292**:1169–1171.

Einstein, L. P., Schneeberger, E. E., and Colten, H. R., 1976, Synthesis of the second component of complement by long-term primary cultures of human monocytes, *J. Exp. Med.* **143**:114–126.

Ellman, L., Green, I., and Frank, M. M., 1970, Genetically controlled total deficiency of the fourth component of complement in the guinea pig, *Science* **170**:74–75.

Fireman, P., Zuchowski, D. A., and Taylor, P. M., 1969, Development of human complement system, *J. Immunol.* **103**:25–31.

Fougere, C., Reinze, F., and Ephrussi, B., 1972, Gene dosage dependence of pigment synthesis in melanoma × fibroblast hybrids, *Proc. Nat. Acad. Sci. U.S.A.* **69**:330–334.

Frank, M. M., May, J., Gaither, T., Ellman, L., 1971, *In vitro* studies of complement function in sera of C4-deficient guinea pigs, *J. Exp. Med.* **134**:176–187.

Fu, S. M., Kunkel, H. G., Brusman, H. P., Allen, F. H., and Fotino, M., 1974, Evidence for linkage between HL-A histocompatability genes and those involved in the synthesis of the second component of complement, *J. Exp. Med.* **140**:1108–1111.

Füst, G., and Surján, M., 1971, Effect of antimacrophage sera on the *in vivo* synthesis of guinea pig complement components, *Boll. Inst. Sieroter. Milan.* **50**:488–494.

Füst, G., Surján, M., and Keresztes, M., 1972, Studies on the synthesis of the fourth component of rat complement *in vivo*, *Boll. Inst. Sieroter. Milan.* **51**:304–313.

Gabrielsen, A. E., Linna, T. J., Wertekamp, D. P., and Pickering, R. J., 1974, Reduced haemolytic C1 activity in serum of hypogammaglobulinaemic chickens, *Immunology* **27**:463–468.

Geiger, H., Day, N., and Good, R. A., 1972, Ontogenetic development and synthesis of hemolytic C8 by piglet tissues, *J. Immunol.* **108**:1092–1097.

Gewurz, H., Pickering, R. J., Christian, C. L., Synderman, R., Mergenhagen, S. E., and Good, R. A., 1968, Decreased C1q protein concentrations and agglutinating activity in agammaglobulinemia syndromes: an inborn error reflected in the complement system, *Clin. Exp. Immunol.* **5**:437–445.

Gitlin, D., and Biasucci, A., 1969, Development of γG, γA, γM, B_1C/B_1A, C1 esterase inhibitor, cerruloplasmin transferrin hemopexin, haptoglobin fibrinogen, plasminogen α1 antitrypsin orosomucoid β lipoprotein α2 macroglobulin and prealbumin in the human conceptus, *J. Clin. Invest.* **48**:1433–1446.

Glade, P. R., and Chessin, L. N., 1968, Synthesis of $B_1C/1A(C'3)$ by human lymphoid cells, *Int. Arch. Allergy Appl. Immunol.* **34**:181–187.

Gordon, P., 1955, Complement activity in the eviscerate rat, *Proc. Soc. Exp. Biol. Med.* **89**:607–608.

Gordon, S., Ripps, C. S., and Cohn, Z., 1971, The preparation and properties of macrophage-L cell hybrids, *J. Exp. Med.* **134**:1187–1199.

Hartveit, F., Børve, W., and Thunold, S., 1973, Serum complement levels and response to turpentine inflammation in mice, *Acta Pathol. Microbiol. Scand. Sec. A Suppl.* **236**:54–59.

Hochwald, G. M., Thorbecke, G. J., and Asofsky, R., 1961, Sites of formation of immune globulins and of a component of C'3. I A new technique for the demonstration of synthesis of individual serum proteins by tissues *in vitro*, *J. Exp. Med.* **114**:459–470.

Hunsicker, L. G., Ruddy, S., Carpenter, C. B., Schur, P. H., Merrill, J. P., Müller-Eberhard, H. J., and Austen, K. F., 1972, Metabolism of third complement component (C3) in nephritis: role of the classical and alternate (properdin) pathways for complement activation, *N. Engl. J. Med.* **287**:835.

Hurlimann, J., Thorbecke, G. J., and Hochwald, G. M., 1966, The liver as the site of C-reactive protein formation, *J. Exp. Med.* **123**:365–378.

Ilgen, C. L., and Burkholder, P. M., 1974, Isolation of C4 synthesizing cells from guinea pig liver by ficoll density gradient centrifugation, *Immunology* **26**:197–203.

Ingraham, J. S., and Bussard, A., 1964, Application of a localized hemolysin reaction for specific detection of individual antibody forming cells, *J. Exp. Med.* **119**:667–682.

Jensen, J. A., Garces, M. C., and Iglesias, E., 1971, Specific inactivation of the fourth complement component. I. *In vivo* studies, *Infect. Immuno.* **4**:12–19.

Jerne, N. K., and Nordin, A. A., 1963, Plaque formation in agar by single antibody producing cells, *Science* **140**:405.

Johnson, A. M., Alper, C. A., Rosen, F. S., and Craig, J. M., 1971a, C1 inhibitor: evidence for decreased hepatic synthesis in hereditary angioneurotic edema, *Science* **173**:553–554.

Johnson, A. M., Alper, C. A., Rosen, F. S., and Craig, J. M., 1971b, Immunofluorescent hepatic localization of complement proteins: evidence for a biosynthetic defect in hereditary angioneurotic edema (HANE), *J. Clin. Invest.* **50**:50a (abstract).

Jungeblut, C. W., and Berlot, J. A., 1926, The role of the reticuloendothelial system in immunity. II. The complement titer after blockade and the physiological regeneration of the reticuloendothelial system as measured by the reduction tests, *J. Exp. Med.* **43**:797–806.

Kashiwagi, N., Groth, C. G., and Starzl, T. E., 1968, Changes in serum haptoglobin and group specific component after orthotopic liver homotransplantation in humans, *Proc. Soc. Exp. Biol. Med.* **128**:247–250.

Kohler, P. F., 1973, Maturation of the human complement system. I. Onset time and sites of fetal C1q, C4, C3, and C5 synthesis, *J. Clin. Invest.* **52**:671–677.

Kohler, P. F., and Müller-Eberhard, H. J., 1969, Complement immunoglobulin relation: deficiency of C1q associated with impaired immunoglobulin G Synthesis, *Science* **163**:474.

Kohler, P. F., Müller-Eberhard, H. J., 1972, Metabolism of human C1q. Studies in hypogammaglobulinemia myeloma and systemic lupus erythematosis, *J. Clin. Invest.* **51**:868–875.

Lai A Fat, R. F. M., and van Furth, R., 1975, *In vitro* synthesis of some complement components (C1q, C3 and C4) by lymphoid tissues and circulating leukocytes in man, *Immunology* **28**:359–368.

Lamm, L. U., Friedrich, U., Petersen, G. B., Jorgensen, J., Nielsen, J., Therkelsen, A. J., and Kissmeyer-Nielsen, F., 1974, Assignment of the major histocompatibility complex to chromosome #6 in a family with a pericentric inversion, *Hum. Hered.* **24**:273–284.

Leddy, J. P., Frank, M. M., Gaither, T., Baum, T., and Klemperer, M. R., 1974, Hereditary deficiency of the sixth component of complement in man. I. Immunochemical, biological and family studies, *J. Clin. Invest.* **53**:544–553.

Lepow, I. H., 1965, *Ciba Found. Symp. Complement* (G. E. W. Wolstenholme and J. Knight, eds.), p. 117, Churchill, London.

Levisohn, S. R., and Thompson, E. B., 1973, Contact inhibition and gene expression in HTC/L cell hybrid lines, *J. Cell Physiol.* **81**:225–232.

Levy, N. L., and Ladda, R. L., 1971, Restoration of haemolytic complement activity in C5-deficient mice by gene complementation in hybrid cells. *Nature New Biol.* **229**:51–52.

Levy, N. L. Synderman, R., Ladda, R. L., and Lieberman, R., 1973, Cytogenetic engineering *in vivo:* restoration of biological complement activity to C5-deficient mice by intravenous innoculation of hybrid cells, *Proc. Nat. Acad. Sci. U.S.A.* **70**:3125–3129.

Littleton, C., Kessler, D., and Burkholder, P. M., 1970, Cellular basis for synthesis of the fourth component of guinea pig complement as determined by a haemolytic plaque technique, *Immunology* **18**:691–702.

Mathews, C. M. E., 1957, The theory of tracer experiments with ^{131}I-labeled plasma proteins, *Phys, Med. Biol.* **2**:36–53.

Merrill, D. A., Kirkpatrick, C. A., Wilson, W. E. C., and Riley, C. M., 1964, Change in serum haptoglobin type following human liver transplantation, *Proc. Soc. Exp. Biol. Med.* **116**:748–751.

O'Connell, R. M., Enriquez, P., Linman, J. W., Gleich, G. J., and McDuffie, F. C., 1967, Absence of activity of first component of complement in man: association with thymic alymphoplasia and defective inflammatory response, *J. Lab. Clin. Med.* **70**:715.

Peters, D. K., Martin, A., Weinstein, A., Cameron, J. S., Barrett, T. M., Ogg, C. S., and Lachmann, P. J., 1972, Complement studies in membranoproliferative glomerulonephritis, *Clin. Exp. Immunol.* **11**:311–320.

Peterson, J. A., and Weiss, M. C., 1972, Expression of differentiated functions in hepatoma cell hybrids: induction of mouse albumin production in rat hepatoma-mouse fibroblast hybrids, *Proc. Nat. Acad. Sci. U.S.A.* **69**:571–578.

Pickering, R. J., Naff, G. B., Stroud, R. M., Good, R. A., and Gewurz, H., 1970, Deficiency of C1r in human serum. Effects on the structure and function of macromolecular C1, *J. Exp. Med.* **131**:803–815.

Phillips, M. E., and Thorbecke, G. J., 1965, Serum protein formation of donor type in rat-into-mouse chimeras, *Nature London* **207**:376–378.

Phillips, M. E., Rother, U. A., Rother, K. O., and Thorbecke, G. J., 1969, Studies on the serum proteins of chimeras. III. Detection of donor type C5 in allogeneic and congenic post-irradiation chimeras, *Immunology* **17**:315–321.

Propp, R. P., and Alper, C. A., 1968, C'3 synthesis in the human fetus and lack of transplacental passage, *Science* **162**:672–673.

Rapp, H. J., and Borsos, T., 1970, Molecular basis of complement action; Appleton-Century-Crofts, New York.

Rommel, F. A., Goldlust, M. B., Bancroft, F. C., Mayer, M. M., and Tashjian, A. H., Jr., 1970, Synthesis of the ninth component of complement by a clonal strain of rat hepatoma cells, *J. Immunol.* **105**:396–403.

Rosenberg, L. T., and Tachibana, D. K., 1962, Activity of mouse complement, *J. Immunol.* **89**:861–867.

Rother, K., Rother, U., Müller-Eberhard, H. J., and Nilsson, U. R., 1966, Deficiency of the sixth component of complement in rabbits with an inherited complement defect, *J. Exp. Med.* **124**:773–785.

Rother, U., Thorbecke, G. J., Stecher-Levin, V. J., Hurlimann, J., and Rother, K., 1968, Formation of C′6 by rabbit liver tissue *in vitro, Immunology* **14**:649–655.

Rubin, D. J., Borsos, T., Rapp, H. J., and Colten, H. R., 1971, Synthesis of the second component of guinea pig complement *in vitro, J. Immunol.* **106**:295–303.

Ruddy, S., and Colten, H. R., 1974, Rheumatoid arthritis: biosynthesis of complement proteins by synovial tissues, *N. Engl. J. Med.* **290**:1284–1288.

Siboo, R., and Vas, S. I., 1965, Studies on *in vitro* antibody production. III. Production of complement, *Can. J. Microbiol.* **11**:415–425.

Sliwinski, A. J., and Zvaifler, N. J., 1972, Decreased synthesis of the third component of complement (C3) in hypocomplementemic systemic lupus erythematosis, *Clin. Exp. Immunol.* **11**:21–29.

Stecher, V. J., and Thorbecke, G. J., 1967a, Sites of synthesis of serum proteins. I. Serum proteins produced by macrophages *in vitro, J. Immunol.* **99**:643–652.

Stecher, V. J., and Thorbecke, G. J., 1967b, Sites of synthesis of serum proteins. II. Medium requirements for serum protein production by macrophages, *J. Immunol.* **99**:653–659.

Stecher, V. J., and Thorbecke, G. J., 1967c, Sites of synthesis of serum proteins. III. Production of B1C, B1E, and transferrin by primate and rodent cell lines, *J. Immunol.* **99**:660–668.

Stecher, V. J., Morse, J. H., and Thorbecke, G. J., 1967, Sites of production of primate serum proteins associated with the complement system, *Proc. Soc. Exp. Med.* **124**:433–438.

Stroud, R. M., and Donaldson, V., 1974, Genetic defects of complement (Workshop), in: *Progress in Immunology II*, Vol. 1 (L. Brent and J. Holbrow, eds.), p. 288, North Holland, Amsterdam.

Stroud, R. M., Nagaki, K., Pickering, R. J., Gewurz, H., Good, R. A., and Cooper, M. D., 1970, Subunits of first complement component in immunological deficiency: independence of C1s and C1q, *Clin. Exp. Immunol.* **7**:133.

Strunk, R. S., Tashjian, A. H., and Colten, H. R., 1975, Complement biosynthesis *in vitro* by rat hepatoma cell strains, *J. Immunol.* **114**:331–335.

Terry, W. D., Borsos, T., and Rapp, H. J., 1964, Differences in serum complement activity among inbred strains of mice, *J. Immunol.* **92**:576–578.

Thorbecke, G. J., Hochwald, G. M., van Furth, R., Müller-Eberhard, H. J., and Jacobson, E. B., 1965, Problems in determining the sites of synthesis of complement components, in: *Ciba Symposium "Complement"* (G. E. W. Wolstenholme and J. Knight, eds.), pp. 99–119, J & A Churchill, London.

Urbach, G., and Cinader, B., 1966, Hormonal control of MuB1 concentration, *Proc. Soc. Exp. Biol. Med.* **122**:779–782.

van Someren, H., Westerveld, A., Hagemeijer, A., Mees, J. R., Meera Khan, P., and Zaalberg, O. B., 1974, Human antigen and enzyme markers in man-chinese hamster somatic cell hybrids: evidence for synteny between the HL-A, PGM_3, ME_1, and IPO-B loci, *Proc. Nat. Acad. Sci. U.S.A.* **71**:962–965.

van Zaipel, G., 1970, Separation from HeLa cell cultures of three esterases, one of which resembles human activated C1s, *Acta Pathol. Microbiol. Scand.* **78**:258–260.

Williams, C. A., Jr., Asofsky, R., and Thorbecke, G. J., 1963, Plasma protein formation *in vitro* by tissues from mice infected with staphylococci, *J. Exp. Med.* **118**:315–326.

Wyatt, H. V., 1974, Synthesis of the second and fourth components of complement by tissue culture cell lines, *Eur. J. Immunol.* **4**:34–38.

Wyatt, H. V., Colten, H. R., and Borsos, T., 1972, Production of the second (C2) and fourth (C4) components of guinea pig complement by single peritoneal exudate cells. Evidence that one cell may produce both components, *J. Immunol.* **108**:1609–1614.

Yount, W. J., Utsinger, P. D., Gatti, R. A., and Good, R. A., 1974, Immunoglobulin classes, IgG subclasses, Gm genetic markers and C1q following bone marrow transplantation in x-linked combined immunodeficiency, *J. Pediat.* **84**:193–199.

4

Plasma Membrane Receptors for Complement

CELSO BIANCO

1. Introduction

The understanding of the relationship between complement and other elements of the immune system has undergone a radical change in recent years. Complement (C) was previously defined only as one of the final effectors of the humoral defense system, which is able to cooperate with antibodies in the lysis of target cells. The discovery of complement's anaphylatoxic activities and later of the plasma membrane receptors for complement in several blood cells stimulated the search for other functional roles for this complex set of serum proteins. It is the purpose of this chapter to review some interactions of blood cells with complement components, especially C3, in terms of the nature of the cells binding these complement components, the nature of the components bound, and the consequences of this binding.

Plasma membrane receptors for complement have been described in many cell types. The specificity of these receptors for certain C components and for certain fragments of C components vary among these cells, and the same cell may simultaneously carry separate receptors for different components or fragments.

Complement receptors on lymphocytes have been extensively reviewed in terms of both their interactions with immune complexes and their properties as markers for bone marrow–derived, thymus-independent (B) lymphocytes (Nussenzweig, 1974). Clinical studies of this receptor have also been reviewed (Shevach *et al.,* 1973). See these articles for more extensive bibliographies.

2. Definitions and Nomenclature

The widespread use of the term *membrane receptor* has led to some confusion. For the purpose of this chapter, a plasma membrane receptor is a structure that is

CELSO BIANCO • The Rockefeller University, New York, New York.

operationally defined as having the ability (1) to interact specifically and with high affinity with the ligand (in our case a complement component); and (2) to be saturated by the ligand, demonstrable by competitive binding studies.

The following nomenclature will be used throughout this chapter: *binding site*—the domain of a complement component or IgG molecule that interacts with a plasma membrane receptor; *indicator erythrocyte* (or *particle*)—an erythrocyte (or particle) used in agglutination and rosette assays. It has no receptors for IgG or for complement and carries, strongly attached to its surface, the complement component being studied; *b receptors*—plasma membrane receptors for C3b and C4b; and *d receptors*—plasma membrane receptors for C3d.

The existence of plasma membrane receptors for complement on blood cells is very well documented, and the above requirements specified for the operational definition have been fulfilled in most instances. Table 1 has a list of the cells on which complement receptors have been detected.

Most of the studies performed with these receptors utilized agglutination or rosette formation between cells bearing the receptor and indicator erythrocytes, having on their surface the complement component to be studied. For example, C3 binds strongly to the indicator erythrocyte membrane by an active, short-lived site, which appears during C3 cleavage. Other portions of the C3 molecule carry stable binding sites that interact reversibly with the plasma membrane receptors on blood cells. It should be noted that the portion of the indicator erythrocyte membrane that interacts with the short-lived site is not considered to be a receptor for the purpose

TABLE 1. Receptors for Complement and for Fc of IgG on Blood Cells

| | | Receptor type | |
| | | *b* (C4b, C3b) | *d* (C3d) |
Cell type	Species		
Erythrocytes	Human and primates	+	−
	Other mammals	−	−
Platelets	Human and primates	−	−
	Other mammals	+	−
B lymphocytes	Mammals	+	+
T lymphocytes	Mammals	−	−
Granulocytes	Mammals	+	−
Monocytes	Mammals	+	−[a]
Macrophages (lung)	Human	+	−[a]
Macrophages (resident peritoneal cavity)	Mouse Guinea pig	+	−[a]
Activated macrophage (peritoneal cavity)	Mouse Guinea pig	+	−

[a] Many authors have detected receptors of type *d* on monocytes and macrophages. Please refer to the discussion in Section 6.4.

of this discussion. In several assays, zymosan (Mendes *et al.,* 1974) and latex (Hoffman, personal communication) have been used as indicator particles. Other means of detecting complement receptors include the use of radiolabeled soluble immune complexes carrying complement (Eden *et al.,* 1973a) and the use of radiolabeled complement components or fragments (Theofilopoulos *et al.,* 1974). Direct examination has also been possible by the use of fluorescent antisera directed against C components (Ross and Polley, 1975). The sensitivity of these methods varies widely.

The biochemical nature of the various membrane receptors for complement is unknown. The operational definition employed here does not imply that the receptor is a single molecular species that remains intact upon disorganization of the plasma membrane. Semantic excesses in interpreting the "receptor" concept may lead either to naïve approaches to receptor fractionation or, even, to the total denial of the existence of receptors. The general problem of receptor purification is very complex and has been recently reviewed (Cuatrecasas, 1974). This complexity is further attested to by the studies of Dierich and Reisfeld (1975). Their attempts to recover C3 binding activity from soluble materials obtained after treatment of lymphoid cells with detergents were unsuccessful. Activity from cell lysates (detected by hemagglutination) was retained only by larger membrane fragments obtained by nitrogen cavitation and treatment with 2 M KBr.

Complement receptors of all cells tested have several properties in common. For example, they are inactivated by trypsin digestion. This protease sensitivity is especially useful in distinguishing binding via complement from binding via the Fc portion of immunoglobulin in cells carrying receptors for both, since the receptor for Fc is insensitive to trypsin (Lay and Nussenzweig, 1968).

Lymphocytes of all species tested and granulocytes, monocytes and macrophages of animals other than the mouse do not require divalent cations for binding. Mouse phagocytes, however, have a requirement for Mg^{2+} ions (Lay and Nussenzweig, 1968). Binding is better initiated at 37°C, and at 0°C, rosette formation and the binding of soluble immune complexes are reduced. However, if binding is allowed to occur at 37°C and the cells are then placed at 0°C, the complexes do not subsequently dissociate. Cells killed by heat or metabolic poisons show near-normal complement receptor activity (Lay and Nussenzweig, 1968).

3. Molecular Structure of C3 and C4

Analysis of the various complement receptors requires some understanding of the molecular structure of C3 and C4. More detailed information on the biochemistry of complement activation is presented in Chapters 1 and 2.

C3 is a protein with a molecular weight of 190,000. Its structure is being intensively studied by several investigators (Bokisch *et al.,* 1975; Gitlin *et al.,* 1975; Nilsson and Beisswenger, 1975; Stossel *et al.,* 1975). Figure 1 is a graphic representation, which is compatible with most of the available information. C3 is constituted of two chains, α and β, linked by disulfide bonds. Both the classical and the alternate pathways of complement fixation generate enzymatic activities that cleave the modecule sequentially into smaller fragments, each with distinct biological properties. Initially, a C3-convertase (classical pathway) (Müller-Eberhard *et al.* 1967) or a C3 activator (alternate pathway) (Götze and Müller-Eberhard, 1971) cleave the C3 molecule into C3a, anaphylatoxin (Silva *et al.,* 1967), with a molecular weight of 9000, and C3b, the remainder of the molecule. C3a is very active pharmacologically, being able to induce smooth muscle contraction, histamine release from mast cells, increased vascular permeability, and chemotactic activity. (Silva *et al.,* 1967). It is inactivated by a serum carboxypeptidase (Bokisch *et al.,* 1969). The amino acid composition, partial sequence, and circular dichroism spectrum have been reported (Hugli *et al.,* 1975a; Hugli *et al.,* 1975b).

The cleavage of C3a simultaneously exposes several active sites on the C3 molecule. This is represented in Figure 1 by the unfolding of the α chain. A short-lived site (or labile site) is generated, which allows C3b to interact strongly with many cell walls and cell membranes. C3b can further activate the complement sequence, as well as bind to *b* and *d* receptors on cells. Some of its activities can be inhibited by a heat-stable serum enzyme, the C3b inactivator (Tamura and Nelson, 1967), or KAF, conglutinogen activating factor (Lachmann and Müller-Eberhard, 1968), which initially cleaves a small fragment of the α chain of C3b, abolishing the ability of the molecule to activate other complement components (Gitlin *et al.,* 1975). The cleavage occurs rapidly (3 min), and the product has been called C3b^i. C3b^i is extremely sensitive to proteases. It is possible that C3b^i is the "opsonic" fragment of C3 (Stossel *et al.,* 1975). These interpretations require further confirmation because in one of the systems studied (Gitlin *et al.,* 1975), the fragments were not analyzed for their ability to bind to cell receptors. In the other study, Stossel *et al.* (1975) used whole serum instead of purified complement components, which led

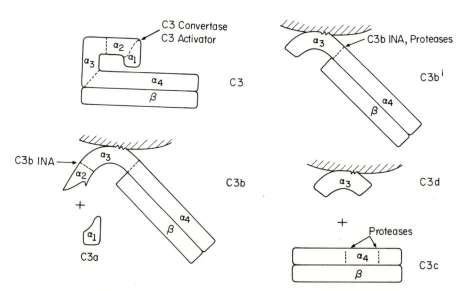

Figure 1. Schematic representation of the C3 molecule and the fragments produced during complement activation. Activation of the classical pathway (C3-convertase) or the alternate pathway (C3 activator) induces the cleavage of C3a, represented in the upper left-hand corner of the figure. A short-lived nonspecific site is generated in α_3, which then binds to cell membranes and walls (hatched), as represented in the lower left-hand corner of the figure. Subsequently, the C3b inactivator, C2bINA, cleaves the molecule initially to C3b^i and later to C3c (released into the fluid phase) and C3d (lower right-hand corner). The binding properties of the plasma membrane receptors for these fragments are summarized in Table 2.

to a complex picture of the effects of C3b inactivator, other proteases, and serum proteins (such as IgG) with opsonic activity, which could also affect the particles used. C3b^i may also correspond to the C3x fragment described by Spitzer *et al.* (1971).

The second cleavage by C3b inactivator occurs more slowly, producing two fragments. With erythrocyte-bound C3b, a large fragment, C3c, is released into the medium, while a smaller fragment, C3d, remains associated with the cell membrane (Ruddy and Austen, 1971). It is not known whether C3d is the final product that remains associated with the membrane or whether further degradation occurs. The diagram in Figure 1 differs somewhat from the model of the C3 molecule recently published (Bokisch *et al.*, 1975). Instead of α_2, the α_3 segment corresponds to C3d. This allows the schematic representation of the initial fast cleavage of α_2 by the C3b inactivator, leaving α_3, α_4, and β behind as a unit attached to the cell membrane. The second cleavage by C3b inactivator releases the fragment $\alpha_4\beta$.

In summary, the biological activities of each fragment are as follows: α_1 has anaphylatoxin activity, α_2 can activate complement, α_3 can bind via its short-lived site to cell membranes and walls and via a stable site to the *d* receptor of leukocytes; $\alpha_4\beta$ contains the site that binds to the *b* receptors.

One of the described receptors for complement on erythrocytes and leukocytes can bind C4b. C4 is a globular protein with a molecular weight of 200,000. It is composed of three chains—α, β, and γ—linked by disulfide bonds (Schreiber and Müller-Eberhard, 1974). It is cleaved by C1$\bar{s}$ into two fragments, C4a and C4b. C4b binds to cell membranes through its labile site. Another site of C4b binds to leukocytes and erythrocytes and is inactivated by a C4b inactivator present in serum. The cleavage sequence and binding abilities of C4 resemble those of C3. Actually, the C4b and the C3b inactivators may be the same enzyme (Cooper, 1975). As will be discussed, C4b and C3b seem to bind to the same receptor (type *b*).

Cooper (1975) also made the observation that when C2 is added to the EAC14 complex, it protects C4b from cleavage by C4b inactivator. This fact may, in some instances, complicate the study of receptors, since the binding site of C4b for blood cells remains available after exposure of the complex to the serum inactivator.

4. Complement Receptors

The following specificities of plasma membrane receptors for complement components have been well characterized:

4.1. Receptor for C3b (*b* Receptor)

This receptor is also called an *immune adherence receptor* when it is present on human (and other primate) erythrocytes and on platelets of nonprimate mammals. It is present on many leukocytes, and it binds C3 after cleavage by C3-convertase or by C3 activator. Indicator erythrocytes carrying C3b lose their ability to bind to this receptor when treated with C3b inactivator. The binding site on the C3b molecule may be located in the $\alpha_4\beta$ fragment. Binding can be inhibited by fluid-phase C3b, C4b, and C3c, but not by C3d.

4.2. Receptor for C4b

There are several indications that this receptor is identical to the *b* receptor just described. In cocapping experiments done with lymphocytes, the receptors seem to be indistinguishable (Ross and Polley, 1975). After cleavage by C1s̄, C4 binds to the indicator erythrocyte membrane through the short-lived site and exposes the C4b binding site. As previously mentioned, C4b is susceptible to digestion by an inactivator to a form of C4 not recognized by the C3b receptor. Binding can be inhibited by fluid-phase C3b, C4b, and C3c, but not by C3d.

4.3. Receptor for C3d (*d* Receptor)

This receptor is specific for the C3d fragment of C3 (after the molecule of C3 has been cleaved by the C3b inactivator). In Figure 1, the binding site is located in the α_3 fragment to represent the fact that it remains associated with the erythrocyte membrane after cleavage by the inactivator. Binding to the *d* receptor can be inhibited by fluid-phase C3b and C3d, but not by C3c. Table 2 summarizes the correlation between C3 fragments and receptor specificities.

Other receptors for complement have been described, including a receptor for native C3 on a lymphoid cell line, Raji (Theofilopoulos *et al.*, 1974) and a receptor for C1q on some lymphocytes (Sobel and Bokisch, 1975).

Since leukocytes show definite responses to the anaphylatoxins C3a and C5a, receptors for these fragments could be postulated. However, the requirements for a receptor stated in the operational definition have not yet been fulfilled for these fragments.

5. Reagents for the Detection of *b* and *d* Receptors

The ability to define the specificities of the several complement receptors depends directly on the quality of the reagents employed. Since rosette formation is the most widely used method, some of the characteristics of the several erythrocyte complexes routinely employed will be described. In all these studies, to avoid interactions with receptors for the Fc segment of IgG, antibodies against erythrocytes should be of the IgM class.

TABLE 2.   Correlation Between Fragments of C3 and Binding to Plasma Membrane Receptors for Complement

Form of C3	Possible chain composition (Figure 1)	Binds to receptors type	
		b	*d*
C3	$\alpha_1, \alpha_2, \alpha_3, \alpha_4, \beta$	−	−
C3a	α_1	−	−
C3b	$\alpha_2, \alpha_3, \alpha_4, \beta$	+	+
C3b^i	$\alpha_3, \alpha_4, \beta$	+	+
C3c	α_4, β	+	−
C3d	α_3	−	+
C3b	−	+	−

5.1. Indicator Complexes Prepared with Whole Serum

Since mouse serum is poorly lytic, it has been widely used in studies of C receptors. The availability of many inbred strains deficient in C5 provides a good reagent for the preparation of EIgMC1423 (Cinader *et al.*, 1964). Since whole serum contains C3b inactivator, the time of incubation with the complement source is critical. In the first 10 min, the predominant activity found that is associated with the erythrocytes is C3b-like. After this period, gradual cleavage of the molecule makes it behave like C3d (Griffin *et al.*, 1975). Suramin, a drug that interferes with the action of the C3b inactivator, partially prevents the loss of C3b activity. Thus, EIgMC, which is prepared by incubating EIgM with C5-deficient mouse complement for short periods of time, detects *b* (C3b and C4b) and *d* (C3d) receptors. After long incubation periods with C, it detects mostly *d* receptors. Complement and leukocytes from different animal species can often be used interchangeably. Among the several combinations tested in mammals, the only one that does not seem to work well is mouse complement components and human leukocytes (Bianco *et al.*, 1970).

5.2. Indicator Complexes Prepared with Purified C Components

The commercial availability of functionally purified human and guinea pig C components (Cordis Corporation, Miami, Florida) allows the widespread use of purified C components in the preparation of EAC. There are a few cautions, however: (1) these components are pure in terms of the absence of other active C components in the mixture; they are not biochemically pure; (2) large amounts of the purified components are required to obtain an effective number of C3 molecules bound; (3) most or all C3 bound is in the form of C3b, and thus would be expected to bind to both C3b and C3d receptors.

The ability to use the EIgMC14 complex for the detection of *b* receptors without simultaneous binding to the *d* receptors is one definite advantage of the use of purified C components for certain studies, as suggested by Ross and Polley (1975).

The further cleavage by C3b inactivator of the C4b and C3b, prepared utilizing purified C components, may, as we will discuss later, lead to some discrepancies. The C4b, if large amounts of C2 are present, may not be cleaved by the C3b inactivator, and the complex will still bind to *b* receptors (Cooper, 1975). Or, one may encounter a situation like the one described by Reynolds *et al.* (1975), where the EAC3d prepared with human purified components binds to human macrophages while the EAC3d prepared with whole serum does not.

6. Cells Bearing Plasma Membrane Receptors for Complement

6.1. Erythrocytes

Several phenomena of "serological adhesion" with human erythrocytes or platelets have been described (reviewed by Nelson, 1963). The phenomenon of immune adherence was first defined clearly by Nelson in 1953 when he showed that opsonized microorganisms bound to human red cells. Since that description, a whole variety of antigens carrying attached complements has been utilized. The initial studies showed that C3 was the complement component involved (Nishioka and Linscott, 1963), the later components being unnecessary.

The form of C3 that binds is C3b, and treatment of the complex with C3b inactivator abolishes the immune adherence phenomenon (Ruddy and Austen, 1971). C3b generated by the alternate pathway is also efficient in immune adherence, as shown by May *et al*. (1972).

The initial studies on immune adherence always focused on C3. Cooper (1969) demonstrated, however, that C4b is also able to participate in immune adherence. Similar numbers of molecules of C4b, compared to C3b, had to be present on the indicator particles (sheep erythrocytes coated with C14). More recently, Cooper (1975) showed that like C3b, C4b is cleaved by a serum enzyme to a form that is inactive in immune adherence. As previously mentioned, C3b and C4b may be cleaved by the same enzyme.

6.2. Platelets

Platelets from guinea pigs, rabbits, mice and other nonprimates bind immune complexes containing complement. The phenomenon is usually detected by agglutination of the platelets upon addition of immune complexes. Platelets from man and other primates do not show this type of adherence (reviewed by Nelson, 1963). The participation of complement in the reaction and the trypsin sensitivity of the platelet membrane receptor were demonstrated by Siqueira and Nelson (1961).

The specificity of the receptor in terms of the fragment of the C3 molecule involved has not been formally studied in platelets. However, the phenomenon is very similar to the one observed with human erythrocytes, leading to the belief that it is a *b*-type receptor.

The binding of immune complexes containing C3 to rabbit platelets induces the release of vasoactive amines and nucleotides without cell lysis (reviewed by Osler and Siraganian, 1972, and by Henson, 1972). Human platelets, which do not carry immune adherence receptors, have also been shown to release vasoactive amines in a complement-dependent phenomenon not involving cell lysis (Zucker *et al.*, 1974). Cell destruction without involvement of *b* receptors, as observed during antibody-mediated platelet lysis is a second mechanism of release of active substances involving complement (Osler and Siraganian, 1972; Henson, 1972).

6.3. Granulocytes

Receptors for complement were demonstrated in mouse granulocytes by Lay and Nussenzweig (1968). These authors showed that the binding of indicator erythrocytes was probably mediated by C3. Gigli and Nelson (1968), using purified guinea pig C components, showed that the phagocytosis of sheep erythrocytes by guinea pig granulocytes required C3b. Their assay was based on measurement of total cell-associated hemoglobin and did not distinguish attachment of the erythrocytes to the cell membrane from internalization. As will be discussed later, C3 does not seem to mediate ingestion in granulocytes. The ingestion observed by Gigli and Nelson was probably mediated by IgG present in their antibody preparation. Using purified human complement components, Eden *et al.* (1973b) confirmed that C3b, and not C3d, binds to granulocytes.

C4b binds to granulocytes very efficiently. Among the various blood cells studied by Ross and Polley (1975), granulocytes were the cells requiring the smallest amount of C4b for significant binding.

6.4. Monocytes and Macrophages

The initial observations on receptors for complement on mouse monocytes and macrophages were made by Lay and Nussenzweig (1968). Human monocytes were shown to carry C3 receptors by Huber *et al.* (1968). Both groups have shown that the C3 receptors can be distinguished from the Fc receptor, as the latter could be inhibited by soluble IgG while the former could not. Lay and Nussenzweig (1968) also showed that trypsin affected the binding via C3 without altering the Fc binding. The presence of antibody molecules on the indicator erythrocytes is not necessary because (1) treatment of the complement-coated indicator erythrocyte with F(ab) fragments of rabbit antiserum to mouse IgG did not reduce binding to macrophages (Mantovani *et al.*, 1972) and (2) erythrocytes prepared with cold agglutinins and complement still bind after removal of the cold agglutinins by washing in warm medium (Huber and Douglas, 1970).

The specificity of the receptor on monocytes and macrophages for the fragments C3b or C3d is controversial. Human peripheral blood monocytes have been shown to bind both C3b- and C3d-coated erythrocytes (Ehlenberger and Nussenzweig, 1975). Starch-elicited guinea pig peritoneal macrophages (Wellek *et al.*, 1975) also bound both forms of E(IgM)C1423, either untreated or treated by a purified C3 inactivator. On the other hand, mouse peritoneal macrophages bind only C3b (Griffin *et al.*, 1975). These differences may be explained in two ways:

1. The criterion of EIgMC3d used by all authors was lack of adherence to human erythrocytes. It is possible that adherence to erythrocytes requires more C3b than does adherence to leukocytes.
2. Reynolds *et al.* (1975), studying C3 receptors on human alveolar macrophages, observed that when purified components of complement were used to sensitize the erythrocytes, both forms, C3 inactivator–treated (C3d) and untreated (C3b) complexes, were bound to the macrophages. When whole serum was used as a source of complement, only C3b was bound. In short, the products obtained after digestion by the C3 inactivator, of complexes prepared with purified complement components, or with whole serum are different; and only the C3d product of indicator cells prepared with purified components binds to macrophages. The discrepancy seems not to be related to late components of the classical pathway or to the alternate pathway of complement fixation (Reynolds *et al.*, 1975). Such an explanation would account for the different findings reported in the literature. All the authors who found both C3b and C3d binding used purified components (Ehlenberger and Nussenzweig, 1975; Ross and Polley, 1975; Wellek *et al.*, 1975). Griffin *et al.* (1975) used whole mouse serum. Whatever the interpretation, in the model closest to the *"in vivo"* situation, i.e., utilizing whole serum, there exists a form of C3 that is not recognized by monocytes and macrophages. It is clear that during the *in vitro* construction of the complexes with purified C components, some event with major significance for the fate of the complex *"in vivo"* is either failing to occur or not being detected. Only a full understanding of the structure of C3 will resolve the differences.

6.5. Lymphocytes

Bone marrow–derived, thymus-independent B lymphocytes carry a membrane receptor for complement (Bianco *et al.,* 1970). This receptor is not found on plasma cells. There is overwhelming evidence showing the absence of C receptors on thymus and thymus-derived lymphocytes. This evidence has been recently reviewed (Nussenzweig, 1974).

A study performed by Arnaiz-Villena (1975) did report C3 receptors on "T cells." However, these authors utilized an unconventional marker for T cells: a rabbit antiserum to mouse brain (preabsorbed with several nonthymic tissues to eliminate nonspecific antibodies) (Gyongyossy and Playfair, 1974). The cytotoxicity against C-receptor-bearing cells can also be interpreted as lack of T cell specificity of this antiserum in the absence of an independent correlation with other T cell markers.

The specificity of the receptors for both C3b and for C3d on lymphocytes is well demonstrated using purified C components (Ross *et al.,* 1973a; Eden *et al.,* 1973b). The results obtained with purified components or whole serum are similar. Both human and mouse lymphocytes bind E(IgM)C (prepared with mouse serum), which probably contains only C3d (Pincus *et al.,* 1972; Griffin *et al.,* 1975). The sensitized erythrocytes did not bind to human or mouse monocytes or macrophages.

Antisera that blocked *b* and *d* receptors of human lymphoid cells have been prepared. (Ross *et al.,* 1973a). The complement receptors are present in many chronic lymphatic leukemia cells (Pincus *et al.,* 1972) and in various cell lines (Shevach *et al.,* 1972). Among the leukemias and the cell lines, most of the receptors are of the *d* type (Ross *et al.,* 1973a). The *b* and *d* receptors on the cell membrane are independent entities. Ross *et al.* (1973a), using antisera that are specific for *b* or *d* receptors, could inhibit either the binding of C3b or C3d, respectively. More recently, Ross and Polley (1975) performed cocapping experiments in which a fluoresceinated rabbit antiserum to C3 was used to cap C3 fragments previously bound to lymphocytes. Indicator erythrocytes were also allowed to cap at 37°C. Distinct *b* and *d* caps formed over different areas of the cell membrane.

7. Functional Significance of the Receptors for Complement

The wide distribution of C receptors among blood cells reflects the importance of the recognition and handling of immune complexes. At least three different functions can be ascribed to the receptors for complement: control of the traffic of immune complexes and cells, control of the fate of immune complexes, and triggering of cellular functions.

An important functional consequence of the interaction of complement products (C3a and C5a) with leukocytes is chemotaxis. This subject is considered in other chapters of this book. Platelets, as mentioned earlier, release vasoactive amines upon interaction with immune complexes containing complement.

7.1. Control of the Traffic of Immune Complexes and Cells

Cells bearing C receptors may carry specific types of immune complexes, and sites where immune complexes are found can become areas of accumulation of C-receptor-bearing cells. Trapping of antigen-retaining cells was used to explain such phenomena as antigen localization in B areas of lymphoid organs and follicle formation (Bianco *et al.,* 1971).

The identification of the *b* and *d* receptors clarified previous observations. For example, it was unclear why, if antigen could be localized by C receptors in lymphoid organs, this same antigen was not retained by erythrocytes or platelets as well. It is now clear that antigen–antibody–complement complexes bind to platelets *in vivo,* but are subsequently released (Miller and Nussenzweig, 1974). The released complexes are probably attacked by the C3b inactivator, losing their ability to bind to the *b* receptor, but remaining capable of binding to cells carrying *d* receptors. Thus, complexes containing C3b can be transported or retained by cells carrying these receptors, but after cleavage of C3 by the C3b inactivator, only a more select group of cells, such as B lymphocytes, is still able to combine with these complexes.

7.2. Control of the Fate of Immune Complexes

It is clear that the form of C3 and the presence or absence of IgG in immune complexes will determine the fate of these complexes. Table 3 summarizes the *in vitro* fate of erythrocytes coated with several C components, with or without IgG.

Complement has long been considered capable of acting as an opsonin to promote phagocytosis. However, recent evidence has accumulated showing that, in many cases, it is really the IgG portion of the immune complex, via its Fc component, that is the opsonin. IgM antibodies, which do not bind to the Fc receptor of cells, cannot form opsonizing complexes after exposure to complement. Erythrocytes allowed to fix complement after exposure to a cold agglutinin and then warmed to elute the antibody are no longer opsonized (Huber and Douglas, 1970). Antibody–complement-coated erythrocytes treated with F(ab) fragments of a rabbit anti-immunoglobulin to block the Fc portion of the opsonizing antibody are not phagocytized by mouse macrophages (Mantovani *et al.,* 1972) or granulocytes (Mantovani, 1975). Human granulocytes will not ingest indicator erythrocytes

TABLE 3. Fate of Erythrocyte Complexes Added to Blood Cells *in Vitro*

Cell type	Form of C3 in complexes	Ig class in complexes	Fate
Erythrocytes (primates)	C3b	Irrelevant	Attachment
Platelets (nonprimates)	C3b	Irrelevant	Attachment
B lymphocytes (mammals)	C3b or C3d	Irrelevant	Attachment
Granulocytes (human, guinea pig)	C3b	Other than IgG / IgG	Attachment / Ingestion
Monocytes (human)	C3b	Other than IgG / IgG	Attachment / Ingestion
Resident peritoneal macrophages (mouse)	C3b	Other than IgG / IgG	Attachment / Ingestion
Activated macrophages (mouse)	C3b	Other than IgG / IgG	Ingestion / Ingestion

coated with IgM and complement (Ross and Polley, 1974). However, the addition of as few as 60 molecules of IgG to EIgMC complexes leads to their phagocytosis by human granulocytes or monocytes (Ehlenberger and Nussenzweig, 1975). This amount of IgG on erythrocytes is insufficient to promote ingestion alone, clearly demonstrating cooperation, in the case of EIgG, between IgG and C3b (Huber *et al,* 1968). Complement, promoting better contact between the particle and the phagocyte, allowed for this cooperation. The presence of IgG in complexes was not ruled out in many of the examples in the literature that claim to show complement-mediated ingestion.

There is, however, one example of a cell in which ingestion can be mediated by C3, namely, the activated mouse peritoneal macrophage. The intraperitoneal injection of thioglycollate medium or bacterial endotoxin, as well as chronic infection with BCG, originates a population of "activated" macrophages that show increased metabolic and bactericidal activity and secrete certain enzymes, such as a plasminogen activator. The ingestion of E(IgM)C provides a convenient marker for macrophage activation at the individual cell level. Thus there is extensive evidence *"in vitro,"* that the C receptors mediate attachment and not ingestion, with the sole exception of the activated macrophages.

These findings provide an explanation at the cellular level for the *in vivo* observations of Schreiber and Frank (1972) and Atkinson and Frank (1974). They showed that IgM-coated homologous erythrocytes injected intravenously into normal guinea pigs were briefly sequestered by the liver and then were released back into the circulation, where they had a half-life similar to that of nonopsonized erythrocytes. The presence of IgG on the cells induced their rapid clearance. On the other hand, guinea pigs infected with BCG, which is known to activate macrophages, cleared with IgM coated cells rather efficiently. These experiments are also informative in showing that, despite the controversy on C3b or C3d binding sites *"in vitro,"* there is a form of C3 that is not recognized by phagocytic cells. When an antigen is introduced into an organism, the initial antibodies produced are usually of the IgM class. The complexes formed are not cleared from the circulation even if, in the case of cellular antigens, the cell is lysed by the full sequence of complement components. Only the production of IgG, the general activation of macrophages, or the existence of properties intrinsic to the antigen that make it ingestible by nonimmunological phagocytosis provide for antigen elimination.

7.3. Cell Triggering

Besides the contact interaction between immune complexes and cells and bridging cells via complexes, the interaction with complement receptors may trigger other cellular functions. As mentioned before, platelets release vasoactive amines upon interaction with C3-bearing immune complexes. The release of chemotactic substances for monocytes by guinea pig B lymphocytes has also been attributed to the interaction with C3 and Fc receptors (Wahl *et al.,* 1974). The release of this lymphokine can also be obtained by direct incubation of the lymphocytes with guinea pig C3b obtained by trypsin digestion (Sandberg *et al.,* 1975).

B lymphocytes have been reported to be stimulated to undergo mitosis interacting with complement (Hartmann and Bokisch, 1975). Dukor and Hartmann (1973) have proposed the interesting hypothesis that the C receptor provides a second signal for B cell activation. They postulate that thymus-independent antigens can activate complement via the alternate pathway and, consequently, can directly activate the B cell by combining simultaneously with membrane Ig and C receptors. T cells would provide the complement-activating factors for thymus-dependent antigens. This hypothesis has not been experimentally supported, and several investigators have demonstrated that C3 is not an absolute requirement for an *in vitro* response to thymus-independent antigens (Janossy *et al.,* 1973; Moller and Coutinho, 1975; Pryjma and Humphrey, 1975; Waldmann and Lachmann, 1975). Actually, many of the thymus-independent antigens have been shown to be polyclonal mitogens for B cells (Coutinho, 1975). However, *in vivo* depletion of complement by cobra venom factor leads to a delay in the immune response to sheep erythrocytes (Pepys, 1972) and *in vitro* responses to thymus-dependent antigens may be blocked by depletion of C3 (Feldman and Pepys, 1974).

More recently, Hartmann and Bokisch (1975) have shown that soluble human C3b is mitogenic for mouse B lymphocytes. A more detailed confirmation is necessary in homologous systems since human C3b, when bound to indicator erythrocytes, interacts poorly with mouse lymphocytes (Bianco *et al.,* 1970). While *in vitro* responses to several antigens can be obtained in the absence of complement, this does not necessarily represent the *in vivo* mechanisms. Furthermore, several alternative mechanisms of antigenic stimulation may operate. The many contradictory findings on the role of C3 in B lymphocyte triggering, however, do not rule out the participation of complement or of receptors for complement in this important function.

8. Conclusion

Two types of receptors for complement have been identified on the plasma membrane of certain leukocytes, erythrocytes, and platelets: *b* receptors, which recognize the complement proteins C3b and C4b, and *d* receptors, which bind C3d, a fragment produced by enzymatic cleavage of C3b. A cell may carry one or both types of receptors. Mouse peritoneal macrophages carry only *b* receptors. B lymphocytes carry both *b* and *d* receptors.

The plasma membrane receptors for complement are absent from T cells, and consequently constitute a useful market for B lymphocytes. Complement interaction with lymphocytes may be necessary for certain immune responses.

Receptors for complement are also useful as markers for macrophage activation. Normal macrophages bind, but do not ingest, particles coated with C3b. On the other hand, activated macrophages bind and ingest opsonized particles via the *b* receptors. In the absence of IgG antibodies, the fate of immune complexes depends on the state of activation of the macrophage.

Note: This review was written in July, 1975.

ACKNOWLEDGMENT

Celso Bianco is a scholar of the Leukemia Society of America, Inc. This work was supported, in part, by grant #A.I.07012 to Z. A. Cohn.

The author is grateful to Drs. Aline Eden, Nadia Nogueira, and Paul Edelson for reading the manuscript.

References

CELSO BIANCO

Arnaiz-Villena, A., and Hay, F. C., 1975, Complement receptor lymphocytes. Analysis of immunoglobulin on their surface and further evidence of heterogeneity, *Immunology* **28**:719–729.

Atkinson, J. P., and Frank M. M., 1974, The effect of bacillus Calmette-Guerin-induced macrophage activation on the *in vivo* clearance of sensitized erythrocytes, *J. Clin. Invest.* **53**:1742–1749.

Bianco, C., Patrick, R., and Nussenzweig, V., 1970, A population of lymphocytes bearing a membrane receptor for antigen–antibody–complement complexes, 1. Separation and characterization, *J. Exp. Med.* **132**:702–720.

Bianco, C., Dukor, P., and Nussenzweig, V., 1971, Follicular localization of antigen: possible role of lymphocytes bearing a receptor for antigen-antibody-complement complexes, in: *Morphological and Functional Aspects of Immunity* (K. Lindahl-Kiessling, G. Alm, and M. G. Hanna Jr., eds.), pp. 251–256, Plenum Press, New York.

Bianco, C., Griffin, F. M., and Silverstein, S. C., 1975, Studies of the macrophage complement receptor. Alteration of receptor function upon macrophage activation, *J. Exp. Med.* **141**:1278–1290.

Bokisch, V. A., Müller-Eberhard, H. J., and Cochrane, C. G., 1969, Isolation of a fragment (C3a) of the third component of human complement containing anaphylatoxin and chemotactic activity and description of an anaphylatoxin inactivator of human serum, *J. Exp. Med.* **129**:1109–1130.

Bokisch, V. A., and Sobel, A. T., 1974, Receptor for the fourth component of complement on human B lymphocytes and cultured human lymphoblastoid cells, *J. Exp. Med.* **140**:1336–1347.

Bokisch, V. A., Dierich, M. P., and Müller-Eberhard, H. J., 1975, Third component of complement (C3): structural properties in relation to functions, *Proc. Nat. Acad. Sci. U.S.A.* **12**:1989–1993.

Cinader, B., Dubiski, S., and Wardlaw, A. C., 1964, Distribution, inheritance, and properties of an antigen, MuB1 and its relation to hemolytic complement, *J. Exp. Med.* **120**:897–924.

Cooper, N. R., 1969, Immune adherence by the fourth component of complement, *Science* **165**:396–398.

Cooper, N., 1975, Isolation and analysis of the mechanism of action of an inactivator of C4b in normal human serum, *J. Exp. Med.* **141**:890–903.

Coutinho, A., 1975, The theory of the "one nonspecific signal" model for B cell activation, *Transplant. Rev.* **23**:49–65.

Cuatrecasas, P., 1974, Membrane receptors, *Annu. Rev. Biochem.* **43**:169–214.

Dierich, M. P., and Reisfeld, R. A., 1975, C3 receptors on lymphoid cells: isolation of active membrane fragments and solubilization of receptor complexes, *J. Immunol.* **114**:1676–1682.

Dukor, P., and Hartmann, K. H., 1973, Bound C3 as the second signal for B-cell activation, *Cell. Immunol.* **7**:349–356.

Eden, A., Bianco, C., and Nussenzweig, V., 1973a, Mechanism of binding of soluble complexes to lymphocytes, *Cell. Immunol.* **7**:459–473.

Eden, A., Miller, G. W., and Nussenzweig, V., 1973b, Human lymphocytes bear membrane receptors for C3b and C3d, *J. Clin. Invest.* **52**:3239–3242.

Ehlenberger, A. G., and Nussenzweig, V., 1975, Synergy between receptors for Fc and C3 in the induction of phagocytosis by human monocytes and neutrophils, *Fed. Proc. Fed. Amer. Soc. Exp. Biol.* **34**:854.

Feldmann, M., and Pepys, M. B., 1974, Role of C3 in *in vitro* lymphocyte cooperation, *Nature London* **249**:159–161.

Gigli, I., and Nelson, Jr., R. A., 1968, Complement dependent immune phagocytosis, 1. Requirements for C'1, C'4, C'2, C'3, *Exp. Cell Res.* **51**:45–67.

Gitlin, J. D., Rosen, F. S., and Lachmann, P. J., 1975, The mechanism of action of the C3b inactivator (conglutinogen-activating factor) on its naturally occurring substrate, the major fragment of the third component of complement (C3b), *J. Exp. Med.* **141**:1221–1226.

Götze, O., and Müller-Eberhard, H. J., 1971, The C3 activator system: an alternate pathway of complement activation, *J. Exp. Med.* **134**:905–1085.

Grey, H. M., Kubo, R. T., and Cerrotini, J.-C., 1972, Thymus-derived (T) cell immunoglobulins:presence of a receptor site for IgG and absence of large amounts of "buried" Ig determinants on T cells, *J. Exp. Med.* **136**:1323–1328.

Griffin, Jr., F. M., Bianco, C., and Silverstein, S. C., 1975, Characterization of the macrophage receptor for complement and demonstration of its functional independence from the receptor for the Fc portion of immunoglobulin G, *J. Exp. Med.* **141**:1269–1277.

Gyongyossy, M. I. C., and Playfair, J. H. L., 1974, Rosette formation by mouse lymphocytes. 1. Demonstration by indirect immunofluorescence of T cells binding sheep erythrocytes, *Clin. Exp. Immunol.* **18**:169–176.

Hartmann, K.-V., and Bokish, V. A., 1975, Stimulation of murine B lymphocytes by purified human C3b, *Fed. Proc. Fed. Amer. Soc. Exp. Biol.* **34**:854.

Henson, P. M., 1972, Complement-dependent adherence of cells to antigen and antibody. Mechanisms and consequences, in: *Biological Activities of Complement* (D. G. Ingram, ed.) pp. 173–201, Karger, Basel.

Huber, H., and Douglas, S. D., 1970, Receptor sites on human monocytes for complement: binding of red cells sensitized by cold autoantibodies, *Br. J. Haematol.* **19**:19–26.

Huber, H., Polley, M. J., Linscott, W. D., Fudenberg, H. H., and Müller-Eberhard, H. J., 1968, Human monocytes: distinct receptor sites for the third component of complement and for immunoglobulin G, *Science* **162**:1281–1283.

Hugli, T. E., Morgan, W. T., and Müller-Eberhard, H. J., 1975a, Circular dicroism of C3a anaphylatoxin, *J. Biol. Chem.* **250**:1479–1483.

Hugli, T. E., Vallota, E. H., and Müller-Eberhard, H. J., 1975b, Purification and partial characterization of human and porcine C3a anaphylatoxin, *J. Biol. Chem.* **250**:1472–1478.

Janossy, G., Humphrey, J. H., Pepys, M. B., and Greaves, M. F., 1973, Complement independence of stimulation of mouse splenic B lymphocytes by mitogens, *Nature (London) New Biol.* **245**:108–112.

Lachmann, P. J., and Müller-Eberhard, H. J., 1968, The demonstration in human serum of "conglutinogen-activating factor" and its effect on the third component of complement, *J. Immunol.* **100**:691–698.

Lay, W. H., and Nussenzweig, V., 1968, Receptors for complement of leukocytes, *J. Exp. Med.* **128**:991–1009.

Mantovani, B., 1975, Different roles of IgG and complement receptors in phagocytosis by polymorphonuclear leukocytes, *J. Immunol.* **115**:15–17.

Mantovani, B., Rabinovitch, M., and Nussenzweig, V., 1972, Phagocytosis of immune complexes by macrophages. Different roles of the macrophage receptor sites for complement (C3) and for immunoglobulin (IgG), *J. Exp. Med.* **135**:780–792.

May, J. E., Kane, M. A., and Frank, M. M., 1972, Immune adherence by the alternate complement pathway, *Proc. Soc. Exp. Biol. Med.* **141**:287–290.

Mendes, N. F., Mike, S. S., and Peixinho, Z. F., 1974, Combined detections of human T and B lymphocytes by rosette formation with sheep erythrocytes and zymosan-C3 complexes, *J. Immunol.* **113**:531–536.

Miller, G. W., and Nussenzweig, V., 1974, Complement as a regulator of interactions between immune complexes and cell membranes, *J. Immunol.* **113**:464–469.

Moller, G., and Coutinho, A., 1975, Role of C3 and Fc receptors in B-lymphocyte activation, *J. Exp. Med.* **141**:647–663.

Müller-Eberhard, H. J., Polley, M. J., and Calcott, M. A., 1967, Formation and functional significance of a molecular complex derived from the second and the fourth component of the human complement, *J. Exp. Med.* **125**:359–380.

Nelson, D. S., 1963, Immune adherence, *Adv. Immunol.* **3**:131–80.

Nelson, R. A., 1953, The immune adherence phenomenon: an immunologically specific reaction between microorganisms and erythrocytes leading to enhanced phagocytosis, *Science* **118**:733–737.

Nilsson, V. R., and Beisswenger, J., 1975, Isolation and characterization of the α and β subunits of human C3, *Fed. Proc. Fed. Amer. Soc. Exp. Biol.* **35**:955.

Nishioka, K., and Linscott, W. D., 1963, Components of guinea pig complement. I. Separation of a serum fraction essential for immune hemolysis and immune-adherence, *J. Exp. Med.* **118**:767–793.

Nussenzweig, V., 1974, Receptors for immune complexes on lymphocytes, *Adv. Immunol.* **19**:217–258.

Osler, A. G., and Siraganian, R. P., 1972, Immunologic mechanisms of platelet damage, *Prog. Allergy* **16**:450–498.

Pepys, M. D., 1972, Role of complement in induction of the allergic response, *Nature London New Biol.* **237**:157–159.

Pincus, S., Bianco, C., and Nussenzweig, V., 1972, Increased proportion of complement-receptor lymphocytes in the peripheral blood of patients with chronic lymphocytic leukemia, *Blood* **40**:303–310.

Pryjma, J., and Humphrey, J. H., 1975, Prolonged C3 depletion by cobra venom factor in thymus-deprived mice and its implications for the role of C3 as an essential second signal for B-cell triggering, *Immunology* **28**:569–576.

Reynolds, H. Y., Atkinson, J. P., Newball, H. H., and Frank, M. M., 1975, Receptors for immunoglobulin and complement on human alveolar macrophages, *J. Immunol.* **114**:1813–1819.

Ross, G. D., and Polley, M. J., 1974, Human lymphocyte and granulocyte receptors for the fourth component of complement (C4) and the role of granulocyte receptors in phagocytosis, *Fed Proc. Fed. Amer. Soc. Exp. Biol.* 33:759.

Ross, G. D., and Polley, M. J., 1975, Specificity of human lymphocyte complement receptors, *J. Exp. Med.* 141:1163–1180.

Ross, G. D., Polley, M. J., Rabellino, E. M., and Grey, H. M., 1973a, Two different complement receptors on human lymphocytes, one specific for C3b and one specific for C3b inactivator–cleaved C3b, *J. Exp. Med.* 138:798–811.

Ross, G. D., Rabellino, E. M., Polley, M. J., and Grey, H. M., 1973b, Combined studies of complement receptor and surface immunoglobulin-bearing cells and sheep erythrocyte rosette-forming cells in normal and leukemic human lymphocytes, *J. Clin. Invest.* 52:377–385.

Ruddy, S., and Austen, K. F., 1971, C3b inactivator of man. II. Fragments produced by C3b inactivator cleavage of cell-bound or fluid phase C3b, *J. Immunol.* 107:742–750.

Sandberg, A. L., and Wahl, S. M., and Mergenhagen, S. E., 1975, Lyphokine production by C3b-stimulated B cells, *J. Immunol.* 115:139–144.

Schreiber, A. D., and Frank, M. M., 1972, Role of antibody and complement in the immune clearance and destruction of erythrocytes. I. *In vivo* effects of IgG and IgM complement-fixing sites, *J. Clin. Invest.* 51:575–589.

Schreiber, R. D., and Müller-Eberhard, H. J., 1974, Fourth component of human complement: description of a three polypeptide chain structure, *J. Exp. Med.* 140:1324–1335.

Shevach, E. M., Herberman, R., Frank, M. M., and Green, I., 1972, Receptors for complement and immunoglobulin on human leukemic cells and human lumphoblastoid cell lines, *J. Clin. Invest.* 51:1933–1938.

Shevach, E. M., Jaffe, E. S., and Green, I., 1973, Receptors for complement and immunoglobulin on human and animal lymphoid cells, *Transplant. Rev.* 16:3–28.

Silva, W. D., Eisele, J. W., and Lepow, I. H., 1967, Complement as a mediator of inflammation. III. Purification of the activity with anaphylatoxin properties generated by interaction of the first four components of complement and its identification as a cleavage product of C'3, *J. Exp. Med.* 126:1027–1048.

Siqueira, M., and Nelson, Jr., R. A., 1961, Platelet agglutination by immune complexes and its possible role in hypersensitivity, *J. Immunol.* 86:516–525.

Sobel, A. T., and Bokisch, V. A., 1975, Receptor for C1q on peripheral human lymphocytes and human lymphoblastoid cells, *Fed. Proc. Fed. Amer. Soc. Exp. Biol.* 34:965.

Spitzer, R. E., Stitzel, A. E., Pauling, V. L., Davis, N. C., and West, C. D., 1971, The antigenic and molecular alterations of C3 in the fluid phase during an immune reaction in normal human serum. Demonstration of a new conversion product, *J. Exp. Med.* 134:656–680.

Stossel, T. P., Field, R. J., Gitlin, J. D., Alper, C. A., and Rosen, F. S., 1975, The opsonic fragment of the third component of human complement (C3), *J. Exp. Med.* 141:1329–1347.

Tamura, N., and Nelson, Jr., R. A., 1967, Three naturally occuring inhibitors of components of complement in guinea pig and rabbit serum, *J. Immunol.* 99:582–589.

Theofilopoulos, A. N., Bokisch, V. A., and Dixon, F. J., 1974, Receptor for soluble C3 and C3b on human lymphoblastoid (Raji) cells, *J. Exp. Med.* 139:696–711.

Wahl, S. M., Iverson, G. M., and Oppenheim, J. J., 1974, Induction of guinea pig B-cell lymphokine synthesis by mitogenic and non-mitogenic signals to Fc, Ig, and C3 receptors, *J. Exp. Med.* 140:1631–1645.

Waldmann, H., and Lachmann, P. J., 1975, The failure to show a necessary role for C3 in the *in vitro* antibody response, *Eur. J. Immunol.* 5:185–193.

Wellek, B., Hahn, H. H., and Opferkuch, W., 1975, Evidence for macrophage C3d-receptor active in phagocytosis, *J. Immunol.* 114:1643–1645.

Zucker, M. B., Grant, R. A., Alper, C. A., Goodkovsky, I., and Lepow, I. H., 1974, Requirement for complement components and fibrinogen in the zymosan-induced release reaction of human blood platelets, *J. Immunol.* 113:1744–1751.

5

Opsonization

FRANK M. GRIFFIN, JR.

1. Introduction

Opsonin is a term introduced by Wright and Douglas (1903) to designate a factor (or factors) in serum that interacts with particles in a manner that renders the particles more readily ingested by phagocytic cells. In this chapter, we will consider the mechanisms by which opsonins interact with the particles they coat and with the phagocytic cells to which they bind and the role opsonization plays in host defense against invasion by microorganisms.

The importance of phagocytic cells—polymorphonuclear leukocytes and mononuclear phagocytes—in host defense against microbial invasion has been appreciated since the studies of Metchnikoff (1887). During the last decade of the nineteenth century, there was much controversy over the relative importance of phagocytic cells and serum factors in defending an organism against infection. The classical studies of Wright and Douglas (1903) made it apparent not only that both were essential, but also that they exerted cooperative effects in the eradication of invading microbes.

Wright and Douglas's studies did much to resolve the conflict between proponents of phagocytes and proponents of serum factors and determined the direction of research that has continued for more than 70 years. Because of the elegance and importance of these studies, it is worth examining them in some detail. These authors used human leukocytes, human serum, and staphylococci to determine the effect of serum on the interaction of leukocytes with the bacteria. The key difference between their studies and all that preceded them is that they separated cells from serum, and were therefore able to alter the serum without altering the cells and to pre-incubate bacteria and phagocytic cells separately with serum. Their assay was the number of bacteria ingested per 20 leukocytes, as judged by examining stained smears. Their findings were that fresh, but not heat-inactivated, serum is opsonic; that treatment of serum with cobra venom or pre-incubation of serum at

FRANK M. GRIFFIN, JR. • The Rockefeller University, New York, New York. Present address: Division of Infectious Diseases, Department of Medicine, University of Alabama in Birmingham, Birmingham, Alabama.

37°C with *Salmonella typhi* eliminates its opsonic capacity; that the effect of opsonins is upon the bacteria; and that immunization increases the opsonic capacity of serum. Unfortunately, they did not examine the effect of heating on the opsonic capacity immune serum, and therefore did not establish that opsonins in immune serum are different from those in nonimmune serum.

These are remarkable studies, especially for that era. They demonstrated that the effect of opsonins is on bacteria, not on phagocytic cells; that the opsonic activity of nonimmune serum is heat-labile; that the opsonic activity of nonimmune serum is not specific for one organism; and that the effect of immunization is upon serum. Thus, the core of what we now know about immune and nonimmune opsonins was determined in 1903. The work that has followed has been directed at characterizing immunospecific and nonspecific opsonins, discerning antibody structure and function, identifying heat-labile opsonins, defining complement components and their reactions, and determining the mechanisms by which opsonins interact with particles and with phagocytic cells.

Clearly, the two most important, if not the only important, serum factors that serve to opsonize particles are IgG and the particle-bound component of cleaved C3, C3b. We will first consider IgG.

2. Immunoglobulin G

It has been known for many years that the combination of antigen-specific, heat-stable antibody with the appropriate antigen on the surface of an organism promotes the ingestion of, or markedly enhances the rate of ingestion of, the organism (Bulloch and Western, 1906; Cowie and Chapin, 1907a,b; Zinsser *et al.*, 1939; Dubos, 1945). As the structure of immunoglobulins was deciphered, it became apparent that IgG is the heat-stable serum factor responsible for antigen-specific opsonization.

2.1. Mechanism of Opsonization by IgG

IgG combines by its two antigen-binding pieces, Fab, with antigenic determinants on the surface of the microorganism (or other particle). This binding is independent of the presence of divalent cations and occurs at 4°C as well as at 37°C (Pillemer *et al.*, 1954). Upon combination with antigen, the IgG molecule undergoes certain conformational and configurational changes in the $F(ab)_2$ hinge region *(vide infra)*, but there is no evidence to suggest that these changes influence the bond between antigen and antibody.

Phagocytic cells of all types have receptors for the IgG molecule on their plasma membranes. The number of these receptors on each mouse peritoneal macrophage (Berken and Benacerraf, 1966; Phillips-Quagliata *et al.*, 1971) and rabbit alveolar macrophage (Arend and Mannik, 1973) has been estimated at 1–2 million. These receptors are resistant to tryptic proteolysis and mediate binding of IgG-coated particles at 4°C as well as at 37°C and in the absence of divalent cations (Huber and Fudenberg, 1968; Huber *et al.*, 1968; Lay and Nussenzweig, 1968; Henson, 1969; Messner and Jelinek, 1970).

Even though all four subclasses of human IgG bind to antigen, only IgG_1 and IgG_3 are capable of binding to receptors on phagocytic cells. This has been shown directly by coupling myeloma IgG of various subclasses to erythrocytes and assaying the binding and uptake of these erythrocytes by human monocytes (Huber and Fudenberg, 1968; Abramson et al., 1970a). In indirect assays, "free" IgG (IgG not bound to antigen) of different subclasses has been added to the incubation medium to compete for receptor sites on human phagocytic cells; only IgG$_1$ and IgG$_3$ bind to these receptors and block binding and ingestion of IgG-coated erythrocytes (Huber and Fudenberg, 1968; Messner and Jelinek, 1970; Abramson et al, 1970a).

The phagocytic cell's receptors for IgG bind only to the Fc portion of the molecule (Uhr, 1965; Berken and Benacerraf, 1966; Huber and Fudenberg, 1968; Quie et al., 1968; Abramson et al., 1970 a,b; Messner and Jelinek, 1970; Lawrence et al., 1975), and are therefore known as *Fc receptors*. Antigens coated with Fab or F(ab')$_2$ fragments of IgG fail to bind to mouse peritoneal macrophages (Uhr, 1965), human monocytes (Huber and Fudenberg, 1968), or human neutrophils (Quie et al., 1968), and mouse peritoneal macrophages fail to ingest erythrocytes or horseradish peroxidase coated with pepsin-digested IgG (Rabinovitch, 1967; Steinman and Cohn, 1972; Griffin and Silverstein, 1974). Inclusion of rheumatoid factor, a macroglobulin that binds to the Fc portion of IgG, in an incubation mixture of staphylococci, antistaphylococcal IgG, and human leukocytes prevented ingestion of the organism, presumably by blocking Fc–Fc receptor interaction (Messner et al., 1968).

Competitive inhibition studies have also demonstrated that the Fc portion of the IgG molecule is the site by which IgG-coated particles bind to phagocytic cells. Ingestion of IgG-coated particles by human neutrophils (Messner and Jelinek, 1970) and human monocytes (Lo Buglio et al., 1967; Abramson et al., 1970a) could be blocked by including Fc fragments of IgG in the incubation medium. Neither Fab nor F(ab')$_2$ fragments affected particle ingestion.

Two studies have been directed toward defining the chemical structure of the Fc piece responsible for binding to the cells' Fc receptors. Quie et al. (1968) treated IgG with periodate and found that its opsonic activity was abolished. However, the Gm(b) locus was also abolished, some amino acids were removed, and the electrophoretic mobility and Svedberg constant of IgG were also changed. These authors were unable to define, from these studies, the carbohydrate or amino acid structure required for Fc binding. Abramson et al. (1970a) demonstrated that IgG$_1$ H cahins and IgG$_3$ H chains could block the uptake of IgG-coated erythrocytes by human monocytes. Cleavage of the Fc disulfide bridges with dithiothreitol abolished the ability of Fc fragments to inhibit binding, but treatment with 8 M urea did not. Pepsin fragments II, III, and IV had no inhibitory activity. They concluded that the site on the Fc portion that is critical for mediating binding of IgG-coated particles to the cell's surface is located on the amino terminal end of the Fc piece and requires intact disulfide bonds but does not require intact tertiary structure.

As indicated previously, the IgG molecule undergoes conformational and configurational changes when it combines with antigen. These changes include optical rotatory changes (Ishizaka and Campbell, 1959; Henney and Stanworth, 1966), an altered susceptibility to chymotrypsin digestion (Grossberg et al., 1965), exposure of new antigenic determinants (Henney et al., 1965; Henney and Stanworth, 1966), and structural changes detected by electron microscopy (Feinstein and Rowe, 1965; Valentine and Green, 1967). The changes appear to be in the H chains of the Fab portions of the molecule (Henney *et al.*, 1965) and to result in a widening of the angle at the F(ab)$_2$ hinge region (Feinstein and Rowe, 1965; Valentine and Green, 1967). Warner *et al.* (1970) have disputed the finding of widening of the F(ab)$_2$ hinge angle, however, for they have found from physical data that the IgG molecule becomes more globular on interaction with antigen.

Despite the occurrence of these conformational and/or configurational changes in antigen-bound IgG, there is no direct evidence that they affect the interaction of IgG-coated particles with phagocytic cells. Binding of antigen–antibody complexes to Fc receptors of phagocytic cells is stronger than the binding of antibody alone, but this increased strength of complex binding may be due to summation of IgG–Fc receptor interactions rather than to allosteric changes in the IgG molecule. There is some evidence that summation of these interactions may be more important than allosteric changes. Pooled IgG, i.e., IgG that is not directed toward one specific antigen, has been coupled by chromic chloride to erythrocytes and found to promote the erythrocytes' binding to human monocytes (Huber and Fudenberg, 1968; Abramson *et al.*, 1970a). Presumably, these IgG molecules, since they had not bound to antigen immunologically, had not undergone allosteric changes. Also, polyvalent hapten–antibody complexes were found to bind much more strongly to rabbit alveolar and peritoneal macrophages than did mono- or oligovalent complexes (Phillips-Quagliata *et al.*, 1971). Finally, antigen–antibody complex binding to phagocytic cells can be competitively blocked by "free" IgG or Fc fragments, as discussed above.

While the foregoing paragraphs express the current views of many investigators regarding the mechanisms by which IgG-coated particles are recognized by the plasma membrane of phagocytic cells, there are other concepts that should be mentioned. Monoclonal (myeloma) and polyclonal IgG have been found to opsonize some nonencapsulated organisms for ingestion by human leukocytes as effectively as did antigen-specific IgG, as judged by examination of stained smears (van Oss and Stinson, 1970; Stinson and van Oss, 1971). Interpretation of these results is difficult, however, for serum was present in the incubation medium and therefore complement could have been exerting the opsonic effect; also, it is difficult to determine which organisms are ingested and which are only attached to cells by examining stained smears. Formerly, a popular notion was that antibody (and other opsonins) rendered particles more hydrophobic (van Oss and Singer, 1966; Davis *et al.*, 1968) or reduced their net negative surface charges (Mudd *et al.*, 1934), thereby making them more palatable to phagocytic cells. However, the relatively low number of IgG molecules, 10^3 to 10^4, required to opsonize an erythrocyte for ingestion by a human monocyte (Huber *et al.*, 1969) or by a mouse peritoneal macrophage (Mantovani *et al.*, 1972) makes these proposed mechanisms unlikely.

2.2. Opsonization of Microorganisms by IgG

Opsonization by specific IgG appears to be most important in defense against infection with most encapsulated bacteria and some of the more virulent strains of nonencapsulated organisms. Smooth strains of *Diplococcus pneumoniae* (Ward and Enders, 1933; Johnston *et al.*, 1969); groups A, B, and C meningococci (Roberts, 1967, 1970); type b *Hemophilus influenzae* (Anderson *et al.*, 1972a, b; Johnston *et al.*, 1973); M-typable streptococci (Rothbard, 1945; Hirsch and Church,

1960); type C *Klebsiella* (Boyden *et al.*, 1965); and some strains of staphylococci (Cohn and Morse, 1959; Quie *et al.*, 1968; Nickerson *et al.*, 1969; Messner and Jelinek, 1970; Wheat *et al.*, 1974) and *Pseudomonas aeruginosa* (Young, 1972; Young and Armstrong, 1972) require opsonization by IgG in order for efficient ingestion to occur. With most of these organisms, ingestion is still further enhanced by the presence of both IgG and complement, as we will see. The critical role of IgG in defense against invasion by encapsulated organisms is demonstrated by the frequency and severity of infections caused by these bacteria in individuals with agammaglobulinemia (Rosen and Janeway, 1966).

IgG antibody may also be important in the pathogenesis of some autoimmune hemolytic anemias and thrombocytopenias (Handin and Stossel, 1974) and in defense against malaria (Cohen and Butcher, 1970). In malaria, the proposed role of IgG is unusual, for, rather than serving as an opsonin, antiplasmodial IgG appeared to prevent infection of monkey erythrocytes by *Plasmodium knowlesi*.

3. Complement

The most important heat-labile opsonin, and perhaps the most important opsonin of all, is C3b.* C3b is the fragment of C3 that binds to particles when C3 is cleaved by a C3-convertase (Müller-Eberhard *et al.*, 1967). C3 can be cleaved by two pathways of complement activation.

3.1. Mechanisms of Generation of C3b Opsonic Activity

The classical pathway begins with binding of IgG or IgM molecules to antigen, which results in binding and activation of the C1 complex. Binding of only one IgM molecule to the particle surface is sufficient to initiate complement fixation (Borsos and Rapp, 1965a). Approximately 800 IgG molecules must bind, however, in order to produce one IgG doublet, which is required to initiate the complement cascade (Borsos and Rapp, 1965b: Cohen, 1968). C1q binds to a site on the Fc portion of the immunoglobulin molecule (Müller-Eberhard, 1968), and then C4 and C2 are cleaved to their active forms, C4b and C2a, which bind to the particle surface. The $\overline{C4b2a}$ complex then cleaves C3, resulting in the deposition of hundreds of C3b molecules on the surface of the particle (Müller-Eberhard *et al.*, 1967). Both Ca^{2+} and Mg^{2+} ions are required for the function of the classical pathway.

C3 may also be cleaved and C3b may be deposited on the particle surface by the alternate, or properdin, pathway first described by Pillemer *et al.* (1954). Several substances can initiate complement fixation by this route. These include antigen–IgG and antigen–IgM complexes; aggregated IgG, IgM, and IgA (Götze and Müller-Eberhard, 1971); the $F(ab')_2$ fragment of IgG (Schur and Becker, 1963; Sandberg *et al.*, 1971a,b); and naturally occurring polysaccharides (Dukor and Hartmann, 1973) and lipopolysaccharides (Gewurz *et al.*, 1968; Marcus *et al.*, 1971). These activating substances convert an as yet unidentified factor, initiating factor (IF), to its activated form ($\overline{IF}$). $\overline{IF}$, in the presence of another unidentified factor (X), converts properdin (P) to its activated form ($\overline{P}$) (Götze and Müller-

---

*Stossel *et al.* (1975) have recently presented evidence that a smaller fragment of C3, rather than the entire C3b molecule, may be sufficient to mediate C3 opsonic activity.

Eberhard, 1974). $\overline{P}$, in the presence of C3b and Mg^{2+} ions, permits C3 proactivator convertase (C3PAse) to cleave C3 proactivator (C3PA) to C3 activator (C3A) (Götze and Müller-Eberhard, 1971; Müller-Eberhard and Götze, 1972). C3A then cleaves C3 to C3b and a smaller fragment, C3a. It is C3b that binds to the surface of the particle and serves as an opsonin (Gigli and Nelson, 1968; Huber *et al.*, 1968). Mg^{2+} ions, but not Ca^{2+} ions, are essential for the function of the alternate pathway (Pillemer *et al.*, 1954; Sandberg and Osler, 1971). Thus, treatment of serum with EGTA, which binds Ca^{2+} but not Mg^{2+}, prohibits complement activation by the classical pathway but leaves the alternate pathway intact and can be used to determine the relative importance of each pathway in generating C3b opsonic activity (Fine *et al.*, 1972).

C3b opsonic activity is destroyed by a protein found in the serum of several species (Lachmann and Müller-Eberhard, 1968; Ruddy and Austen, 1969, 1971). This enzyme, C3b inactivator, cleaves C3b into two fragments, fluid-phase C3c and particle-bound C3d, neither of which appears to be opsonic (Logue *et al.*, 1973; Griffin *et al.*, 1975a).

3.2. Binding and Ingestion of C3b-Coated Particles by Phagocytic Cells

Once a particle is coated with C3b, it must then be recognized by, and bound to, the surface of a phagocytic cell before it can be ingested. The mechanisms by which these events occur have been partially characterized. All mononuclear phagocytes and polymorphonuclear leukocytes thus far studied have receptors on their plasma membranes for C3b (Gigli and Nelson, 1968; Lay and Nussenzweig, 1968: Huber *et al.*, 1968; Henson, 1969; Huber and Douglas, 1970; Mantovani *et al.*, 1972; Logue *et al.*, 1973; Ehlenberger and Nussenzweig, 1975; Bianco *et al.*, 1975; Griffin *et al.*, 1975a; Ross and Polley, 1975). Unlike the receptors for the Fc portion of IgG, these complement receptors can be cleaved by tryptic proteolysis (Lay and Nussenzweig, 1968; Henson, 1969; Huber and Douglas, 1970; Mantovani *et al.*, 1972; Griffin *et al.*, 1975a); antimacrophage antibodies, which completely block Fc receptor function, have no affect on C3b receptors (Bianco *et al.*, 1975); binding of C3b-coated particles to C3b receptors of some cells requires the presence of divalent cations in the medium (Lay and Nussenzweig, 1968; Henson, 1969; Huber and Douglas, 1970).

That C3b receptors mediate ingestion as well as binding of particles is implied by the many studies in which opsonization of microorganisms by fresh serum enhances their ingestion and killing by phagocytic cells. And some cells have been shown to ingest C3b-coated erythrocytes, prepared by coating the erythrocytes with anti-erythrocyte IgM and the first four complement components. These include guinea pig neutrophils (Gigli and Nelson, 1968), human monocytes (Huber *et al.*, 1968; Huber and Douglas, 1970), bacillus Calmette-Guerin (BCG)–activated guinea pig hepatic macrophages (Atkinson and Frank, 1974a), and thioglycollate-induced mouse peritoneal macrophages (Bianco *et al.*, 1975). However, in many studies it has been found that most types of phagocytic cells bind, but do not ingest, C3b-coated erythrocytes. These cells include human neutrophils (Ross and Polley, 1975; Ehlenberger and Nussenzweig, 1975), human monocytes (Ehlenberger and Nussenzweig, 1975), human hepatic macrophages (Atkinson and Frank, 1974b), guinea pig hepatic macrophages (Schreiber and Frank, 1972a,b), and mouse peritoneal macrophages (Lay and Nussenzweig, 1968; Mantovani *et al.,* 1972; Bianco *et al.,* 1975). Two recent studies have, in fact, suggested that C3b serves to bind erythrocytes to the cell's surface, but that it is IgG, even in minute quantities, that then prompts ingestion of these erythrocytes (Mantovani *et al.,* 1972; Ehlenberger and Nussenzweig, 1975). It should be emphasized, however, that activated macrophages do appear to ingest particles coated with C3b without the participation of immunoglobulin (Atkinson and Frank, 1974a; Bianco *et al.,* 1975; Griffin *et al.,* 1975b). These results suggest that activation of macrophages by lymphocyte products (lymphokines) may be essential for optimal clearance of C3b-coated microorganisms and other C3b-coated particles *in vivo.*

Several mechanisms by which C3b may directly mediate ingestion have recently been proposed. Stossel (1973) has found that the opsonic fragment of C3 eliminates the requirement for divalent cations in the binding and ingestion of paraffin oil particles that have been coated with *Escherichia coli* lipopolysaccharide and then with C3. C3b is known to have enzymatic activity for aromatic dipeptides (Basch, 1965; Cooper and Müller-Eberhard, 1967; Cooper and Becker, 1967; Cooper, 1967). Johnston and his coworkers (Johnston *et al.,* 1969, 1973) have found that preincubation of C3b-coated pneumococci or C3b-coated type b *Hemophilus influenzae* with aromatic dipeptides, or inclusion of aromatic dipeptides in the incubation medium with organisms and neutrophils, blocks the uptake of these bacteria. They proposed that cleavage of aromatic dipeptides on the neutrophil's plasma membrane may be a means by which C3b mediates phagocytosis of particles to which it is bound. However, Griffin *et al.* (unpublished observation) have found that C3 peptidase activity is not essential in the uptake of C3b-coated erythrocytes by thioglycollate-induced mouse peritoneal macrophages. Pearlman *et al.* (1969) found that preincubating guinea pig neutrophils with *p*-nitrophenylethyl phosphate esters, or inclusion of these esters in the incubation medium, markedly reduced the uptake of C3b-coated erythrocytes, but had no effect on their binding to the neutrophils. These workers interpreted the results as evidence that a serine esterase, located on the surface of the neutrophil, must act upon complement-coated particles in order for these particles to be ingested. Woodin (1974) has cautioned against interpreting data obtained when cells are treated with organophosphorus compounds, however, for these agents in doses commonly employed act as detergents. Griffin *et al.* (1975b) have recently defined another possible role for C3b in the ingestion phase of phagocytosis. These results are discussed in detail in Section 7.

3.3. Opsonization of Microorganisms by C3b

We will now examine some of the studies in which complement has been found to be opsonic for microorganisms, and we will try to determine the importance of C3b opsonization in host defense against a variety of bacteria and fungi and the relative importance of the classical and the alternate pathways in opsonization *in vivo.*

3.3.1. Pneumococci

The complement system has been shown by several groups to be important in the ingestion of encapsulated pneumococci. Ward and Enders (1933) first demonstrated that heat-labile factors, while not capable of inducing phagocytosis of virulent pneumococi by themselves, markedly enhanced the rate of ingestion of antibody-coated organisms by human neutrophils. The importance of complement in opsonization of virulent strains of pneumococci has been confirmed by the observations that serum depleted of complement activity by heat inactivation, EDTA treatment, cobra venom factor treatment (Johnston *et al.*, 1969; Shin *et al.*, 1969), or anticomplement antibody (Jeter *et al.*, 1961) is no longer opsonic. Some studies have implicated the classical complement pathway in depositing C3b on the surface of pneumococci. Serum depleted of either C2 or C4 failed to opsonize types 1, 2, and 25 organisms preincubated with small quantities of antipneumococcal polysaccharide antibody (Smith and Wood, 1969; Johnston *et al.*, 1969). However, in other *in vitro* systems, the importance of the alternate pathway has been emphasized. The purified capsular polysaccharide of type 3 pneumococcus has been shown to fix complement by the alternate pathway (Dukor and Hartmann, 1973). A recent study has revealed that guinea pig IgG2, or its F(ab')$_2$ fragment, hastens the fixation of C3 to type 25 pneumococci; the alternate pathway is responsible for this fixation, which was demonstrated by using C4 deficient serum as the source of complement components (Winkelstein and Shin, 1974). Serum depleted of either C4 or C2, but containing all alternate pathway components, has been shown to be as opsonic as normal serum for several types of pneumococci (Smith and Wood, 1969; Johnston *et al.*, 1972; Root *et al.*, 1972; Winkelstein *et al.*, 1972).

Thus, C3b can be fixed to the surface of the pneumococcus in three ways. Immunoglobulins bound to the surface of the organism can initiate complement fixation by the classical pathway; the pneumococcal capsular polysaccharide can initiate complement fixation directly by the alternate pathway; and immunoglobulins, or their F(ab')$_2$ fragments, can initiate fixation, also by the alternate pathway. The pathway most important in opsonizing the organisms appears to depend on the *in vitro* system employed.

3.3.2. Staphylococci

The requirement for heat-labile opsonins for the enhancement of uptake of staphylococci has been repeatedly demonstrated (Wright and Douglas, 1903; Cohn and Morse, 1959; Williams *et al.*, 1969; Williams and Quie, 1971; Wheat *et al.*, 1974). Forsgren and Quie (1974) suggested that opsonization requires the classical complement pathway, for *Staphylococcus aureus* 502A did not fix complement and was not ingested when preincubated in EGTA-treated, Mg^{2+}-supplemented serum. Others, however, have demonstrated opsonization of staphylococci by the alternate complement pathway. C2-deficient serum (Johnson *et al.*, 1972), C4-deficient serum (Root *et al.*, 1972), and serum depleted of both C1q and immunoglobulins (Jasin, 1972) were found to opsonize *S. aureus* as well as, or nearly as well as, normal serum. Heat inactivation destroyed the opsonic capacity of all these sera, and, in the one case so studied, the addition of purified C3PA to heat-inactivated serum completely restored its opsonic capacity (Jasin, 1972). Therefore, the alternate pathway of complement activation appears to be more important than the classical pathway in generating C3b opsonic activity on the surface of staphylococci.

Many investigators have determined the ability of heat-labile factors to opsonize gram-negative bacilli. Two studies have demonstrated the importance of complement components in the clearance of an intravenously administered load of *E. coli* (Spiegelberg *et al.,* 1963; Gilbert *et al.,* 1973). Animals decomplemented by injection of either antigen–antibody complexes or cobra venom factor cleared the organisms from the circulation at a slower rate than animals with normal complement levels. However, in at least one of these studies (Gilbert *et al.,* 1973), the organisms employed could be killed *in vitro* by fresh serum. Thus, these results cannot be interpreted to mean that complement was opsonic for the organism, for *in vivo* complement-mediated bacterial lysis could have accounted for these results. The results of two studies argue for the importance of the classical complement pathway in opsonization of gram-negative bacilli. Agammaglobulinemic human sera were found not to contain heat-labile opsonic activity for *E. coli, P. aeruginosa,* or *Bacillus proteus* (Williams and Quie, 1971). And antigen-specific guinea pig IgG2, C1, C4, and C2 were required to lyse erythrocytes coated with lipopolysaccharides of *S. typhi* or *Veillonella alcalescens* (Phillips *et al.,* 1972).

However, many investigators have found that the alternate pathway is sufficient and perhaps necessary to fix C3b to the surfaces of gram-negative bacilli. Incubation of *V. alcalescens* lipopolysaccharide in serum depleted of C2 by anti-C2 antibody results in cleavage of C3 (Marcus *et al.,* 1971). Serum deficient in C2 (Johnson *et al.,* 1972) or C4 (Root *et al.,* 1972) opsonized *E. coli* or *E. coli* lipopolysaccharide-coated paraffin oil particles (Stossel *et al.,* 1973a) as well as, or nearly as well as, normal serum. EGTA-treated, Mg^{2+}-supplemented serum was maximally opsonic for *E. coli* (Forsgren and Quie, 1974) and for *Shigella* (Reed, 1975). Sera depleted of C1q and immunoglobulins opsonized *E. coli* normally (Jasin, 1972). Properdin and a heat-labile serum factor (presumably C3PA) have been found necessary for opsonization of *P. aeruginosa* (Bjornson and Michael, 1973), and C3PA was necessary for maximal opsonization of *Shigella* (Reed, 1975). Also, addition of purified C3PA to heat-inactivated serum has been found to restore completely the opsonic capacity for *E. coli* (Jasin, 1972) and for paraffin oil particles coated with *E. coli* lipopolysaccharide (Stossel *et al.,* 1973a). That the alternate pathway of complement activation may be physiologically important in the opsonization of gram-negative bacilli was suggested by the finding that serum of human newborns deficient in C3PA is deficient in opsonizing these lipopolysaccharide-coated particles (Stossel *et al.,* 1973b).

3.3.4. Other Organisms

Opsonization of other organisms by C3b has also been demonstrated, but has not been studied as extensively as those above. *Candida albicans* was found to require heat-labile serum factors for optimal ingestion (Lehrer and Cline, 1969), but to be opsonized normally by EGTA-treated, Mg^{2+}-supplemented serum (Forsgren and Quie, 1974). Both normal and C4 deficient guinea pigs survived challenge with *Cryptococcus neoformans* better than did animals depleted of complement components by cobra venom factor. *In vitro,* normal, but not cobra-venom-factor treated, serum was found to opsonize the organism for uptake by guinea pig neutrophils and monocytes (Diamond *et al.*, 1973). Uptake of streptococci by human leukocytes was found to be enhanced by both normal and C2 deficient sera, but not by properdin-depleted serum (Stollerman *et al.*, 1963, 1967). And heat-labile serum factors were found to enhance the ingestion and killing of groups A, B, and C meningococci above the level of opsonization achieved with IgG alone (Roberts, 1967, 1970).

Thus, C3b opsonization enhances the uptake of most organisms by phagocytic cells. It is likely to be clinically important, especially in the early, pre-antibody phase of infections, and it may be the chief means of opsonization of gram-negative bacilli.

3.4. C3-Deficiency States

The central role of C3 in opsonization has been emphasized by the increased susceptibility to infection of a few patients who lack C3. Two individuals have been described who had undetectable levels of C3, apparently due to an inherited absence of the gene responsible for coding for the molecule (Alper *et al.*, 1972; Ballow *et al.*, 1975). Both had histories of repeated infections with both gram-positive and gram-negative bacteria. One kindred with half-normal levels of C3 has been studied. These individuals had no history of repeated infections, and their serum C3–mediated functions were normal when tested *in vitro* (Alper *et al.*, 1969).

A patient has been described in whom C3b inactivator activity was markedly diminished. Such a deficiency would lead to depletion of C3, for circulating C3b would continually activate the alternate complement pathway (Götze and Müller-Eberhard, 1971). The patient had a history of repeated infections. Studies of his serum revealed low C3 levels, most of which was C3b; increased catabolic rate of C3; failure of C3b to be converted to C3c and C3d by his serum; and diminished opsonic capacity of his serum when tested *in vitro* (Alper *et al.*, 1970a,b). Infusion of purified C3b inactivator restored C3-mediated functions to normal (Ziegler *et al.*, 1975). Another patient, also with a history of frequent infections, was found to have low C3 but elevated C3c levels and increased C3 catabolism. The defect is not clear, but he may have a qualitative abnormality of C3b inactivator (Alper *et al.*, 1973).

Finally, patients with some auto-immune diseases and low serum C3 levels have an increased susceptibility to infections (Estes and Christian, 1971), but they usually have many defects that predispose to infection, and it is difficult to judge the significance of low C3 levels in these individuals.

There is considerable evidence from *in vitro* studies, as we have seen, to suggest that the alternate complement pathway may be sufficient to generate C3b opsonic activity, especially for gram-negative bacilli. This impression is borne out clinically. Several kindreds have been described who have a complete absence of C2. Some did not have a history of repeated infections, and complement-mediated functions, including opsonization, were normal when tested *in vitro* (Silverstein, 1960; Gewurz *et al.*, 1966; Klemperer *et al.*, 1966, 1967; Cooper *et al.*, 1968; Ruddy *et al.*, 1970). C4-deficient guinea pigs do not have, under conditions of ideal husbandry, shortened life spans or predisposition to infection (Ellman *et al.*, 1970). And a recent report suggests that, in humans with gram-negative bacteremia and shock, activation of complement may occur by the alternate, and not by the classical, pathway (Fearon *et al.*, 1975).

Some investigators have found an apparent opsonic requirement for C5 under certain conditions. C5-deficient mouse serum was found not to be so opsonic as normal mouse serum for pneumococci, and mice deficient in C5 were killed by a smaller inoculum of pneumococci than were normal mice (Shin *et al.*, 1969; Smith *et al.*, 1969). Miller and his co-workers (Miller *et al.*, 1968; Miller and Nilsson, 1970; Jacobs and Miller, 1972; Nilsson *et al.*, 1974) have evaluated three individuals with recurrent infections and found that their serum failed to opsonize yeast particles. Their isolated C5 was physicochemically and quantitatively normal, but addition of normal human or mouse serum, but not C5-deficient mouse serum, corrected the opsonic defect. The patients appeared to improve clinically on treatment with normal human serum. A defect in opsonization of yeast particles has been shown to develop in normal human serum that has been allowed to stand at 4°C for 36 hr (Miller and Nilsson, 1974). The C5 in this serum is also physicochemically and quantitatively normal, but addition of purified human C5 restores its opsonic capacity. Recently, however, a kindred with C5 deficiency was reported by other investigators, who found that their sera opsonized baker's yeast normally (Rosenfeld and Leddy, 1974).

Finally, three recent papers report C4b-mediated particle binding to human B lymphocytes, monocytes, neutrophils (Bokisch and Sobel, 1974; Ross and Polley, 1975), and erythrocytes (Cooper, 1969). Future investigation may reveal that C4b has direct opsonic activity.

4. Other Opsonins

4.1. Immunoglobulin M

As we have seen, IgM is indirectly opsonic by its ability to generate C3b on the surfaces of particles. Whether IgM can opsonize directly has not been resolved.

Several investigators have reported that IgM is directly opsonic for some bacteria. Pre-incubating organisms with the IgM fraction of immune serum was found to enhance the clearance of the organisms when injected intrevenously or intraperitoneally into mice (Robbins *et al.*, 1965; Rowley and Turner, 1966), pigs (Turner and Rowley, 1963; Knop *et al.*, 1971), or rabbits (Eddie *et al.*, 1971). These results cannot be interpreted to mean that IgM was directly responsible for opsonizing these organisms, however, for it is likely that complement-mediated bacterial lysis and complement-mediated phagocytosis were the factors responsible for the increased clearance observed.

Two *in vitro* studies have provided evidence for IgM mediated ingestion of bacteria. The IgM fraction of serum from heroin addicts was found to be directly opsonic for some strains of gram-negative bacilli (Nickerson *et al.*, 1970). It should be noted that less than 90% of organisms opsonized with IgM were ingested and killed by human neutrophils in the absence of serum after a 2-hr incubation period, while 99.9% were killed when both IgM and a complement source (fresh serum) were present. So even here, the direct opsonic capacity of IgM was meager when compared with its indirect opsonic capability. *P. aeruginosa* coated with IgM were found to be ingested by mouse peritoneal macrophages (Bjornson and Michael, 1971). However, again only about 90% of the inoculum were ingested.

In a few studies, IgM has been found to mediate binding of erythrocytes to macrophages. Sheep crythrocytes coated with the IgM fraction of immune mouse serum bound to mouse peritoneal macrophages (Lay and Nussenzweig, 1969). Unlike IgG-mediated binding, IgM-mediated binding required the presence of Ca^{2+} ions in the medium. Mouse erythrocytes coated with Vi antigen of *S. typhi* bound to mouse peritoneal macrophages when "early" anti-Vi-antigen antiserum or the IgM fraction of this serum was present in the incubation medium (Levenson *et al.*, 1970). Erythrocytes coated with 8 S IgM have recently been found to form rosettes around 0.8% of guinea pig spleen cells (Rhodes, 1973). The rosette-forming cells were felt to be macrophages because the percentage of rosette-forming cells dropped to 0.3% when glass-adherent cells were removed.

Most investigators using experimental systems that eliminate the participation of complement and IgG have found IgM not to be directly opsonic. Antiproteus IgM failed to enhance the uptake of the organisms by rabbit neutrophils (Smith *et al.*, 1967). Neither has IgM been found to be directly opsonic for *S. aureus* (Laxdal *et al.*, 1968; Dosset *et al.*, 1969), *E. coli* (Laxdal *et al.*, 1968; Dossett *et al.*, 1969), *Shigella* (Reed, 1975), or type b *H. influenzae* (Johnston *et al.*, 1973) when tested in the Maaloe (1946) system. Human monocytes failed to interact at all with IgM-coated human erythrocytes (Lo Buglio *et al.*, 1967; Huber and Fudenberg, 1968; Abramson *et al.*, 1970b; Zipursky *et al.*, 1973). Mouse macrophages failed to ingest previously attached horse erythrocytes when anti-erythrocyte IgM was added to the cultures (Rabinovitch, 1967). Mantovani *et al.* (1972) and Griffin *et al.* (1975a) found that IgM-coated sheep erythrocytes did not interact with mouse macrophages. 8 S IgM has been found not to bind to human monocytes (Lawrence *et al.*, 1975). *In vivo*, C4 deficient guinea pigs failed to clear IgM-coated guinea pig erythrocytes from the circulation (Schreiber and Frank, 1972a).

In summary, IgM probably has no direct opsonic function *in vivo*.

4.2. Immunoglobulin A

In two studies, opsonic effects of 11 S secretory IgA (Knop *et al.*, 1971; Kaplan *et al.*, 1972) and of 7 S serum IgA (Kaplan *et al.*, 1972) have been found. In the first study, *E. coli* coated with secretory IgA were cleared from the mouse peritoneal cavity more readily than *E. coli* coated with either IgG or IgM. In the other study, human neutrophils and monocytes ingested human erythrocytes coated with either 7 S or 11 S IgA in the presence of fresh serum, but not in the absence of serum. Most investigators, however, have found no opsonic effect of either 7 S or 11 S IgA. Coating gram-positive bacteria (Quie *et al.*, 1968; Wilson, 1972), gram-negative bacteria (Quie *et al.*, 1968; Eddie *et al.*, 1971; Reed, 1975), or erythrocytes (Huber *et al.*, 1971; Zipursky *et al.*, 1973) with IgA was found not to enhance particle uptake by human neutrophils or monocytes or by rabbit neutrophils, whether or not fresh serum was included in the incubation medium.

Thus, there is no evidence for direct, i.e., complement-independent, opsonization by IgA. The mechanism by which IgA might be indirectly opsonic is not immediately apparent either, for most investigators have found that IgA–antigen complexes do not fix complement (Ishizaka *et al.*, 1966; Smith *et al.*, 1966), although aggregated myeloma IgA appears to fix complement by the alternate pathway (Müller-Eberhard, 1971). As pointed out by Zipursky *et al.* (1973), it is difficult to obtain IgA fractions that are free of contamination by IgM or IgG, and even small quantities of these immunoglobulins may be opsonic. Perhaps undetected contamination of IgA fractions with other immunoglobulins accounts for the findings of opsonization by IgA in some studies. It is unlikely that opsonization is the chief means by which IgA is protective or that IgA opsonization, if it occurs at all, is physiologically important.

4.3. C-Reactive Protein

Only limited data are available concerning the ability of C-reactive protein to function as an opsonin. It is known that this protein can bind to several types of organisms (Kindmark, 1972) and that it can combine with some compounds, including lecithin and sphingomyelin, to initiate complement fixation (Kaplan and Volanakis, 1974; Siegel *et al.*, 1974). So it would not be surprising if C-reactive protein were to serve as an indirect opsonin, i.e., by fixing C3b to the particle surface in the presence of complement components.

The experimental data are conflicting. In one study, the rate of ingestion of carbonyl iron particles, pneumococci, and *Serratia* by human and rabbit peripheral blood leukocytes in the presence of fresh serum was increased when the particles were pretreated with C-reactive protein (Hokama *et al.*, 1962). In another study, however, the ingestion of staphylococci, streptococci, and *Serratia* by human leukocytes in the presence of either fresh or immune serum was not influenced by the presence of C-reactive protein in the incubation mixture (Williams and Quie, 1968). In two other studies, the uptake of several gram-positive and gram-negative organisms by human neutrophils in the absence of serum was enhanced by preincubating the organisms with C-reactive protein (Ganrot and Kindmark, 1969; Kindmark, 1971).

Whether this acute phase reactant is physiologically important as either a direct or an indirect opsonin must be determined by future investigation.

4.4 Noncomplement Heat-Labile Opsonins

Several heat-labile substances that appear not to be involved in either complement-activation pathway have been proposed as having opsonic activity. A heat-labile factor present in normal rabbit and guinea pig serum was found to be opsonic for several bacteria (Hirsch, 1964; Hirsch and Strauss, 1964). Its characteristics were those of the complement system with the single exception of its ability to be absorbed onto the surfaces of bacteria in the absence of divalent cations. Johnston and his co-workers (Johnston *et al.*, 1969) have found that a heat-labile, dialyzable factor and a heat-labile 5–6 S β-pseudoglobulin appear to be necessary for maximal opsonization of pneumococci. They (Johnston *et al.*, 1972) also found that patients with sickle cell disease have a defect in heat-labile opsonization, which can be restored by the addition of the pseudoglobulin to their sera. Patients with sickle cell disease appeared to have diminished heat-labile opsonic activity for pneumococci in another study (Winkelstein and Drachman, 1968). The only evidence presented to suggest that this deficient activity was not involved in complement activation was

FRANK M. GRIFFIN,
JR.

that the CH_{50} levels of these individuals were normal. That some such patients have a deficiency in Factor B of the alternate complement pathway has, however, been observed (Day,* unpublished observation).

The identity and physiological importance of these heat-labile factors are not known.

5. Cytophilic Antibody

The term *cytophilic antibody* was introduced by Boyden and Sorkin (1960) to describe a factor in the serum of immunized rabbits that bound to rabbit and guinea pig spleen cells and promoted binding of the immunizing antigen to these cells. The cytophilic substance was antigen specific and heat stable, bound to cells more avidly at 37°C than at 4°C, and could be absorbed from the serum by spleen cells (Boyden and Sorkin, 1961). Subsequent investigation has been directed at characterizing the cytophilic immune factors that promote binding of antigen to cells, the cell type(s) for which these factors are cytophilic, and the plasma membrane structures to which binding occurs.

It has recently been shown that both specific (Leslie and Cohen, 1974b) and nonspecific (Leslie and Cohen, 1974a; Lawrence *et al.*, 1975) immunoglobulins of various classes can bind to the surfaces of lymphocytes, mononuclear phagocytes, neutrophils, basophils, and mast cells (Ishizaka *et al.*, 1970; Ishizaka, 1970; Lawrence *et al.*, 1975). And IgE on the surface of mast cells and basophils has been shown to bind antigen (Ishizaka, 1970). In this discussion, I will consider only the interaction of cytophilic antibody with phagocytic cells and will use the term *cytophilic antibody* as it was originally defined by Boyden and Sorkin (1960), i.e., those substances that not only bind to the cell but also mediate antigen binding to the cell surface.

Only macrophages have been demonstrated to be capable of expressing cytophilic antibody activity, i.e., cell surface antibody that can promote antigen binding; neutrophils have not (Boyden, 1964; Parish, 1965; Nickerson *et al.*, 1969). Berken and Benacerraf (1966) demonstrated that mouse cytophilic antibody mediated both binding and phagocytosis of sheep erythrocytes by mouse peritoneal macrophages; most investigators, however, have assayed only antigen binding.

Binding of antigen to cells by cytophilic antibody has been assayed by measuring uptake of radiolabeled soluble antigen, by determining binding of particulate antigens (usually erythrocytes) microscopically, and by determining binding of erythrocytes coated with soluble antigens. Macrophages from immunized animals have been shown to display, on their surfaces, a factor that promotes binding of the immunizing antigen to the cells' plasma membranes (Boyden, 1964; Berken and Benacerraf, 1966; Hoy and Nelson, 1969). More often, passive sensitization of macrophages from nonimmunized animals with serum or serum fractions from immunized animals has been used to demonstrate cytophilic antibody.

Some investigators have found that only IgG antibody is cytophilic (Sorkin, 1963; Jonas *et al.*, 1965; Berken and Benacerraf, 1966, 1968; Nelson and Mildenhall, 1968; Askenase and Hayden, 1974) and that, in guinea pigs, IgG_2 has cytophilic activity but IgG_1 does not (Berken and Benacerraf, 1966). The Fc portion of the IgG

---

*Day, 1976, unpublished observation.

molecule is essential in mediating cytophilia, for pepsin digests of IgG [F(ab')$_2$] do not promote antigen binding (Berken and Benacerraf, 1966; Tizard, 1969; Ishizaka *et al.*, 1970) and "free" Fc pieces can block binding of cytophilic antibody to guinea pig macrophages (Inchley *et al.*, 1970).

Other investigators, however, have presented evidence that IgM may be able to bind to macrophages and promote antigen binding. Rowley *et al.* (1964) found that peritoneal cells from mice immunized with *S. typhimurium,* or a 19 S, 2-mercaptoethanol sensitive extract of these cells, when injected intraperitoneally into nonimmunized mice, conferred upon the recipients an increased capacity to kill an intraperitoneal challenge of that organism. They suggested that anti-*S. typhimurium* IgM was bound to the peritoneal macrophages of the donor animals and was responsible for the observed effect. However, anti-*S. typhimurium* IgM could well have been either on or in lymphoid cells contained in the donor peritoneal population, and bacterial killing could have been due to complement-mediated bacterial lysis or to complement-mediated phagocytosis.

In other studies, mouse and guinea pig cytophilic antibody was found in the IgM fraction of immune serum (Hoy and Nelson, 1969; del Guercio *et al.*, 1969; Tizard, 1971) and could be inactivated by Na_2SO_4 precipitation or by 2-mercaptoethanol treatment (Parish, 1965; del Guercio *et al.*, 1969). "Early" cytophilic antibody, i.e., cytophilic activity in mouse serum obtained a few days after a single injection of antigen, was present in the β or fast γ region on electrophoresis and was 2-mercaptoethanol sensitive; "late," hyperimmune cytophilic activity was present only in the γ region and was 2-mercaptoethanol resistant (Tizard, 1969). In another study, however, neither early nor late mouse cytophilic antibody could be affected by 2-mercaptoethanol treatment (Nelson *et al.*, 1967).

Cytophilic antibody activity has been found in non-γ-globulin fractions of serum (Nelson *et al.*, 1967; Hoy and Nelson, 1969), but it is difficult to be certain that these fractions may not have been contaminated with immunoglobulin.

An important question is whether cytophilic antibodies are qualitatively different from opsonic antibodies. Both have some features in common. They are resistant to heating at 56°C for 30 min (Boyden and Sorkin, 1960; Berken and Benacerraf, 1966); both bind to macrophages in the absence of divalent cations (Berken and Benacerraf, 1966); most, if not all, cytophilic antibodies are immunoglobulins, as are heat-stable opsonic antibodies; the same subclass of guinea pig IgG is opsonic and cytophilic (Berken and Benacerraf, 1966); both opsonic and "late" cytophilic antibodies bind to a trypsin-resistant structure on the cell's plasma membrane (del Guercio *et al.*, 1969); and both opsonic and cytophilic IgG antibodies bind to the cell by the Fc portion of the immunoglobulin molecule (Berken and Benacerraf, 1966; Tizard, 1969).

Nonetheless, the results of some studies have suggested that some cytophilic antibodies may be qualitatively different from opsonic antibody. Cytophilic activity could be absorbed by macrophages, while opsonic activity could not (Parish, 1965). Treatment of antisera with 2 mercaptoethanol or Na_2SO_4 could remove cytophilic, but not opsonic activity (Parish, 1965), especially when "early" antisera were employed (Tizard, 1969). Cytophilic antibody mediates antigen binding only to macrophages, while opsonic antibody coats particles for binding and ingestion by neutrophils as well (Tizard, 1971). Trypsin treatment of macrophages appears to cleave receptors for "early" cytophilic antibody but not those for either opsonic antibody or "late" cytophilic antibody (del Guercio *et al.*, 1969; Hoy and Nelson, 1969; Askenase and Hayden, 1974).

All these differences could be due to quantitative differences between the number of antibody molecules required to opsonize a particle in suspension and the number required to bind to Fc receptors in order to promote particle binding to the cell. It has yet to be convincingly demonstrated that those substances that bind to macrophages and mediate antigen binding are different from, or function in a different manner from, opsonic antibody. The importance of cytophilic antibody in promoting particle ingestion *in vivo* is entirely unknown.

6. Intracellular Effects of Opsonins

While opsonins clearly alter the rates of ingestion of many organisms by phagocytic cells, it is not clear that they can affect the rate of intracellular killing or intracellular degradation of ingested bacteria.

Many investigators have found that opsonization has no effect on the intracellular fate of ingested organisms. Rabbit monocytes ingested *S. aureus* at a higher rate when the incubation medium contained fresh serum than when the medium contained heat-inactivated serum; but the rates of intracellular killing of the organisms were the same in both preparations (Shayegani and Mudd, 1966). *P. aeruginosa* coated with IgG from immune animals were killed by rabbit alveolar macrophages at the same rate as those incubated with IgG from nonimmune animals (Reynolds and Thompson, 1973). IgG-coated proteus were killed by human neutrophils at the same rate as IgM-coated proteus even though the rates of ingestion of the two groups were markedly different (Smith *et al.*, 1967). Heat-labile serum factors were found to be necessary for optimal ingestion of *C. albicans* by human leukocytes but did not alter the intracellular fate of the organisms (Lehrer and Cline, 1969); and killing of ingested *C. albicans* by mouse peripheral blood leukocytes was the same whether the organisms were opsonized with normal or with C5 deficient mouse serum, even though the ingestion rates were different (Morelli and Rosenberg, 1971). *E. coli* were ingested and killed at the same rate by rabbit neutrophils in the presence of either immune or nonimmune serum (Cohn, 1963); immune serum appeared to retard somewhat the rate of intracellular degradation of the organisms.

Some workers, however, believe that opsonins may enhance intracellular killing or degradation of ingested bacteria. Jenkin (1963) found that the rate of ingestion of *S. typhimurium* by mouse peritoneal macrophages was the same in cultures containing normal mouse serum as in those containing serum that had been previously adsorbed with the test organisms. However, intracellular killing occurred only when nonadsorbed serum was used. In other studies, heat-inactivated immune serum has been found to increase both the rate of ingestion and the rate of intracellular killing of *Salmonella* (Jenkin and Benacerraf, 1960) and *E. coli* (Rowley, 1958). Both heat-stable and heat-labile immune serum factors were found to be important in the intracellular killing of *Brucella melitensis* by rabbit peritoneal macrophages (Ralston and Elberg, 1969).

Heat-labile components appeared to enhance the intracellular digestion of *Histoplasma capsulatum* by mouse peritoneal macrophages (Miya and Marcus, 1961; Wu and Marcus, 1963). Subsequent studies revealed that either "complement" (fresh guinea pig serum) or partially purified calf properdin, either fresh or heated, could enhance intracellular killing of these organisms and that the combination of "complement" and properdin was better than either alone (Wu and Marcus, 1964). It is difficult to understand how properdin could have had such an effect in the absence of a source of complement components, however. The assay for intracellular killing was performed by radiolabeling histoplasmas with ^{32}P and determining the total radioactivity released into the medium at various times after ingestion was completed. It is possible that some organisms that were considered ingested were merely bound to the macrophage surface in some preparations. If so, a difference in total radioactivity subsequently released into the medium would be difficult to interpret.

In all the studies discussed above, differences in intracellular killing between experimental and control cultures were relatively small. Separating phagocytosis from intracellular killing by using either colony counts or radiolabeled organisms is very difficult, for the range of experimental error is great; some organisms counted as phagocytized may, in fact, be only attached to the surface of the phagocytic cell; phagocytic loads may differ between experimental and control preparations; and the cell's handling of ingested material may vary depending on the size of the ingested load. Therefore, one must be very cautious in ascribing differences in colony counts or amounts of recovered label to differences in intracellular killing rates.

There are three situations in which opsonic factors clearly appear to alter the intracellular fate of organisms. *Rickettsia typhi,* when coated with methylated albumin, are ingested by human monocyte-derived macrophages, but they grow and destroy the monolayer. When coated with immune serum, however, the organisms are killed intracellularly (Gambrill and Wisseman, 1973). *Toxoplasma gondii* are ingested by mouse peritoneal macrophages, but somehow they prevent lysosomal fusion with the phagosome and subsequently multiply within the cells (Jones and Hirsch, 1972). When opsonized with immune serum, however, lysosomal fusion occurs and the organisms are destroyed (Jones *et al.,* 1975). *Vaccinia virions* are interiorized by mouse peritoneal macrophages and by strain L cells, but they escape from the phagocytic vacuoles and multiply in the cytosol. Virus particles that have been ingested in the presence of antiserum, on the other hand, appear in the lysosomes and are subsequently degraded by the cells (Dales and Kajioka, 1964; Silverstein and Castle, 1970).

7. Mechanism of Action of Opsonins in the Ingestion Phase of Phagocytosis

As indicated in the preceding sections, investigation over the past 70 years has done much to characterize factors in immune and nonimmune serum which interact with particles to render them more readily ingested by phagocytic cells. The mechanism by which these opsonins, chiefly IgG and C3b, are generated and bind to the surface of particles has been defined. And some requirements for binding of opsonized particles to the plasma membranes of phagocytic cells have been identified. Opsonins enhance the rate of binding of particles to the surfaces of phagocytic cells. However, the mechanisms by which these bound particles are then ingested are not known and have until recently not been explored.

We (Griffin *et al.,* 1975b) have attempted to determine whether the binding of a particle coated with opsonins (IgG or C3b) to appropriate receptors on the plasma membrane of the phagocytic cell is sufficient to trigger intracellular events that result in ingestion of the bound particle or whether opsonins have a further role in the ingestion of the bound particle. In order to answer this question, we needed to create a particle with opsonins on only one arc of its circumference and determine whether the binding of the particle to the cell by these localized opsonins would predestine the particle for ingestion or whether opsonins must be present over the entire surface of the particle in order for ingestion to occur. We have been able to create such a particle in two ways.

C3b-coated sheep erythrocytes were prepared by incubating the erythrocytes first with anti-erythrocyte IgM and then with C5 deficient mouse serum. Under these conditions, erythrocytes are first coated with IgM, an immunoglobulin that mediates neither binding nor ingestion of erythrocytes. C5 deficient mouse serum provides the first four complement components, which are activated by the erythrocyte–IgM complex and bind to the surface of the erythrocyte. The complement-component-mediating interaction of these erythrocytes with phagocytic cells is C3b. These C3b-coated erythrocytes were then incubated at 4°C with thioglycollate-induced mouse peritoneal macrophages. Under these conditions, an average of 20 erythrocytes bound to the C3b receptors of each macrophage, but ingestion was prevented by the low temperature of incubation. Trypsin, in a concentration of 750 μg/ml, was then added to these preparations and incubation was continued, also at 4°C. The effect of trypsin was to remove C3b from the "free" surface of the bound erythrocyte, i.e., from the surface not bound to C3b receptors of the macrophage plasma membrane. Trypsin had no effect on the macrophage C3b receptors or on the C3b–C3b receptor bonds in the zone of attachment of the erythrocyte to the macrophage. When these preparations were washed with trypsin inhibitor to terminate the enzyme's activity and then incubated in fresh medium at 37°C, the bound erythrocytes were not ingested but remained attached to the macrophage C3b receptors. These results demonstrate that binding of the erythrocyte to the macrophage by opsonin-receptor bonds is not sufficient to trigger intracellular events that result in ingestion of the bound particle, but that opsonins (C3b molecules) must be present over the entire surface of the erythrocyte in order for ingestion to occur.

We have also demonstrated that IgG molecules must be present over the entire surface of the particle in order for IgG-coated particles to be ingested. In these studies (Griffin et al., 1976), we used mouse lymphocytes as the indicator particles and mouse peritoneal macrophages as the phagocytic cells. Mouse B lymphocytes display surface immunoglobulin, which can be made to migrate to one pole of the cell. This phenomenon is called capping and can be effected by treating lymphocytes at room temperature with antibody to immunoglobulin. Under these conditions, both the surface immunoglobulin of the lymphocyte and the antibody to immunoglobulin migrate to one pole of the cell. We treated mouse lymph node lymphocytes with rabbit IgG directed against mouse immunoglobulin. The initial incubation was performed at 4°C. Under these conditions, IgG binds to surface immunoglobulin over the entire lymphocyte surface. When these lymphocytes, with anti-immunoglobulin IgG present over their entire surfaces, were incubated with macrophages at 37°C, they were readily ingested. Other IgG-coated lymphocytes were warmed to room temperature for 20 min before being incubated with macrophages. These capped lymphocytes, with anti-immunoglobulin IgG located only at one pole of the cell, bound to Fc receptors of the macrophage plasma membrane but were not ingested.

These results also demonstrate that attachment of a particle to a phagocytic cell by opsonins (IgG molecules) located over only a small arc of the particle surface is not sufficient to trigger ingestion of the bound particle but that opsonins must be present over the entire particle surface in order for the particle to be ingested. We believe that the ingestion of bound particles requires that specific receptors on the plasma membrane of the phagocytic cell bind to opsonins over the entire particle surface in a sequential, circumferential manner until the leading edges of membrane fuse to form the phagocytic vacuole.

The experiments described suggest that Fc receptors or C3b receptors located outside the zone of particle attachment must bind sequentially to opsonins (IgG or C3b) located on the "free" surface of the bound particle in order for ingestion to proceed. We were able to demonstrate that the functional integrity of Fc receptors lying outside the zone of particle attachment is required for the ingestion of IgG-coated erythrocytes (Griffin *et al.,* 1975b). IgG-coated sheep erythrocytes were bound to Fc receptors of the macrophage plasma membrane at 4°C. An average of 14 erythrocytes attached to each macrophage, but ingestion was inhibited by the low temperature of incubation. The Fc receptors not involved in the attachment process were then blocked by incubating the preparations at 4°C with an antimacrophage IgG fraction, which specifically blocks Fc receptor function but has no effect on other phagocytic receptors or on the cell's phagocytic capacity in general (Holland *et al.,* 1972; Bianco *et al.,* 1975). When these preparations were then incubated at 37°C, the erythrocytes were not ingested but remained attached to the macrophages' Fc receptors. These results indicate that phagocytic receptors not involved in the initial binding of an opsonin-coated particle to the surface of the phagocytic cell are necessary for ingestion of the bound particle.

We conclude from the studies just described that the simultaneous presence of opsonins covering the entire surface of a particle and of functional receptors for these opsonins on the surface of the phagocytic cell are required for ingestion of the particle and that the process of phagocytosis requires the sequential, circumferential attachment of phagocytic receptors on the plasma membrane of the cell to opsonins located over the entire surface of the particle.

Our studies demonstrate that opsonins on the particle surface act as guides along which phagocytic cells can extend pseudopods. Receptors on the pseudopods attach to the opsonins until the plasma membrane projections completely encompass the particle and fuse to form the phagocytic vacuole. The mechanisms by which the pseudopod is extended are not known, but roles for the actin–myosin system (Boxer *et al.,* 1974; Stossel and Pincus, 1975) and microfilaments (Allison *et al.,* 1971) have been proposed. We offer the following hypothesis for the mechanism by which opsonins and these intracellular structures may cooperate to effect particle ingestion. Opsonins coat a particle and promote its binding to plasma membrane receptors for the opsonin (C3b or IgG). The initial binding of opsonins to receptors triggers local intracellular events—microfilament rearrangement, actin-myosin binding, and/or actin polymerization—which result in the extension of a pseudopod. Receptors on the pseudopod bind to opsonins on the surface of the particle until the leading edges meet and fuse to form a phagosome. The entire phagocytic event may occur in recycling steps in which opsonin-receptor binding triggers local intracellular events, which result in extension of a pseudopod, and extension of a pseudopod then leads to further opsonin-receptor binding.

8. Conclusions

Opsonization, to paraphrase the definition of Wright and Douglas, is the process by which serum factors interact with particles in a manner that renders the particles more readily ingested by phagocytic cells. Abundant work by numerous investigators has done much to elucidate the structure of opsonins and many of the molecular mechanisms involved in opsonin function. IgG and C3b are clearly the most important, perhaps the only important, opsonic factors. These molecules bind initially to particle surfaces and then bind the particles to specific receptors (Fc receptors and C3b receptors) on the surfaces of phagocytic cells.

It is becoming increasingly apparent that the function of opsonins does not end once they bind particles to cell surfaces. The interaction of opsonins with receptors almost certainly generates a signal that is transmitted intracellularly. While the nature of this putative signal is completely unknown, there is growing evidence that it effects changes in the state of actin polymerization, in actin–myosin interactions, and/or in microfilament arrangement—leading to extension of pseudopods adjacent to the attached particle. Opsonins distributed over the entire particle surface serve as guides to which receptors on the plasma membrane of these pseudopods bind sequentially until the particle is enclosed within a phagocytic vacuole.

Finally, it is clear that in a few situations, opsonins enhance lysosomal fusion with phagosomes and, consequently, enhance intracellular killing of ingested micro-organisms. Technical difficulties have hampered previous efforts at determining the influence opsonins may have on intracellular killing of bacteria. However, techniques are being developed that may overcome these problems, and it will be of considerable interest to follow the progress of studies designed to define the role of opsonins in intracellular bacterial killing.

Thus, although the chief opsonins, IgG and C3b, have been well characterized and the mechanisms by which they bind particles to phagocytic cells have been well defined, there are many other aspects of opsonin function that may be important in determining the outcome of a microorganism's encounter with a phagocytic cell.

ACKNOWLEDGMENTS

This work was supported in part by grants AI 08697, AI 07012, and AI 01831 from the National Institutes of Health, and by grant PF-867 from the American Cancer Society.

References

Abramson, N., Gelfand, E. W., Jandl, J. H., and Rosen, F. S., 1970a, The interaction between human monocytes and red cells. Specificity for IgG subclasses and IgG fragments, *J. Exp. Med.* **132**:1207–1215.

Abramson, N., Lo Buglio, A. F., Jandl, J. H., and Cotran, R. S., 1970b, The interaction between human monocytes and red cells. Binding characteristics, *J. Exp. Med.* **132**:1191–1206.

Allison, A. C., Davies, P., and de Petris, S., 1971, Role of contractile microfilaments in macrophage movement and endocytosis, *Nature London New Biol.* **232**:153–155.

Alper, C. A., Propp, R. P., Klemperer, M. R., and Rosen, F. S., 1969, Inherited deficiency of the third component of human complement (C'3), *J. Clin. Invest.* **48**:553–557.

Alper, C. A., Abramson, N., Johnston, R. B., Jr., Jandl, J. H., and Rosen, F. S., 1970a, Increased susceptibility to infection associated with abnormalities of complement-mediated functions and of the third component of complement (C3), *N. Engl. J. Med.* **282**:349–354.

Alper, C. A., Abramson, N., Johnston, R. B., Jr., Jandl, J. H., and Rosen, F. S., 1970b, Studies *in vivo* and *in vitro* on an abnormality in the metabolism of C3 in a patient with increased susceptibility to infection, *J. Clin. Invest.* **49**:1975–1985.

Alper, C. A., Colten, H. R., Rosen, F. S., Rabson, A. R., Macnab, G. M., and Gear, J. S. S., 1972, Homozygous deficiency of C3 in a patient with repeated infections, *Lancet* **2**:1179–1181.

Alper, C. A., Bloch, K. J., and Rosen, F. S., 1973, Increased susceptibility to infection in a patient with type II essential hypercatabolism of C3, *N. Engl. J. Med.* **288**:601–606.

Anderson, P., Johnston, R. B., Jr., and Smith, D. H., 1972a, Human serum activities against *Hemophilus influenzae*, type by, *J. Clin. Invest.* **51**:31–38.

Anderson, P., Peter, G., Johnston, R. B., Jr., Wetterlow, L. H., and Smith, D. H., 1972b, Immunization of humans with polyribophosphate, the capsular antigen of *Hemophilus influenzae*, type b, *J. Clin. Invest.* **51**:39–44.

Arend, W. P., and Mannik, M., 1973, The macrophage receptor for IgG: number and affinity of binding sites, *J. Immunol.* **110**:1455–1463.

Askenase, P. W., and Hayden, B. J., 1974, Cytophilic antibodies in mice contactsensitized with oxazolone. Immunochemical characterization and preferential binding to a trypsin-sensitive macrophage receptor, *Immunology* **27**:563–576.

Atkinson, J. P., and Frank, M. M., 1974a, The effect of bacillus Calmette-Guérin-induced macrophage activation on the *in vivo* clearance of sensitized erythrocytes, *J. Clin. Invest.* **53**:1742–1749.

Atkinson, J. P., and Frank, M. M., 1974b, Studies of the *in vivo* effects of antibody. Interaction of IgM antibody and complement in the immune clearance and destruction of erythrocytes in man, *J. Clin. Invest.* **54**:339–348.

Ballow, M., Yang, S. Y., and Day, N. K., 1975, Complete absence of the third component of complement, *Fed. Proc. Fed. Amer. Soc. Exp. Biol.* **34**:853.

Basch, R. S., 1965, Inhibition of the third component of the complement system by derivatives of aromatic amino acids, *J. Immunol.* **94**:629–640.

Berken, A., and Benacerraf, B., 1966, Properties of antibodies cytophilic for macrophages, *J. Exp. Med.* **123**:119–144.

Berken, A., and Benacerraf, B., 1968, Sedimentation properties of antibodies cytophilic for macrophages, *J. Immunol.* **100**:1219–1222.

Bianco, C., Griffin, F. M., Jr., and Silverstein, S. C., 1975, Studies of the macrophage complement receptor. Alteration of receptor function upon macrophage activation, *J. Exp. Med.* **141**:1278–1290.

Bjornson, A. B., and Michael, J. G., 1971, Contribution of humoral and cellular factors to the resistance to experimental infection by *Pseudomonas aeruginosa* in mice. I. Interaction between immunoglobulins, heat-labile serum factors, and phagocytic cells in the killing of bacteria, *Infect. Immun.* **4**:462–467.

Bjornson, A. B., and Michael, J. G., 1973, Factors in normal human serum that promote bacterial phagocytosis, *J. Infect. Dis.* **128**:S182–S186.

Bokisch, V. A., and Sobel, A. T., 1974, Receptor for the fourth component of complement on human B lymphocytes and cultured human lymphoblastoid lines, *J. Exp. Med.* **140**:1336–1347.

Borsos, T., and Rapp, H. J., 1965a, Hemolysin titration based on fixation of the activated first component of complement: evidence that one molecule of hemolysin suffices to sensitize an erythrocyte, *J. Immunol.* **95**:559–566.

Borsos, T., and Rapp, H. J., 1965b, Complement fixation on cell surfaces by 19 S and 7 S antibodies, *Science* **150**:505–506.

Boxer, L. A., Hedley-White, E. T., and Stossel, T. P., 1974, Neutrophil actin dysfunction and abnormal neutrophil behavior, *N. Engl. J. Med.* **291**:1093–1099.

Boyden, S. V., 1964, Cytophilic antibody in guinea-pigs with delayed-type hypersensitivity, *Immunology* **7**:474–483.

Boyden, S. V., and Sorkin, E., 1960, The adsorption of antigen by spleen cells previously treated with antiserum *in vitro*, *Immunology* **3**:272–283.

Boyden, S. V., and Sorkin, E., 1961, The adsorption of antibody and antigen by spleen cells *in vitro*. Some further observations, *Immunology* **4**:244–252.

Boyden, S. V., North, R. J., and Faulkner, S. M., 1965, Complement and the activity of phagocytes, in: *Ciba Foundation Symposium: Complement* (G. E. W. Wolstenholme and J. Knight, eds.), pp. 190–213, Little, Brown and Co., Boston.

Brown, D. L., Lachmann, P.J., and Dacie, J. V., 1970, The *in vivo* behaviour of complement-coated red cells: studies in C6-deficient, C3-depleted and normal rabbits, *Clin. Exp. Immunol.* 7:401–421.

Bulloch, W., and Western, G. T., 1906, The specificity of the opsonic substances in the blood serum, *Proc. Roy. Soc. London Ser. B* 77:531–536.

Cohen, S., 1968, The requirement for the association of two adjacent rabbit γG-antibody molecules in the fixation of complement by immune complexes, *J. Immunol.* 100:407–413.

Cohen, S., and Butcher, G. A., 1970, Properties of protective malarial antibody, *Immunology* 19:369–383.

Cohn, Z. A., 1963, The fate of bacteria within phagocytic cells. II. The modification of intracellular degradation, *J. Exp. Med.* 117:43–53.

Cohn, Z. A., and Morse, S. I., 1959, Interactions between rabbit polymorphonuclear leucocytes and staphylococci, *J. Exp. Med.* 110:419–443.

Cooper, N. R., 1967, Complement associated peptidase activity of guinea pig serum. II. Role of a low molecular weight enhancing factor, *J. Immunol.* 98:132–138.

Cooper, N. R., 1969, Immune adherence by the fourth component of complement, *Science* 165:396–398.

Cooper, N. R., and Becker, E. L., 1967, Complement associated peptidase activity of guinea pig serum. I. Role of complement components, *J. Immunol.* 98:119–131.

Cooper, N. R., and Müller-Eberhard, H. J., 1967, Quantitative relation between peptidase activity and the cell-bound second (C′2), third (C′3) and fourth (C′4) components of human complement (C′), *Fed. Proc. Fed. Amer. Soc. Exp. Biol.* 26:361.

Cooper, N. R., ten Bensel, R., and Kohler, P. F., 1968, Studies of an additional kindred with hereditary deficiency of the second component of human complement (C2) and description of a new method for the quantitation of C2, *J. Immunol.* 101:1176–1182.

Cowie, D. M., and Chapin, W. S., 1907a, On the reaction of heated normal human opsonic serum with fresh diluted serum. A contribution to the study of opsonins, *J. Med. Res.* 17:57–75.

Cowie, D. M., and Chapin, W. S., 1907b, Experiments in favor of the amboceptor–complement structure of the opsonin of normal human serum for the *Staphylococcus albus*, *J. Med. Res.* 17:95–117.

Dales, S., and Kajioka, R., 1964, The cycle of multiplication of vaccinia virus in Earle's strain L cells. I. Uptake and penetration, *Virology* 24:278–294.

Davis, B. D., Dulbecco, R., Eisen, H. N., Ginsberg, H. S., and Wood, W. B., Jr., 1968, *Microbiology*, p. 609, Harper, New York.

Diamond, R. D., May, J. E., Kane, M., Frank, M. M., and Bennett, J. E., 1973, The role of late complement components and the alternate complement pathway in experimental cryptococcosis, *Proc. Soc. Exp. Biol. Med.* 144:312–315.

Dossett, J. H., Williams, R. C., Jr., and Quie, P. G., 1969, Studies on interaction of bacteria, serum factors and polymorphonuclear leukocytes in mothers and newborns, *Pediatrics* 44:49–57.

Dubos, R. J., 1945, *The Bacterial Cell*, pp. 205–212, Harvard University Press, Cambridge, Massachusetts.

Dukor, P., and Hartmann, K. U., 1973, Bound C3 as the second signal for B-cell activation, *Cell. Immunol.* 7:349–356.

Eddies, D. S., Schulkind, M. L., and Robbins, J. B., 1971, The isolation and biologic activities of purified secretory IgA and IgG anti-*Salmonella typhimurium* "O" antibodies from rabbit intestinal fluid and colostrum, *J. Immunol.* 106:181–190.

Ehlenberger, A. G., and Nussenzweig, V., 1975, Synergy between receptors for Fc and C3 in the induction of phagocytosis by human monocytes and neutrophils, *Fed. Proc. Fed. Amer. Soc. Exp. Biol.* 34:854.

Ellman, L., Green, I., and Frank, M. M., 1970, Genetically controlled total deficiency of the fourth component of complement in the guinea pig, *Science* 170:74–75.

Estes, D., and Christian, C. L., 1971, The natural history of systemic lupus erythematosus by prospective analysis, *Medicine* 50:85–95.

Fearon, D. T., Ruddy, S., Schur, P. H., and McCabe, W. R., 1975, Activation of the properdin pathway of complement in patients with gram-negative bacteremia, *N. Engl. J. Med.* 292:937–940.

Feinstein, A., and Rowe, A. J., 1965, Molecular mechanism of formation of an antigen–antibody complex, *Nature (London)* 205:147–149.

Fine, D. P., Marney, S. R., Colley, D. G., Sergent, J. S., and Des Prez, R. M., 1972, C3 shunt activation in human serum chelated with EGTA, *J. Immunol.* 109:807–809.

Forsgren, A., and Quie, P. G., 1974, Opsonic activity in human serum chelated with ethylene glycoltetra-acetic acid, *Immunology* **26**:1251–1256.

Gambrill, M. R., and Wisseman, C. L., Jr., 1973, Mechanisms of immunity in typhus infections. III. Influence of human immune serum and complement on the fate of *Rickettsia mooseri* within human macrophages, *Infect. Immun.* **8**:631–640.

Ganrot, P. O., and Kindmark, C.-O., 1969, C-reactive protein—a phagocytosis-promoting factor, *Scand. J. Clin. Lab. Invest.* **24**:215–219.

Gewurz, H., Pickering, R. J., Muschel, L. H., Mergenhagen, S. E., and Good, R. A., 1966, Complement-dependent biological functions in complement deficiency in man, *Lancet* **2**:356–359.

Gewurz, H., Shin, H. S., and Mergenhagen, S. E., 1968, Interactions of the complement system with endotoxic lipopolysaccharide: consumption of each of the six terminal complement components, *J. Exp. Med.* **128**:1049–1057.

Gigli, I., and Nelson, R. A., Jr., 1968, Complement dependent immune phagocytosis. I. Requirements for C′1, C′4, C′2, C′3, *Exp. Cell Res.* **51**:45–67.

Gilbert, D. N., Barnett, J. A., and Sanford, J. P., 1973, *Escherichia coli* bacteremia in the squirrel monkey. I. Effect of cobra venom factor treatment, *J. Clin. Invest.* **52**:406–413.

Götze, O., and Müller-Eberhard, H. J., 1971, The C3-activator system: an alternate pathway of complement activation, *J. Exp. Med.* **134**:90s–108s.

Götze, O., and Müller-Eberhard, H. J., 1974, The role of properdin in the alternate pathway of complement activation, *J. Exp. Med.* **139**:44–57.

Griffin, F. M., Jr., and Silverstein, S. C., 1974, Segmental response of the macrophage plasma membrane to a phagocytic stimulus, *J. Exp. Med.* **139**:323–336.

Griffin, F. M., Jr., Bianco, C., and Silverstein, S. C., 1975a, Characterization of the macrophage receptor for complement and demonstration of its functional independence from the receptor for the Fc portion of immunoglobulin G, *J. Exp. Med.* **141**:1269–1277.

Griffin, F. M. Jr., Griffin, J. A., Leider, J. E., and Silverstein, S. C., 1975b, Studies on the mechanism of phagocytosis. I. Requirements for circumferential attachment of particle-bound ligands to specific receptors on the macrophage plasma membrane, *J. Exp. Med.* **142**:1263–1282.

Griffin, F. M., Jr., Griffin, J. A., and Silverstein, S. C., 1976, Studies on the mechanism of phagocytosis. II. The interaction of macrophages with anti-immunoglobulin IgG-coated bone-marrow-derived lymphocytes, *J. Exp. Med.* **144**:788–809.

Grossberg, A. L., Markus, G., and Pressman, D., 1965, Change in antibody conformation induced by hapten, *Proc. Nat. Acad. Sci. U.S.A.* **54**:942–945.

del Guercio, P., Tolone, G., Braga Andrade, F., Biozzi, G., and Binaghi, R. A., 1969, Opsonic, cytophilic and agglutinating activity of guinea-pig γ2 and γM anti-*Salmonella* antibodies, *Immunology* **16**:361–371.

Handin, R. I., and Stossel, T. P., 1974, Phagocytosis of antibody-coated platelets by human granulocytes, *N. Engl. J. Med.* **290**:989–993.

Henney, C. S., and Stanworth, D. R., 1966, Effect of antigen on the structural configuration of homologous antibody following antigen–antibody combination, *Nature London* **210**:1071–1072.

Henney, C. S., Stanworth, D. R., and Gell, P. G. H., 1965, Demonstration of the exposure of new antigenic determinants following antigen–antibody combination, *Nature London* **205**:1079–1081.

Henson, P. M., 1969, The adherence of leucocytes and platelets induced by fixed IgG antibody and complement, *Immunology* **16**:107–121.

Hirsch, J. G., 1964, Demonstration by fluorescence microscopy of adsorption onto bacteria of a heat-labile factor from guinea pig serum, *J. Immunol.* **92**:155–158.

Hirsch, J. G., and Church, A. B., 1960, Studies of phagocytosis of group A streptococci by polymorphonuclear leukocytes *in vitro*, *J. Exp. Med.* **111**:309–322.

Hirsch, J. G., and Strauss, B., 1964, Studies on heat-labile opsonin in rabbit serum, *J. Immunol.* **92**:145–154.

Hokama, Y., Coleman, M. K., and Riley, R. F., 1962, *In vitro* effects of C-reactive protein on phagocytosis, *J. Bacteriol.* **83**:1017–1024.

Holland, P., Holland, N. H., and Cohn, Z. A., 1972, The selective inhibition of macrophage phagocytic receptors by anti-membrane antibodies, *J. Exp. Med.* **135**:458–475.

Hoy, W. E., and Nelson, D. S., 1969, Studies on cytophilic antibodies. V. Alloantibodies cytophilic for mouse macrophages, *Aust. J. Exp. Biol. Med. Sci.* **47**:525–539.

Huber, H., and Douglas, S. D., 1970, Receptor sites on human monocytes for complement: binding of red cells sensitized by cold auto-antibodies, *Br. J. Haematol.* **19**:19–26.

Huber, H., and Fudenberg, H. H., 1968, Receptor sites of human monocytes for IgG, *Int. Arch. Allergy Appl. Immunol.* **34**:18–31.

Huber, H., Polley, M. J., Linscott, W. D., Fudenberg, H. H., and Müller-Eberhard, H. J., 1968, Human monocytes: distinct receptor sites for the third component of complement and for immunoglobulin G, *Science* **162**:1281–1283.

Huber, H., Douglas, S. D., and Fudenberg, H. H., 1969, The IgG receptor: an immunological marker for the characterization of mononuclear cells, *Immunology* **17**:7–21.

Huber, H., Douglas, S. D., Huber, C., and Goldberg, L. S., 1971, Human monocyte receptor sites. Failure of IgA to demonstrate cytophilia, *Int. Arch. Allergy Appl. Immunol.* **41**:262–267.

Inchley, C., Grey, H. M., and Uhr, J. W., 1970, The cytophilic activity of human immunoglobulins, *J. Immunol.* **105**:362–369.

Ishizaka, K., 1970, Human reaginic antibodies, *Annu. Rev. Med.* **21**:187–200.

Ishizaka, K., and Campbell, D. H., 1959, Biological activity of soluble antigen–antibody complexes. V. Change of optical rotation by the formation of skin reactive complexes, *J. Immunol.* **83**:318–326.

Ishizaka, T., Ishizaka, K., Borsos, T., and Rapp, H. J., 1966, C′1 fixation by human isoagglutinins: fixation of C′1 by γG and γM but not by γA antibody, *J. Immunol.* **97**:716–726.

Ishizaka, K., Tomioka, H., and Ishizaka, T., 1970, Mechanisms of passive sentivization, I. Presence of IgE and IgG molecules on human leukocytes, *J. Immunol.* **105**:1459–1467.

Jacobs, J. C., and Miller, M. E., 1972, Fatal familial Leiner's disease: a deficiency of the opsonic activity of serum complement, *Pediatrics* **49**:225–232.

Jasin, H. E., 1972, Human heat labile opsonins: evidence for their mediation via the alternate pathway of complement activation, *J. Immunol.* **109**:26–31.

Jenkin, C. R., 1963, The effect of opsonins on the intracellular survival of bacteria, *Br. J. Exp. Pathol.* **44**:47–57.

Jenkin, C. R., and Benacerraf, B., 1960, *In vitro* studies on the interaction between mouse peritoneal macrophages and strains of salmonella and *Escherichia coli*, *J. Exp. Med.* **12**:403–417.

Jeter, W. S., McKee, A. P., and Mason, R. J., 1961, Inhibition of immune phagocytosis of *Diplococcus pneumoniae* by human neutrophils with antibody against complement, *J. Immunol.* **86**:386–391.

Johnson, F. R., Agnello, V., and Williams, R. C., Jr., 1972, Opsonic activity in human serum deficient in C2, *J. Immunol.* **109**:141–145.

Johnston, R. B., Jr., Klemperer, M. R., Alper, C. A., and Rosen, R. S., 1969, The enhancement of bacterial phagocytosis by serum. The role of complement components and two cofactors, *J. Exp. Med.* **129**:1275–1290.

Johnston, R. B., Jr., Struth, G., and Newman, S. L., 1972, Deficient serum opsonins in sickle cell disease, *Pediatr. Res.* **6**:381.

Johnston, R. B., Jr., Anderson, P., Rosen, F. S., and Smith, D. H., 1973, Characteristics of human antibody to polyribophosphate, the capsular antigen of *Hemophilus influenzae*, type b, *Clin. Immunol. Immunopathol.* **1**:234–240.

Jonas, W. E., Gurner, B. W., Nelson, D. S., and Coombs, R. R. A., 1965, Passive sensitization of tissue cells. I. Passive sensitization of macrophages by guinea-pig cytophilic antibody, *Int. Arch. Allergy Appl. Immunol.* **28**:86–104.

Jones, T. C., and Hirsch, J. G., 1972, The interaction between *Toxoplasma gondii* and mammalian cells. II. The absence of lysosomal fusion with phagocytic vacuoles containing living parasites, *J. Exp. Med.* **136**:1173–1194.

Jones, T. C., Len, L., and Hirsch, J. G., 1975, Assessment *in vitro* of immunity against *Toxoplasma gondii*, *J. Exp. Med.* **141**:466–482.

Kaplan, M. H., and Volanakis, J. E., 1974, Interaction of C-reactive protein complexes with the complement system. I. Consumption of human complement associated with the reactions of CRP with pneumococcal C-polysaccharide and with the choline phosphatides, lecithin and sphingomyelin, *J. Immunol.* **112**:2135–2147.

Kaplan, M. E., Dalmasso, A. P., and Woodson, M., 1972, Complement-dependent opsonization of incompatible erythrocytes by human secretory IgA, *J. Immunol.* **108**:275–278.

Kindmark, C.-O., 1971, Stimulating effect of C-reactive protein on phagocytosis of various species of pathogenic bacteria, *Clin. Exp. Immunol.* **8**:941–948.

Kindmark, C.-O., 1972, *In vitro* binding of human C-reactive protein by some pathogenic bacteria and zymosan, *Clin. Exp. Immunol.* **11**:283–289.

Klemperer, M. R., Woodworth, H. C., Rosen, F. S., and Austen, K. F., 1966, Hereditary deficiency of the second component of complement (C′2) in man, *J. Clin. Invest.* **45**:880–890.

Klemperer, M. R., Austen, K. F., and Rosen, F. S., 1967, Hereditary deficiency of the second component of complement (C′2) in man: further observations on a second kindred, *J. Immunol.* **98**:72–78.

Knop, J., Breu, H., Wernet, P., and Rowley, D., 1971, The relative antibacterial efficiency of IgM, IgG and IgA from pig colostrum, *Aust. J. Exp. Biol. Med. Sci.* **49**:405–413.

Lachmann, P. J., and Müller-Eberhard, H. J., 1968, The demonstration in human serum of "conglutinogen-activating factor" and its effect on the third component of complement, *J. Immunol.* **100**:691–698.

Lawrence, D. S., Weigle, W. O., and Speigelberg, H. L., 1975, Immunoglobulins cytophilic for human lymphocytes, monocytes, and neutrophils, *J. Clin. Invest.* **55**:368–376.

Laxdal, T., Messner, R. P., Williams, R. C., Jr., and Quie, P. G., 1968, Opsonic, agglutinating, and complement-fixing antibodies in patients with subacute bacterial endocarditis, *J. Lab. Clin. Med.* **71**:638–653.

Lay, W. H., and Nussenzweig, V., 1968, Receptors for complement on leukocytes, *J. Exp. Med.* **128**:991–1009.

Lay, W. H., and Nussenzweig, V., 1969, Ca^{++}-dependent binding of antigen-19S antibody complexes to macrophages, *J. Immunol.* **102**:1172–1178.

Leddy, J. P., Frank, M. M., Gaither, T., Baum, J., and Klemperer, M. R., 1974, Hereditary deficiency of the sixth component of complement in man. I. Immunochemical, biologic, and family studies, *J. Clin. Invest.* **53**:544–553.

Lehrer, R. I., and Cline, M. J., 1969, Interaction of *Candida albicans* with human leukocytes and serum, *J. Bacteriol.* **98**:996–1004.

Leslie, R. G. Q., and Cohen, S., 1974a, Cytophilic activity of IgG2 from sera of unimmunized guinea-pigs, *Immunology* **27**:577–587.

Leslie, R. G. Q., and Cohen, S., 1974b, Cytophilic activity of IgG2 from sera of guinea-pigs immunized with bovine γ-globulin, *Immunology* **27**:589–599.

Levenson, V. I., Braude, N. I., and Chernokhvostova, E. V., 1970, Adherence-promoting antibodies. The investigation of physicochemical properties of mouse anti-Vi antibodies providing immune fixation of antigen to macrophage surface, *Aust. J. Exp. Biol. Med. Sci.* **48**:417–427.

Lo Buglio, A. F., Cotra, R. S., and Jandl, J. H., 1967, Red cells coated with immunoglobulin G: binding and sphering by mononuclear cells in man, *Science* **158**:1582–1585.

Logue, G. L., Rosse, W. F., and Adams, J. P., 1973, Complement-dependent immune adherence measured with human granulocytes: changes in the antigenic nature of red cell-bound C3 produced by incubation in human serum, *Clin. Immunol. Immunopathol.* **1**:398–407.

Maaloe, O., 1946, *Relation between Alexin and Opsonin,* Elinar Munksgaard, Copenhagen.

Mantovani, B., Rabinovitch, M., and Nussenzweig, V., 1972, Phagocytosis of immune complexes by macrophages. Different role of the macrophage receptor sites for complement (C3) and for immunoglobulin (IgG), *J. Exp. Med.* **135**:780–792.

Marcus, R. L., Shin, H. S., and Mayer, M. M., 1971, An alternate complement pathway: C3 cleaving acitivity, not due to C$\overline{4,2a}$, on endotoxic lipopolysaccharide after treatment with guinea pig serum; relation to properdin, *Proc. Nat. Acad. Sci. U.S.A.* **68**:1351–1354.

Messner, R. P., and Jelinek, J., 1970, Receptors for human γG on human neutrophils, *J. Clin. Invest.* **49**:2165–2171.

Messner, R. P., Laxdal, T., Quie, P. G., and Williams, R. C., Jr., 1968, Serum opsonin, bacteria, and polymorphonuclear leukocyte interactions in subacute bacterial endocarditis. Anti-γ-globulin factors and their interaction with specific opsonins, *J. Clin. Invest.* **47**:1109–1120.

Metchnikoff, E., 1887, Sur la lutte des cellules de l'organismes centre l'invasion des microbes, *Ann. Inst. Pasteur* **1**:321–336.

Miller, M. E., and Nilsson, U. R., 1970, A familial deficiency of the phagocytosis-enhancing activity of serum related to a dysfunction of the fifth component of complement (C5), *N. Engl. J. Med.* **282**:354–358.

Miller, M. E., and Nilsson, U. R., 1974, A major role of the fifth component of complement (C5) in the opsonization of yeast particles. Partial dichotomy of function and immunochemical measurement, *Clin. Immunol. Immunopathol.* **2**:246–255.

Miller, M. E., Seals, J., Kaye, R., and Levitsky, L. C., 1968, A familial, plasma-associated defect of phagocytosis: a new cause of recurrent bacterial infections, *Lancet* **2**:60–63.

Miya, F., and Marcus, S., 1961, Effect of humoral factors on *in vitro* phagocytosis and cytopeptic activities of normal and "immune" phagocytes, *J. Immunol.* **86**:652–668.

Morelli, R., and Rosenberg, L. T., 1971, The role of complement in the phagocytosis of *Candida albicans* by mouse peripheral blood leukocytes, *J. Immunol.* **107**:476–480.

Mudd, S., McCutcheon, M., and Lucké, B., 1934, Phagocytosis, *Physiol Rev.* **14**:210–275.

Müller-Eberhard, H. J., 1968, Chemistry and reaction mechanisms of complement, *Adv. Immunol.* **8**:1–80.

Müller-Eberhard, H. J., 1971, Biochemistry of complement, in: *Progress in Immunology* (B. Amos, ed.), pp. 553–565, Academic Press, New York.

Müller-Eberhard, H. J., and Götze, O., 1972, C3 proactivator convertase and its mode of action, *J. Exp. Med.* **135**:1003–1008.

Müller-Eberhard, H. J., Polley, M. J., and Calcott, M. A., 1967, Formation and functional significance of a molecular complex derived from the second and fourth component of human complement, *J. Exp. Med.* **125**:359–380.

Nelson, D. S., and Mildenhall, P., 1968, Studies on cytophilic antibodies. II. The production by guinea pigs of macrophage cytophilic antibodies to sheep erythrocytes and human serum albumin: relationship to the production of other antibodies and the development of delayed-type hypersensitivity, *Aust. J. Exp. Biol. Med. Sci.* **46**:33–49.

Nelson, D. S., Kossard, S., and Cox, P. E., 1967, Heterogeneity of macrophage cytophilic antibodies in immunized mice, *Experientia* **23**:490–491.

Nickerson, D. S., Kazmierowski, J. A., Dossett, J. H., Williams, R. C., Jr., and Quie, P. G., 1969, Studies of immune and normal opsonins during experimental staphylococcal infections in rabbits, *J. Immunol.* **102**:1235–1241.

Nickerson, D. S., Williams, R. C., Jr., Boxmeyer, M., and Quie, P. G., 1970, Increased opsonic capacity of serum in chronic heroin addiction, *Ann. Intern. Med.* **72**:671–677.

Nilsson, U. R., Miller, M. E., and Wyman, S., 1974, A functional abnormality of the fifth component of complement (C5) from human serum of individuals with a familial opsonic defect, *J. Immunol.* **112**:1164–1176.

van Oss, C. J., and Singer, J. M., 1966, The binding of immune globulins and other proteins by polystyrene latex particles, *J. Reticuloendothel. Soc.* **3**:29–40.

van Oss, C. J., and Stinson, M. W., 1970, Immunoglobulins as aspecific opsonins. I. The influence of polyclonal and monoclonal immunoglobulins on the *in vitro* phagocytosis of latex particles and staphylococci by human neutrophils, *J. Reticuloendothel. Soc.* **8**:397–406.

Parish, W. E., 1965, Differentiation between cytophilic antibody and opsonin by a macrophage phagocytic system, *Nature London* **108**:594–595.

Pearlman, D. S., Ward, P. A., and Becker, E. L., 1969, The requirement of serine esterase function in complement-dependent erythrophagocytosis, *J. Exp. Med.* **130**:745–764.

Phillips, J. K., Snyderman, R., and Mergenhagen, S. E., 1972, Activation of complement by endotoxin: a role for γ2 globulin, C1, C4 and C2 in the consumption of terminal complement components by endotoxin-treated erythrocytes, *J. Immunol.* **109**:334–341.

Phillips-Quagliata, J. M., Levine, B. B., Quagliata, F., and Uhr, J. W., 1971, Mechanisms underlying binding of immune complexes to macrophages, *J. Exp. Med.* **133**:589–601.

Pillemer, L., Blum, L., Lepow, I. H., Ross, O. A., Todd, E. W., and Wardlaw, A. C., 1954, The properdin system in immunity: I. Demonstration and isolation of a new serum protein, properdin, and its role in immune phenomena, *Science* **120**:279–285.

Quie, P. G., Messner, R. P., and Williams, R. C., Jr., 1968, Phagocytosis in subacute bacterial endocarditis. Localization of the primary opsonic site to Fc fragment, *J. Exp. Med.* **128**:553–570.

Rabinovitch, M., 1967, Studies on immunoglobulins which stimulate the ingestion of glutaraldehyde-treated red cells attached to macrophages, *J. Immunol.* **99**:1115–1120.

Ralston, D. J., and Elberg, S. S., 1969, Serum-mediated immune cellular responses to *Brucella melitensis* REVI. II. Restriction of *Brucella* by immune sera and macrophages, *J. Reticuloendothel. Soc.* **6**:109–139.

Reed, W. P., 1975, Serum factors capable of opsonizing *Shigella* for phagocytosis by polymorphonuclear neutrophils, *Immunology* **28**:1051–1059.

Reynolds, H. Y., and Thompson, R. E., 1973, Pulmonary host defenses. II. Interaction of respiratory antibodies with *Pseudomonas aeruginosa* and alveolar macrophages, *J. Immunol.* **111**:369–380.

Rhodes, J., 1973, Receptor for monomeric IgM on guinea-pig splenic macrophages, *Nature London* **243**:527–528.

Robbins, J. B., Kenny, K., and Suter, E., 1965, The isolation and biological activities of rabbit γM- and γG-anti-*Salmonella typhimurium* antibodies, *J. Exp. Med.* **122**:385–402.

Roberts, R. B., 1967, The interaction *in vitro* between group B meningococci and rabbit polymorphonuclear leukocytes. Demonstration of type specific opsonins and bactericidins, *J. Exp. Med.* **126**:795–817.

Roberts, R. B., 1970, The relationship between group A and group C meningococcal polysaccharides and serum opsonins in man, *J. Exp. Med.* **131**:499–513.

Root, R. K., Ellman, L., and Frank, M. M., 1972, Bactericidal and opsonic properties of C4-deficient guinea pig serum, *J. Immunol.* **109**:477–486.

Rosen, F. S., and Janeway, C. A., 1966, The gamma globulins. III. The antibody deficiency syndromes, *N. Engl. J. Med.* **275**:709–715.

Rosenfeld, S. I., and Leddy, J. P., 1974, Hereditary deficiency of fifth component of complement (C5) in man, *J. Clin. Invest.* **53**:67a.

Ross, G. D., and Polley, M. J., 1975, Specificity of human lymphocyte complement receptors, *J. Exp. Med.* **141**:1163–1180.

Rothbard, S., 1945, Bacteriostatic effect of human sera on group A streptococci. II. Comparative bacteriostatic effect of normal whole blood from different animal species in the presence of human convalescent sera, *J. Exp. Med.* **82**:107–118.

Rowley, D., 1958, Bactericidal activity of macrophages *in vitro* against *Escherichia coli, Nature London* **181**:1738–1739.

Rowley, D., and Turner, K. J., 1966, Number of molecules of antibody required to promote phagocytosis of one bacterium, *Nature London* **210**:496–498.

Rowley, D., Turner, K. J., and Jenkin, C. R., 1964, The basis for immunity to mouse typhoid. 3. Cell-bound antibody, *Aust. J. Exp. Biol. Med. Sci.* **42**:237–248.

Ruddy, S., and Austen, K. F., 1969, C3 inactivator of man. I. Hemolytic measurement by the inactivation of cell-bound C3, *J. Immunol.* **102**:533–543.

Ruddy, S., and Austen, K. F., 1971, C3b inactivator of man. II. Fragments produced by C3b inactivator cleavage of cell-bound or fluid phase C3b, *J. Immunol.* **107**:742–750.

Ruddy, S., Klemperer, M. R., Rosen, F. S., Austen, K. F., and Kumate, J., 1970, Hereditary deficiency of the second component of complement (C2) in man: correlation of C2 haemolytic activity with immunochemical measurements of C2 protein, *Immunology* **18**:943–954.

Sandberg, A. L., and Osler, A. G., 1971, Dual pathways of complement interaction with guinea pig immunoglobulins, *J. Immunol.* **107**:1268–1273.

Sandberg, A. L., Oliveira, B., and Osler, A. G., 1971a, Two complement interaction sites in guinea pig immunoglobulins, *J. Immunol.* **106**:282–285.

Sandberg, A. L., Götze, O., Müller-Eberhard, H. J., and Osler, A. G., 1971b, Complement utilization by guinea pig γ1 and γ2 immunoglobulins through the C3 activator system, *J. Immunol.* **107**:920–923.

Schreiber, A. D., and Frank, M. M., 1972a, Role of antibody and complement in the immune clearance and destruction of erythrocytes. I. *In vivo* effects of IgG and IgM complement-fixing sites, *J. Clin. Invest.* **51**:575–582.

Schreiber, A. D., and Frank, M. M., 1972b, Role of antibody and complement in the immune clearance and destruction of erythrocytes. II. Molecular nature of IgG and IgM complement-fixing sites and effects of their interaction with serum, *J. Clin. Invest.* **51**:583–589.

Schur, P. H., and Becker, E. L., 1963, Pepsin digestion of rabbit and sheep antibodies: the effect on complement fixation, *J. Exp. Ed.* **118**:891–904.

Shayegani, M. G., and Mudd, S., 1966, Role of serum in the intracellular killing of staphylococci in rabbit monocytes, *J. Bacteriol.* **91**:1393–1398.

Shin, H. S., Smith, M. R., and Wood, W. B., Jr., 1969, Heat labile opsonins to pneumococcus. II. Involvement of C3 and C5, *J. Exp. Med.* **130**:1229–1241.

Siegel, J., Rent, R., and Gewurz, H., 1974, Interaction of C-reactive protein with the complement system. I. Protamine-induced consumption of complement in acute phase sera, *J. Exp. Med.* **140**:631–647.

Silverstein, A. M., 1960, Essential hypocomplementemia: report of a case, *Blood* **16**:1338–1341.

Silverstein, S. C., and Castle, D., 1970, The effect of antibody on the phagocytosis and processing of vaccinia virus by mouse peritoneal macrophages, *J. Cell Biol.* **47**:192a.

Smith, J. W., Barnett, J. A., May, R. P., and Sanford, J. P., 1967, Comparison of the opsonic activity of γ-G- and γ-M-anti-proteus globulins, *J. Immunol.* **98**:336–343.

Smith, M. A., Cooper, M. D., Wollheim, F. A., Hong, R., and Good, R. A., 1966, The IgA system. I. Studies of the transport and immunochemistry of IgA in the saliva, *J. Exp. Med.* **123**:615–627.

Smith, M. R., and Wood, W. B., Jr., 1969, Heat labile opsonins to pneumococcus. I. Participation of complement, *J. Exp. Med.* **130**:1209–1227.

Smith, M. R., Shin, H. S., and Wood, W. B., Jr., 1969, Natural immunity to bacterial infections: the relation of complement to heat-labile opsonins, *Proc. Nat. Acad. Sci. U.S.A.* **63**:1151–1156.

Sorkin, E., 1963, Cytophilic antibody, in: *Ciba Found. Symp., The Immunologically Competent Cell* (G. E. W. Wolstenholme and M. P. Cameron, eds.), p. 53, Churchill, London.

Speigelberg, H. L., Miescher, P. A., and Benacerraf, B., 1963, Studies on the role of complement in the immune clearance of *Escherichia coli* and rat erythrocytes by the reticuloendothelial system in mice, *J. Immunol.* **90**:751–759.

Steinman, R. M., and Cohn, Z. A., 1972, The interaction of particulate horseradish peroxidase (HRP)-anti HRP immune complexes with mouse peritoneal macrophages *in vitro, J. Cell Biol.* **55**:616–634.

Stinson, M. W., and van Oss, C. J., 1971, Immunoglobulins as aspecific opsonins. II. The influence of specific and aspecific immunoglobulins on the *in vitro* phagocytosis of nonencapsulated, capsulated, and decapsulated bacteria by human neutrophils, *J. Reticuloendothel. Soc.* **9**:503–512.

Stollerman, G. H., Rytel, M., and Ortiz, J., 1963, Accessory plasma factors involved in the bactericidal test for type-specific antibody to group A streptococci. II. Human plasma cofactors(s) enhancing opsonization of encapsulated organisms, *J. Exp. Med.* **117**:1–17.

Stollerman, G. H., Alberti, H., and Plemmons, J. A., 1967, Opsonization of group A streptococci by complement deficient blood from a patient with hereditary angioneurotic edema, *J. Immunol.* **99**:92–97.

Stossel, T. P., 1973, Quantitative studies on phagocytosis. Kinetic effects of cations and heat-labile opsonins, *J. Cell Biol.* **58**:346–356.

Stossel, T. P., and Pincus, S. H., 1975, A new macrophage actin-binding protein: evidence for its role in endocytosis, *Clin. Res.* **23**:407A.

Stossel, T. P., Alper, C. A., and Rosen, F. S., 1973a, Serum-dependent phagocytosis of paraffin oil emulsified with bacterial lipopolysaccharide, *J. Exp. Med.* **137**:690–705.

Stossel, T. P., Alper, C. A., and Rosen, F. S., 1973b, Opsonic activity in the newborn: Role of properdin, *Pediatrics* **52**:134–137.

Stossel, T. P., Field, R. J., Gitlin, J. D., Alper, C. A., and Rosen, F. S., 1975, The opsonic fragment of the third component of human complement (C3), *J. Exp. Med.* **141**:1329–1347.

Tizard, I. R., 1969, Macrophage cytophilic antibody in mice. Differentiation between antigen adherence due to these antibodies and opsonic adherence, *Int. Arch. Allergy Appl. Immunol.* **36**:332–346.

Tizard, I. R., 1971, Macrophage cytophilic antibodies in mice: the adsorption of cytophilic antibodies from solution by mouse peritoneal cells and cooperative interaction between receptors for immunoglobulin, *J. Reticuloendothel, Soc.* **10**:449–460.

Turner, K. J., and Rowley, D., 1963, Opsonins in pig serum and their purification, *Aust. J. Exp. Biol. Med. Sci.* **41**:595–613.

Uhr, J. W., 1965, Passive sensitization of lymphocytes and macrophages by antigen–antibody complexes, *Proc. Nat. Acad. Sci. U.S.A.* **54**:1599–1606.

Valentine, R. C., and Green, N. M., 1967, Electron microscopy of an antibody–hapten complex, *J. Mol. Biol.* **27**:615–617.

Ward, H. K., and Enders, J. F., 1933, An analysis of the opsonic and tropic action of normal and immune sera based on experiments with the pneumococcus, *J. Exp. Med.* **57**:527–547.

Warner, C., Schumaker, V., and Karush, F., 1970, The detection of a conformational change in the antibody molecule upon interaction with hapten, *Biochem. Biophys. Res. Commun.* **38**:125–128.

Wheat, L. J., Humphreys, D. W., and White, A., 1974, Opsonization of staphylococci by normal human sera: the role of antibody and heat-labile factors, *J. Lab. Clin. Med.* **83**:73–78.

Williams, R. C., Jr., and Quie, P. G., 1968, Studies of human C-reactive protein in an *in vitro* phagocytic system, *J. Immunol.* **101**:426–432.

Williams, R. C., Jr., and Quie, P. G., 1971, Opsonic activity of agammaglobulinemic human sera, *J. Immunol.* **106**:51–55.

Williams, R. C., Jr., Dossett, J. H., and Quie, P. G., 1969, Comparative studies of immunoglobulin opsonins in osteomyelitis and other established infections, *Immunology* **17**:249–265.

Wilson, I. D., 1972, Studies on the opsonic activity of human secretory IgA using an *in vitro* pahgocytosis system, *J. Immunol.* **108**:726–730.

Winkelstein, J. A., and Drachman, R. H., 1968, Deficiency of pneumococcal opsonizing activity in sickle-cell disease, *N. Engl. J. Med.* **279**:459–466.

Winkelstein, J. A., and Shin, H. S., 1974, The role of immunoglobulin in the interaction of pneumococci and the properdin pathway: evidence for its specificity and lack of requirement for the Fc portion of the molecule, *J. Immunol.* **112**:1635–1642.

Winkelstein, J. A., Shin, H. S., and Wood, W. B., Jr., 1972, Heat labile opsonins to pneumococcus. III. The participation of immunoglobulin and of the alternate pathway of C3 activiation, *J. Immunol.* **108**:1681–1689.

Woodin, A. M., 1974, Action of organophosphorus compounds on the *p*-nitrophenyl phosphatase of membranes from rabbit and guinea pig polymorphonuclear leucocytes, *Exp. Cell Res.* **89**:15–22.

Wright, A. E., and Douglas, S. R., 1903, An experimental investigation of the role of the body fluids in connection with phagocytosis, *Proc. R. Soc. London* **72**:357–370.

Wu, W. G., and Marcus, S., 1963, Humoral factors in cellular resistance. I. The effects of heated and unheated homologous and heterologous sera on phagocytosis and cytopepsis by normal and "immune" macrophages, *J. Immunol.* **91**:313–322.

Wu, W. G., and Marcus, S., 1964, Humoral factors in cellular resistance. II. The role of complement and properdin in phagocytosis and cytopepsis by normal and "immune" macrophages, *J. Immunol.* **92**:397–403.

Young, L. S., 1972, Human immunity to *Pseudomonas aeruginosa*. II. Relationship between heat-stable opsonins and type-specific lipopolysaccharides, *J. Infect. Dis.* **126**:277–287.

Young, L. S., and Armstrong, D., 1972, Human immunity to *Pseudomonas aeruginosa*. I. *In-vitro* interaction of bacteria, polymorphonuclear leukocytes, and serum factors, *J. Infect. Dis.* **126**:257–276.

Ziegler, J. B., Alper, C. A., Rosen, F. S., Lachmann, P. J., and Sherington, L., 1975, Restoration by purified C3b inactivator of complement-mediated function in vivo in a patient with C3b inactivator deficiency, *J. Clin. Invest.* **55**:668–672.

Zinsser, H., Enders, J. F., and Fothergill, L., 1939, The phenomenon of phagocytosis, in: *Immunity, Principles and Applications in Medicine and Public Health,* pp. 317–319, Macmillan Co., New York.

Zipursky, A., Brown, E. J., and Bienenstock, J., 1973, Lack of opsonization potential of 11 S human secretory γA, *Proc. Soc. Exp. Biol. Med.* **142**:181–184.

6

Killing of Nucleated Cells by Antibody and Complement

SARKIS H. OHANIAN and TIBOR BORSOS

1. Introduction

The ability of antibody–antigen complexes to fix complement (C) has been known since the end of the last century. Up to and including the recent past, complement has been used mainly as a very sensitive indicator to detect the interaction of antibody with antigen. With the development of refined immunochemical methods it has been possible to analyze what complement is and to study its interaction with antigen–antibody complexes and with the surface of the cell (Müller-Eberhard, 1968; Rapp and Borsos, 1970; Humphrey and Dourmashkin, 1965, 1969).

Much of the knowledge concerning the molecular events of complement action has come from studies of a model system consisting of sheep red cells (E) as target cells, rabbit antibody to Forssman antigen of sheep red cells, and guinea pig serum as a source of C.

With this model system, the individual steps of immune hemolysis have been delineated (Figure 1). This system is composed of at least nine components and at least six major phases. In the first phase, C1 binds to antibody and is activated. In the second phase, the enzymatically active complex C42 is assembled on the surface of the cell. In the third phase, C3 binds to the surface of the cell. The fourth phase involves the fixation of the trimolecular complex C567 on the cell membrane, rendering it susceptible to the action of C8 and C9. In the fifth phase, C8 and C9 interact with the cell membrane. The damage-causing steps (phase 6) occur on or in the membrane and require several clearly distinguishable steps. The nature of the damage-causing steps is unknown. In addition to delineating the sequential steps of C fixation and activation, it has been possible with the red cell system to determine

SARKIS H. OHANIAN AND TIBOR BORSOS • Laboratory of Immunobiology, National Cancer Institute, National Institutes of Health, Bethesda, Maryland.

SARKIS H. OHANIAN
AND TIBOR BORSOS

the quantitative aspects of the complement system. Work in this and other groups has shown that one IgM or two or more IgG molecules are capable of fixing and activating one molecule of the first component of C (C1) (Humphrey and Dourmashkin, 1969; Borsos and Rapp, 1965a; Cohen, 1968) and that to achieve cytolysis, the activation of complement must proceed through to the ninth component and must interact with the surface of the target cell (Frank *et al.*, 1965). From these studies, evidence has been accumulated supporting a one-hit mechanism of immuncytolysis (Mayer, 1961). The one-hit theory states that the interaction of an antigen–antibody complex, on the surface of a cell, with the complement components leads to the generation of a single lesion that is sufficient to lyse or kill a cell. Thus, the time to reach an endpoint, i.e., the time when all cells that have reacted with antibody and complement have lysed, depends on the rate of lysis of cells with only one lesion.

The fundamental mechanism of immune hemolysis or cytolysis appears to be the same for all model systems investigated thus far (Kalfayan and Kidd, 1953; Gorer and O'Gorman, 1956; Bickis *et al.*, 1959; Goldberg and Green, 1959; Green and Goldberg, 1960; Ferrone *et al.*, 1971; Levy *et al.*, 1972). Apparent mechanistic differences among the models are probably related to quantitative and qualitative differences, i.e., how many and in what ways C molecules interact with the cell surface.

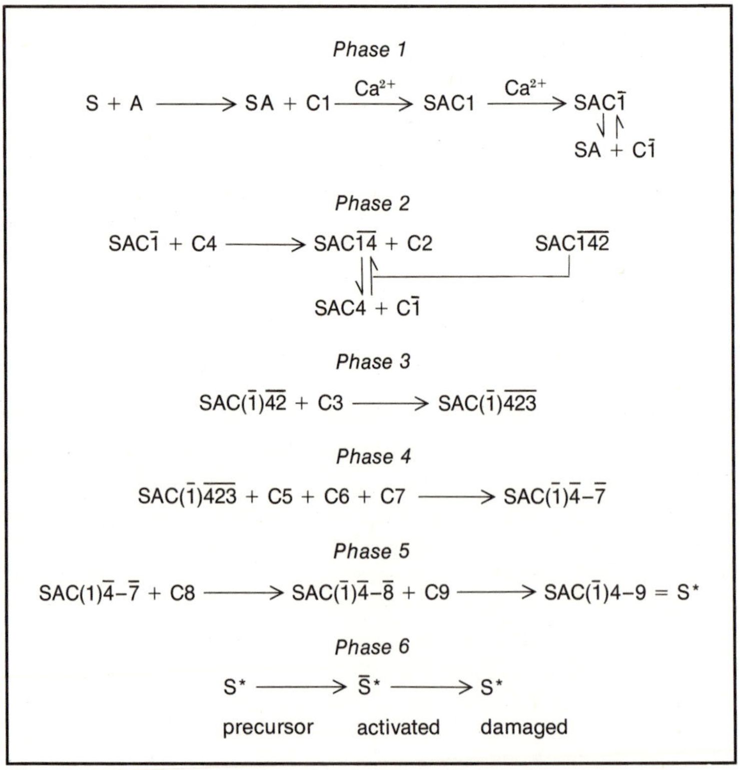

$$\text{Phase 1}$$
$$S + A \longrightarrow SA + C1 \xrightarrow{Ca^{2+}} SAC1 \xrightarrow{Ca^{2+}} SAC\overline{1}$$
$$SAC\overline{1} \rightleftharpoons SA + C\overline{1}$$

$$\text{Phase 2}$$
$$SAC\overline{1} + C4 \longrightarrow SAC\overline{14} + C2 \qquad SAC\overline{142}$$
$$SAC\overline{14} \rightleftharpoons SAC4 + C\overline{1}$$

$$\text{Phase 3}$$
$$SAC(\overline{1})\overline{42} + C3 \longrightarrow SAC(\overline{1})\overline{423}$$

$$\text{Phase 4}$$
$$SAC(\overline{1})\overline{423} + C5 + C6 + C7 \longrightarrow SAC(\overline{1})\overline{4-7}$$

$$\text{Phase 5}$$
$$SAC(1)\overline{4-7} + C8 \longrightarrow SAC(\overline{1})\overline{4-8} + C9 \longrightarrow SAC(\overline{1})4-9 = S^*$$

$$\text{Phase 6}$$
$$S^* \longrightarrow \overline{S}^* \longrightarrow S^*$$
$$\text{precursor} \qquad \text{activated} \qquad \text{damaged}$$

Figure 1. Sequence of reaction step of immune hemolysis. (S) Antigenic site on cell surface; (A) antibody to S. Adapted from Rapp and Borsos (1970).

It is generally accepted that cells of different types are not equally susceptible to the cytotoxic action of antibody and C. This variation in sensitivity to cytotoxicity has been ascribed to differences in the amount and distribution of antigen determinants on the cell surface, class of antibody, and source of C. However, other considerations must be taken into account and include (1) the topographical relationship of cell surface antigen to C binding sites, (2) the lack of activation and binding of sufficient amounts of C components, (3) the lack of surface areas susceptible to C action, (4) the prevention of damage to cell surface areas under attack by C, and (5) the repair of surface sites damaged by C.

We are currently attempting to determine the relative importance of these considerations in the antibody-C-mediated killing of diethylnitrosamine-induced guinea pig hepatoma cell lines, line 1 and line 10 (Rapp *et al.*, 1968; Zbar *et al.*, 1971; Ohanian *et al.*, 1973; Borsos *et al.*, 1973), using the knowledge gained from analysis of the mechanism of lysis of sheep red cells by Forssman antibody and C.

2. Role of Antigen, Antibody, and C in the Killing of Nucleated Cells

In our attempts to study the role of antigen, antibody, and sources of C on the killing of nucleated cells, we chose the Forssman model system because we could (1) identify and isolate antibodies of the various Ig classes, (2) determine their concentration on a molecular basis, (3) determine the number of C fixing antibody–antigen complexes accurately, and (4) identify and measure Forssman antigen activity.

2.1. Antigen

It has generally been concluded that the resistance of cells to antibody-C-mediated killing can be ascribed to differences in the amount and distribution of antigenic determinants on the cell surface (Moller and Moller, 1962; Winn, 1960; Rosse, 1968; Friberg, 1972; Schlesinger, 1965; Moller, 1963; Linscott, 1970).

Thus, in our initial studies, we measured Forssman antigen of sheep red cells and of guinea pig normal liver and line 1 and line 10 tumor cells with quantitative absorption tests. We found that sheep red cells, normal guinea pig liver cells, line 1 cells, and line 10 cells, on a per-cell basis, absorbed equivalent amounts of Forssman antibody (Figure 2) (Ohanian *et al.*, 1973). Analysis of the curves by curve fitting showed that liver, line 1, and line 10 cells were not entirely superimposable on the sheep red cell curve. This suggested the determinants on the nucleated cell were qualitatively different from that of the Forssman antigen of sheep red cells. Using the quantitative C1 fixation and transfer test, a method capable of measuring the number of cell-bound C fixing antigen–antibody complexes, line 1 and line 10 cells were found to have approximately 31,000 and 33,000 C1 fixing sites per cell, respectively (Figure 3) (Ohanian *et al.*, 1973).

When these tumor cells were examined for their sensitivity to killing by antibody plus C, differences were noted (Figure 4). Line 1, but not line 10, cells were efficiently killed when sensitized with anti-Forssman antibody and HuC. In addition, line 1 cells could also be killed with rabbit and GPC, but to a lesser extent

SARKIS H. OHANIAN
AND TIBOR BORSOS

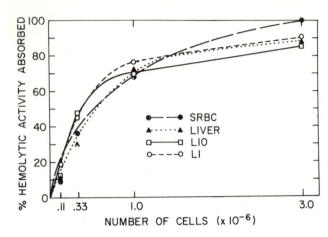

Figure 2. Hemolytic activity absorbed as a function of the number of normal guinea pig liver cells, SRBC, and hepatoma cells (line 1 and line 10) used for absorption.

than with HuC. Line 10 cells, on the other hand, were killed only with HuC (Table 1). It will be noted in this table that similar results were observed with specific antitumor antibody.

Thus, it would appear that resistance to killing could not be ascribed solely to antigen expression. Similar conclusions have been reached by other investigators using cells from different animal species in culture. It has been observed by some investigators that susceptibility of some cell lines to killing by antibody and C changes during the growth cycle (Shipley, 1971; Lerner et al., 1971; Cikes, 1970a,b; Cikes et al., 1972; Cikes and Klein, 1972a,b; Götze et al., 1972; Pellegrino et al., 1974). In some of these studies, the time of maximal susceptibility to antibody-C-

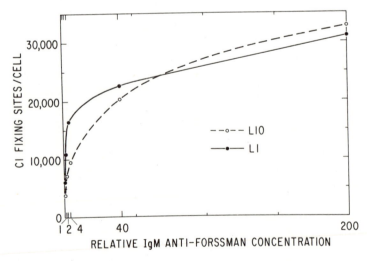

Figure 3. Determination of the number of $C\bar{1}$ fixing sites generated per cell as a function of the relative IgM Forssman antibody concentration; 1 = 1:400.

mediated killing appeared to be correlated with increased expression of cell surface antigens (Cikes, 1970; Cikes and Klein, 1972; Cikes *et al.,* 1972; Götze *et al.,* 1972), whereas in other studies, no correlation with antigen density could be made (Pellegrino *et al.,* 1974; Ferrone *et al.,* 1973; Lerner *et al.,* 1971). Therefore, in general, it would appear that the role of antigen in antibody-C-mediated toxicity must be that of fixation of antibody and the induction of conformation changes in the antibody molecules that are required to interact with C (Henney and Ishizaka, 1968). From these considerations one would expect the nature (e.g., shape, form, size, distribution, etc.) of the antigen or of antigen-determinant groups to be important. Experimental evidence in support of these ideas is available (Ishizaka *et al.,* 1968; Ishizaka *et al.,* 1966; Cuniff and Stollar, 1968). Apart from these considerations, for C killing to occur, it is obvious that antibody must be of the C fixing type and remain effective on the cell surface long enough to activate the C sequence.

2.2. Antibody

In general, in studies of antibody-C-mediated killing of nucleated cells, the class of antibody is not known. Antisera contain a heterogenous population of antibody molecules that vary in affinity and avidity for antigen and complement-fixing ability (Borsos, 1971; Hoyer *et al.,* 1968; Plotz *et al.,* 1968). This variation is a complication in attempts to interpret the reasons for the variability of particular cell types to be killed by antibody and C. A good example of the quantitative aspects involved can be seen in the sheep red cell–Forssman antibody model system. In these studies, it has been determined that one complement-fixing IgM molecule is sufficient to initiate the damage-producing steps and to cause lysis of the cell, whereas hundreds or thousands of IgG molecules must be fixed to produce one complement-fixing site before lysis can occur (Humphrey and Dourmashkin, 1965; Borsos and Rapp, 1965a; Cohen, 1968). The need for large numbers of IgG

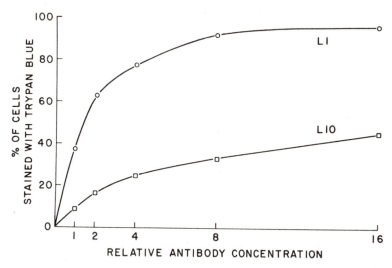

Figure 4. Lysis of IgM Forssman antibody sensitized line 1 and line 10 tumor cells. HuC diluted 1:8, with line 10, 1 = 1:80 dilution of antibody; with line 1, 1= 1:1280 dilution of antibody.

TABLE 1. Sensitivity of Line 1 and Line 10 Cells to Lysis by Human, Rabbit, and Guinea Pig Complement Sources[a]

Cells	Human C[b]	Rabbit C[b]	Rabbit C 2[b]	Guinea pig C[b]
Line 1				
Anti-Forssman[c]	61[d]	53	N.D.[e]	21
Anti-line 1[c]	54	29	N.D.	8
Cell control	15	15	N.D.	15
C control	14	12	N.D.	9
Line 10				
Anti-Forssman[c]	44	18	20	20
Anti-line 10[c]	69	24	63	16
Cell control	19	19	19	19
C control	16	14	14	19

[a]From Ohanian *et al.* (1973).
[b]Complement sources diluted 1:8.
[c]Anti-Forssman, anti-line 1 (R1), and anti-line 10 (RA) at dilutions where approximately 50% of the cells were stained with trypan blue.
[d]Percentage of cells stained with trypan blue.
[e]Not done.

molecules to generate a few complement-fixing sites probably reflects the need for at least two adjacent C fixing IgG molecules to initiate C fixation and the possible interference of this configuration by non-complement-fixing molecules in the antisera (Basch, 1974; Borsos and Rapp, 1965b; Thompson and Hoffmann, 1974; Humphrey and Dourmashkin, 1965).

To overcome the problem of class of antibody, it is necessary to use antibody preparations of known activity. This can be done with the IgM Forssman antibody system, since the number of C1 fixing molecules can be determined accurately for any antibody preparation. Using this antibody with the guinea pig tumor cell system, we have found that resistance of the tumor cells to immune killing cannot be correlated with lack of binding of C fixing antibody. This can be seen most clearly in Table 2. In addition, resistance could not be correlated with loss of C fixing antibody from the cell surface. These facts are further supported by the

TABLE 2. Number of C1 Fixing Sites per Cell Generated at Dilutions of Specific Antibody Giving One Cytolytic Site per Cell[a]

	Line 1	Line 10
R1	780[b]	N.D.[c]
R2	3800	N.D.
RA	N.D.	40,000
R293	N.D.	3,000

[a]Rabbit anti-line 1 (R1 and R2) and rabbit anti-line 10 (RA and R293) at dilutions where 63% of the cells were killed on addition of complement.
[b]Number of C1 molecules bound per cell sensitized with the indicated antibody.
[c]Not done.

observations that the antibody-coated tumor cells can be killed more efficiently by HuC than by rabbit or GPC (See Table 1). It would appear, therefore, that antibody does bind C1 in close proximity to the cell surface and that resistance of nucleated cells to killing may be the result of other factors, such as the paucity or absence of binding sites for some C components, the lack of surface areas susceptible to C action, and the topographical relationship between cell surface antigen and C binding sites. Other considerations include the cell's ability to repair cell surface damage or the prevention of damage to cell surface areas under attack by C.

In all *in vitro* studies concerning lysis of sheep erythrocytes or killing of nucleated cells, antibody alone failed to kill the cells. However, antibody in conjunction with complement can lead to the killing of the target cells. The effects of antibody and complement on nucleated cells include changes in morphology (Goldberg and Green, 1959; Bickis *et al.*, 1959; Latta and Kutsakis, 1957; Miller and Hsu, 1956; Ellem, 1958), permeability (Ellem, 1957; Flax, 1956; Green *et al.*, 1959; Green and Goldberg, 1960), and metabolic processes (Flax, 1956, Bickis *et al.*, 1959).

Studies with cold agglutinins in the lysis of human erythrocytes by C have shown that the only role antibody has in the lytic process is to initiate the fixation of C to the cell surface (Harboe *et al.*, 1963; Harboe, 1964; Rosse, 1968).

It is concluded from these studies that for complement to be effective, the cell must possess binding sites for C and sites susceptible to the effect of C.

2.3. Complement

2.3.1. Paucity or Absence of Binding Sites for C Action

It has generally been found that xenogeneic C is better than allogeneic or syngeneic C in the killing of antibody-coated cells (Fass and Herberman, 1969; Baker *et al.*, 1971; Haughton and McGehee, 1969). Part of the reason may be the presence of natural antibodies in the xenogeneic C source, which are directed against normal tissue antigens of the target cell (Mittal *et al.*, 1973). This, however, does not seem to be the whole reason, for in our studies extensive absorption of the C source with target cells does not change the relative activity of the C to kill the target cells (Ohanian *et al.*, 1973).

In most studies, no attempts were made to determine whether the lack of sensitivity to killing was due to the lack of activation and fixation of C. In our studies, we have measured the fixation of C4 and C3 during killing of the tumor cells by antibody and C (Ohanian and Borsos, 1975). Tables 3 and 4 show the quantitative aspects of killing of line 1 and line 10 tumor cells by antibody and C and the binding of Hu and GP C4 and C3 to the cell surface. In the red cell system, it has been estimated that several hundred molecules of cell-bound C4 and C3 are required to generate one cytolytic site on sensitized erythrocytes (Müller-Eberhard, 1968; Shin and Mayer, 1968). The observation that hundreds of thousands of C4 and C3 molecules are associated with unlysed or partially lysed tumor cells is evidence for the killing inefficiency of the bound components. It would appear, in contrast to the red cell system, that millions of C4 and hundreds of thousands of C3 are required to generate one cytotoxic site (63% killing) per antibody-coated line 1 and line 10 cell.

Other investigators have also found that resistance to killing cannot be attributed to lack of activation and/or fixation of large amounts of C (Table 5) (Lerner *et*

TABLE 3. Quantitation of Hu and GP C4 and C3 on Line 1 Tumor Cells Sensitized with Anti-Forssman IgM Antibody or Specific Anti-Line 1 Antibody[a]

Cell treatment[b]	Trypan blue positive cells (%)[c]	Molecules C4 per cell ($\times 10^{-5}$)[d]	Molecules C3 per cell ($\times 10^{-5}$)[d]
(1) Line 1 + anti-Forssman 1:5 + GPC 1:8	61±4	11.1 ±2.5	7.4 ±0.74
(2) Line 1 + anti-Forssman 1:800 + GPC 1:8	3±3	1.9 ±1.1	1.65±0.8
(3) Line 1 + anti-line 1 1:30 + GPC 1:8	0	N.D.[e]	0.48±0.37
(4) Line 1 + VBS + GPC 1:8	0	0.5 ±0.5	0.27±0.16
(5) Line 1 + anti-Forssman 1:5 + HuC 1:8	95±1.5	10.0 ±2.4	2.6 ±0.56
(6) Line 1 + anti-Forssman 1:800 + HuC	56±0.6	3.2 ±0.84	3.7 ±1.0
(7) Line 1 + anti-line 1 1:30 + HuC	65±2	6.3 ±0.73	3.8 ±0.53
(8) Line 1 + VBS + HuC	0	0.24±0.24	1.53±0.5

[a] From Ohanian and Borsos (1975).
[b] C1 fixing sites generated per cell with dilutions of antibody: anti-Forssman diluted 1:5, $0.56 \times 10^5 \pm 0.03$; anti-Forssman diluted 1:800, $0.011 \times 10^5 \pm 0.002$; anti-line 1 diluted 1:30, $0.171 \times 10^5 \pm 0.05$.
[c] Percent trypan blue positive cells = (1 − percent nonstained in experiment/percent nonstained in cell control) × 100.
[d] Number of molecules per cell calculated from an estimated molecular weight of 230,000 for Hu and GP C4 and 185,000 for Hu and GPC3. Calculations made after subtracting in each experiment the amount of C4 or C3 in control tubes receiving VBS and C 1:8 alone.
[e] Not detected after correcting for control values.

al., 1971; Pellegrino et al., 1974; Cooper et al., 1974). In these studies, cells taken from various phases of their growth cycle were examined for their sensitivity to killing and the quantity of C components bound to their surfaces. While comparable amounts of components were detected on cells examined at the different growth phase, only those from the G_1 or S phase were killed by the antibody and C. In addition, electron-microscopic examination of cells showed that ultrastructural lesions could be detected on cells that were resistant to killing by antibody and C (Cooper et al., 1974).

Thus, it would appear that while activation and fixation of complement are necessary for cell killing, cell killing does not necessarily result from activation and fixation.

2.3.2. Topographical Relationship Between Cell Surface Antigen and C Binding Sites

Part of the reason for the lack of sensitivity to antibody-C-mediated killing, in spite of the fact that large amounts of C components can be detected on the cell

TABLE 4. Quantitation of Hu and GP C4 and C3 on Line 10 Tumor Cells Sensitized with IgM Anti-Forssman Antibody or Specific Anti-Line 10 Antibody[a]

Cell treatment[b]	Trypan blue positive cells (%)[c]	Molecules C4 per cell ($\times 10^{-5}$)[d]	Molecules C3 per cell ($\times 10^{-5}$)[d]
(1) Line 10 + anti-Forssman, undiluted + GPC 1:8	2.5±1.6	19.1 ±3.2	5.4 ±1.4
(2) Line 10 + anti-line-10, 1:20 + GPC 1:8	3.3±2.6	10.8 ±1.8	5.0 ±0.91
(3) Line 10 + VBS + GPC 1:8	0	0.94±0.44	1.34±0.51
(4) Line 10 + anti-Forssman, undiluted + HuC 1:8	33.0±5.3	12.5 ±1.7	3.8 ±0.76
(5) Line 10 + anti-line-10, 1:20 + HuC 1:8	60.0±4.9	17.9 ±0.89	12.4 ±1.36
(6) Line 10 + VBS + HuC 1:8	0	0.82±0.29	1.05±0.66

[a] From Ohanian and Borsos (1975).
[b] C1 fixing sites generated per cell with dilutions of antibody anti-Forssman, undiluted, $1.2 \times 10^5 \pm 0.13$; anti-line 10, 1:20; $2.35 \times 10^5 \pm 0.28$.
[c] Percent trypan blue positive cells calculated as described in Table 3.
[d] Number of molecules per cell calculated as described in Table 3.

surface, may be the fact that the location of the antigen–antibody C1 complex to C binding sites on the cell surface is such that sufficient numbers of cytolytically active clusters of components are not generated on the cell surface. While there is very little, if any, information concerning this point on nucleated cells, there is evidence for it in the sheep red cell model. It has been demonstrated (Müller-Eberhard, 1968) that activated components of complement must bind to the cell surface within a very short time after activation to retain their hemolytic activity. Borsos *et al.* (1970) have demonstrated that C4 molecules bound to sheep red cells may exist in various states of hemolytic activity. In addition, these authors have shown that the rate, but not the extent, of hemolysis is dependent on the number of clusters of SAC142 generated on the cell surface (Opferkuch *et al.,* 1971). In these studies, the C components were quantitated by their functional activity, but not in molecular terms. It is difficult to quantitate functional activity of complement components on nucleated cells; however, it is possible to measure, in molecular terms, the amount of individual components bound to nucleated cells.

Using these methods, we have found that in the guinea pig tumor system, line 1 and line 10 tumor cells coated with anti-Forssman antibody generally have more GPC4 and C3 than HuC4 and C3 bound per cell (see Tables 3 and 4), while the opposite is the case when the tumor cells are coated with specific antitumor antibody. These results strongly suggest that the topographical location of the Forssman antibody binding sites is such that GPC4 and C3 may bind more efficiently than HuC4 and C3. However, the tumor antigen site is located such that HuC4 and C3 may bind more efficiently than GPC4 and C3. This latter observation may be a partial reason why antitumor-antibody-sensitized cells are more sensitive to killing than anti-Forssman sensitized cells.

2.3.3. Lack of Areas Susceptible to C Action

It is proposed that for hemolysis of sheep red cells or killing of nucleated cells to occur, the late-acting C components C8 and C9 interact with some as yet chemically unidentified component of the membrane, subsequently causing the cells to lose their semipermeable qualities (Müller-Eberhard, 1968; Mayer, 1972; Humphrey and Dourmashkin, 1969).

From the available evidence, however, it would appear that the areas suscepti-

TABLE 5. Binding of C5 and C8 and Cytotoxicity on Addition of Anti-Viral Antibody and Complement to a Synchronized Population of YCAB Cells[a]

Time after release from G_1 (hr)	Phase of cell cycle	Molecules per cell[b]		Cytotoxicity[c]
		C5	C8	
0	Early G_1	8,170	16,600	++
16	S	18,150	17,345	0
21	S, G_2, M	20,800	20,620	0

[a]From Cooper *et al.* (1974).
[b]After subtraction of values for nonspecific binding. These values were 10,800, 10,550, and 7,760 molecules of C5, and 19,000, 19,900, and 22,200 molecules of C8 per cell for the 0-, 16-, and 21-hr samples, respectively.
[c]++:>50%; 0: <10%.

ble to C action are distinct from the C9 binding site, since resistance to killing is observed in spite of the activation and fixation of larger amounts of C8 or C9 (Lerner *et al.,* 1971; Cooper *et al.,* 1974). Indeed, electron-microscopic examination of the physical size of "holes" produced in cell membranes by HuC, on the one hand, and GPC, on the other, suggests that the end-products of C from different sources (Humphrey and Dourmashkin, 1969) differ. The damage-causing agent could be generated from the bound C component or could arise by alteration or removal of substances pre-existing in the membrane (Smith and Becker, 1968). At present, it is not possible to determine which of the alternatives is true.

That large amounts of C components are required to kill nucleated cells suggests that resistance to killing may reflect intrinsic properties of the cells. These properties may be the cell's ability to repair C damaged sites and/or to inhibit the action of C. In the next section, we will discuss some of our studies that suggest the existence of such cellular properties.

3. Role of Cell Repair of C Damage or Inhibition of C Action

The relative inefficiency of antibody-C-mediated lysis of nucleated cells compared to red cells may reflect the ability of the nucleated cell to repair damage caused by complement or to inactivate the cell-bound components. At the present time, it is not possible to differentiate between the alternatives.

In our attempts to study the cellular defense mechanism against immune injury, we have employed inhibitors of macromolecule synthesis and drugs commonly used in the treatment of cancer (Segerling *et al.,* 1974, 1975a,b,c). In these studies, both line 1 and line 10 cells can be made sensitive to antitumor-antibody-GPC-mediated killing if they were pretreated with certain of the inhibitors (Table 6). The tumor cells were incubated for 17 hr at 37°C in culture medium containing inhibitor at concentrations that were nontoxic. After this time, the cells were washed and tested for their sensitivity. It will be noted that selected drugs were effective with line 1 cells (5 FU and 6 MP), but not with line 10 cells or vice versa (vincristine). In addition, it was noted that one preparation of tumor cells may not be rendered susceptible to killing following treatment with a particular inhibitor [shown by (+)] even though most other preparations would be rendered susceptible by the same inhibitor. The reason for this variability is not clear at the moment; however, since the tumor cells used in these studies were obtained after growth *in vivo,* such variations may represent the effect of host factors (Evans *et al.,* 1975).

The sensitivity of these tumor cells to antibody and HuC, to which they are normally susceptible, can be further increased by inhibitor treatment. This observation is similar to the findings of other investigators who used cultured human cell lines normally sensitive to HLA alloantibody and rabbit C (Ferrone *et al.,* 1974). These authors found that cycloheximide and puromycin, but not actinomycin D treatment, increased the cell's sensitivity.

While there is no evidence to prove the existence of prevention of damage to cell membranes and/or repair of damaged surface antigen, we have evidence to support the requirement for at least some level of macromolecular synthesis in the resistance of the cells. This comes from our observations that the effect of inhibitors is dose dependent, reversible, and temperature dependent (Segerling *et al.,* 1975b). Figure 5 shows the results obtained with varying concentrations of five effective inhibitors on line 10 tumor cells. It is evident that sensitivity to killing with saturating levels of either anti-Forssman or antitumor antibody plus GPC was dependent on the concentration of inhibitors used to treat the cells. Similar experiments were carried out with line 1 tumor cells, and these also showed that increased sensitivity was dependent on the concentration of inhibitors used to treat the cells.

Figure 6 shows the results of the reversibility tests obtained with puromycin. It will be seen that cells cultured for 17 hr in the presence of the inhibitor begin to show resistance to killing by antitumor antibody or anti-Forssman antibody after culturing for 4–7 hr in medium free of added inhibitor. This figure also shows that untreated cells transferred to medium with puromycin become sensitive to killing within 4–7 hr. Similar results were obtained with other active drugs.

The effectiveness of inhibitors in increasing cell susceptibility also depended on the temperature of incubation; i.e., cells incubated with the inhibitor at 37°C become sensitive to killing, but cells incubated at 4°C do not. Furthermore, reversion of inhibitor-treated cells, from susceptible to resistant, occurred at 37°C but not at 4°C.

TABLE 6.   Effect of Inhibitors on the Killing of Line 1 and Line 10 Cells by Antibody and GPC[a]

Inhibitor	Line 1		Line 10	
	Anti-Forssman	Anti-line 1	Anti-Forssman	Anti-line 10
Actinomycin D (25 μg/ml)	+	+	+	+
Puromycin (25 μg/ml)	+	+	+	+
Mitomycin C (20 μg/ml)	+	+	+	+
Hydroxyurea (500 μg/ml)	+	+	(+)	(+)
Adriamycin (50 μg/ml)	+	+	+	+
Vincristine (20 μg/ml)	0	(+)	+	(+)
Cytosine arabinoside (100 μg/ml)	(+)	0	0	0
Azacytidine (20 μg/ml)	+	(+)	(+)	(+)
Methotrexate (500 μg/ml)	+	(+)	(+)	(+)
Cyclophosphamide (100 μg/ml)	(+)	0	(+)	(+)
5 FU (500 μg/ml)	+	0	0	0
6 MP (500 μg/ml)	+	0	0	0

[a] +: All cell preparations were rendered susceptible to killing by antibody plus GPC. Sensitivity of drug-treated cells to killing by antibody-C was at least two-fold higher than that of the untreated cells. (+): Not all cell preparations were rendered susceptible. 0: No cell preparation was rendered susceptible.

SARKIS H. OHANIAN
AND TIBOR BORSOS

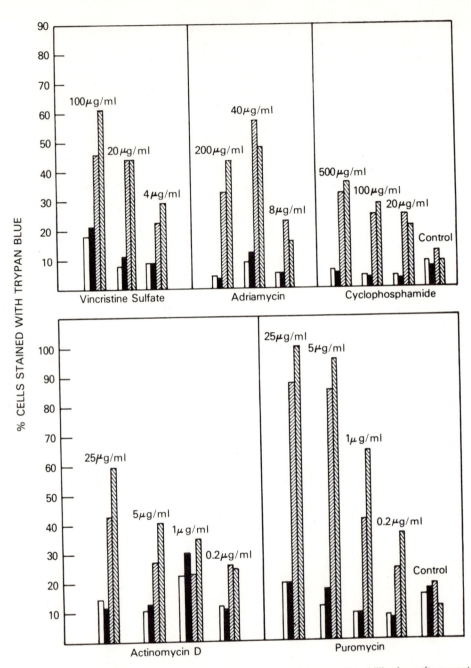

Figure 5. Effect of inhibitor concentration on sensitivity of line 10 tumor cells to killing by antitumor antibody and GPC. Tumor cells were incubated 17 hr at 37°C in air–5% CO_2 in RPMI 1640–20% FCS containing the concentrations of inhibitor indicated above each group of four bars. Controls are results with tumor cells cultured in medium free of inhibitors: (□) Cells plus buffer control; (■) cells plus GPC diluted 1:8 control; (▨) cells plus anti-Forssman antibody diluted 1:2 plus GPC diluted 1:8; (▧) cells plus specific antitumor antibody diluted 1:20 plus GPC diluted 1:8.

In preliminary experiments employing radiolabeled precursors of DNA, RNA, and protein, we have found that the level of drug required to give maximal sensitivity to killing was 2–5 times more than that required to inhibit the synthesis of these macromolecules (Ohanian, unpublished observations). In addition, treated tumor cells that had reverted back to the resistant state after 4 and 7 hr still had not recovered their capacity for macromolecular synthesis. These results suggest that resistance is not solely dependent on the synthesis of macromolecules.

Other investigators have shown that cells treated with some of the inhibitors used in our study either increased, decreased, or had no effect on antigen expression (Cikes and Klein, 1972a; Ferrone *et al.*, 1972). In our studies, the increased sensitivity of the tumor cells to antibody-C-mediated killing cannot be ascribed to

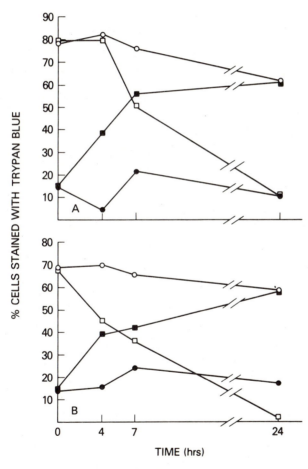

Figure 6. Effect of time of inhibitor treatment on sensitivity of line 10 tumor cells to antibody-C-mediated cytotoxicity. Tumor cells cultured in medium without puromycin (●); cultured 17 hr without puromycin, washed, and cultured in medium with puromycin (■); cultured with puromycin (○); cultured 17 hr with puromycin, washed, and cultured in medium without puromycin (□). (A) Specific anti-line 10 diluted 1:20; (B) anti-Forssman antibody diluted 1:2. Guinea pig complement diluted 1:8.

measurable increases in antigen expression or binding of C4 and C3 to the tumor cell membranes (Tables 7 and 8) (Segerling *et al.*, 1975c). Furthermore, antigen movement used as one measure of membrane properties could not be associated with the change in sensitivity of the cells (Boyle *et al.*, 1975). These results confirm and extend our previous observations and those of others that antigen expression and amount of antibody and C components bound to cells do not correlate in a simple way with the efficiency of cell killing by antibody and C (Cooper *et al.*, 1974; Ferrone *et al.*, 1973; Lerner *et al.*, 1971; Ohanian *et al.*, 1973; Ohanian and Borsos, 1975; Pellegrino *et al.*, 1974).

Studies concerning the variability in the sensitivity of cells taken from different phases of their growth cycle suggest, in agreement with our results, that cellular changes may be responsible for differences in resistance to killing by antibody and C (Cikes, 1970a,b; Cikes and Friberg, 1971; Cooper *et al.*, 1974; Götze *et al.*, 1972; Lerner *et al.*, 1971; Pasternak *et al.*, 1971; Pellegrino *et al.*, 1974; Shipley, 1971). The cells used by the various investigators were from different species and of different morphological types, and some were more sensitive at either the G_1 or S phases and others at G_0 phases of their growth cycle. However, no one phase of the growth cycle appeared to correlate with the sensitivity to killing in all the systems studied.

Enzymes have been used by many investigators to increase the sensitivity of serological reactions on nucleated cells. The increased sensitivity has been ascribed to increased antigen expression and/or increased efficiency of C action. Using enzymes of differing specificity to modify the cell surface of the line 10 guinea pig hepatoma cell, we have found that only cells treated with proteolytic enzymes

TABLE 7. Measurement of Antigen Expression and Sensitivity to Killing by Antibody Plus C of Line 10 Hepatoma Cells Following Treatment with Inhibitors[a]

Experiment	Anti-Forssman antibody		Anti-line 10 antibody	
	Trypan blue stained cells (%)	C1 fixing sites per cell ($\times 10^{-4}$)	Trypan blue stained cells (%)	C1 fixing sites per cell ($\times 10^{-4}$)
Experiment 1				
No treatment	11	4.3	10	4.4
6 MP (500 μg/ml)	25	3.6	32	4.8
Azacytidine (20 μg/ml)	50	2.5	78	6.4
Experiment 2				
No treatment	5	3.0	6	15.4
Adriamycin (40 μg/ml)	57	1.3	53	3.7
Experiment 3				
No treatment	16	8.4	20	36.4
Actinomycin D (25 μg/ml)	40	4.5	59	34.0
Experiment 4				
No treatment	4	5.4	4	10.2
Puromycin (5 μg/ml)	57	3.2	71	3.4
Hydroxyurea (500 μg/ml)	11	5.0	25	6.0

[a] Dilution of anti-Forssman antibody, 1:2; Dilution of anti-line 10 antibody, 1:15.

TABLE 8. Measurement of GP C4 and C3 on Inhibitor-Treated Line 10 Tumor Cells Sensitized with Anti-Forssman or Specific Antitumor Antibody

Experiment	Trypan blue stained cells (%)		Molecules C4 per cell ($\times 10^{-5}$)[a]		Molecules C3 per cell ($\times 10^{-5}$)[a]	
	No treatment	Inhibitor-treated	No treatment	Inhibitor-treated	No treatment	Inhibitor-treated
Experiment 1: Puromycin (5 μg)						
Line 10 + anti-Forssman 1:2 + GPC 1:8	0	63	18.0±0.8	6.8 ±0.5	10.1 ±0.45	6.9±0.35
Line 10 + anti-line 10 1:15 + GPC 1:8	0	63	69.3±2.2	45.0 ±0.2	12.8 ±0	9.8±0.15
Line 10 + buffer + GPC 1:8	11	9	5.2	1.0	N.D.[b]	0.7
Line 10 + buffer + buffer	2	7	N.D.	N.D.	N.D.	1.6
Experiment 2: Adriamycin (50 μg)						
Line 10 + anti-Forssman 1:2 + GPC 1:8	6	52	6.8±0.95	4.0 ±0.8	4.95±0.45	4.7±0.1
Line 10 + anti-line 10 1:15 + GPC 1:8	6	51	45.5±0.5	21.8 ±0.8	15.3 ±0.5	7.0±1.0
Line 10 + buffer + GPC 1:8	0	5	N.D.	N.D.	1.2	1.6
Line 10 + buffer + buffer	1	5	N.D.	N.D.	0.3	3.6
Experiment 3: Actinomycin D (25 μg)						
Line 10 + anti-Forssman 1:2 + GPC 1:8	7	26	22.6±0.95	17.6 ±0.6	14.8 ±0	11.8±0.04
Line 10 + anti-line 10 1:15 + GPC 1:8	11	43	90.0±0.75	76.0 ±1.0	17.3 ±0	17.9±0.7
Line 10 + buffer + GPC 1:8	9	14	3.1	1.2	3.2	1.5
Line 10 + buffer + buffer	13	11	1.3	1.2	3.2	1.3
Experiment 4: Azacytidine (20 μg)						
Line 10 + anti-Forssman 1:2 + GPC 1:8	11	58	10.5±0.5	9.95±0.6	7.0 ±0	9.6±0.16
Line 10 + anti-line 10 1:15 + GPC 1:8	12	63	30.5±0.1	28.3 ±2.0	10.4 ±0	14.1±0.45
Line 10 + buffer + GPC 1:8	0	1	0.91	1.3	2.8	7.0
Line 10 + buffer + buffer	0	2	1.55	1.9	0.7	0.42

[a]Number of molecules per cell calculated from an estimated molecular weight of 230,000 for GPC4 and 185,000 for GPC3. Calculations made after subtracting in each experiment the amount of C4 and C3 in control tubes receiving just GPC diluted 1:8.
[b]None detected after correcting for control tube receiving just GPC diluted 1:8.

showed increased sensitivity to killing by antibody plus HuC or GPC (Table 9). The increased killing could not be ascribed to increased expression of antigen. Treatment with DNAse, RNAse, β-glucuronidase, hyaluronidase, pectinesterase, or lipase were not effective (Boyle, *et al.*, 1976a). An interesting and possibly very important observation was that tumor cells treated with neuraminidase showed increased susceptibility to HuC only. The results would suggest that the site of action of HuC may be chemically different from the site of action of GPC.

As mentioned previously, it is not possible at present to determine whether the nucleated cell is able to repair damage caused by C action and/or to inactivate cell-bound C components. Results from other laboratories have shown that loss of antibody from tumor cells occurs when the cells are cultured under physiological conditions (Chang, 1967; Amos *et al.*, 1970; Chang *et al.*, 1971; Ran *et al.*, 1974). In addition, there is evidence that tumor cells are capable of degrading cell-bound protein molecules and that degradation and release of cell-bound immunoglobulin can occur (Keisari and Witz, 1973; Dauphinee *et al.*, 1974; Fish *et al.*, 1974). In experiments that confirm and extend these observations, we have shown that line 10 tumor cells coated *in vitro* or *in vivo* with antibody and the initial components of GPC, C4, and C3 lose these molecules upon transfer to *in vitro* culture conditions (Segerling *et al.*, 1976). Complement-fixing activity of cell-bound antibody, C4, and C3 disappeared rapidly at 37°C, but significant losses also occurred at 4°C. The continued presence of cell-bound Ig in a noncomplement fixing form could be demonstrated while no complement-fixing activity was released into the medium. On the other hand, both C4 and C3 were released into the medium and could be demonstrated in the medium by immunochemical methods. Treatment of the cells with metabolic inhibitors did not prevent the loss of components. Taken together, the results suggest that either mechanical release and/or release due to enzyme activity of the cell may play an important role in the resistance of nucleated cells to humoral immune attack.

Studies on the terminal stages of immune hemolysis have demonstrated that, in

TABLE 9. Effect of Enzyme Pretreatment on the Killing of Line 10 by Antibody and C[a,b]

Enzyme	Anti-Forssman + GPC	Anti-line 10 + GPC	Anti-Forssman + HuC	Anti-line 10 + HuC
Trypsin	±	±	±	±
Papain	+	+	+	+
Ficin	+	+	+	+
Elastase	+	+	+	+
Collagenase	+	+	+	+
Bromelain	+	+	+	+
Lipase type I[c]	+	+	+	+
Lipase type VI[c]	+	+	+	+
Lipase type VII	0	0	0	0
Neuraminidase *Vibrio cholerea*	0	0	+	+
Neuraminidase *Cl. perfringens*[c]	+	+	+	+
Neuraminidase *Cl. perfringens* (purified)[d]	0	0	+	+
Neuraminidase ex influenza virus	0	0	+	+

[a]From Boyle *et al.* (1976a).
[b]+—Increase in susceptibility compared with untreated cells; ±—Marginal increase in susceptibility; 0—No increase in susceptibility.
[c]Contains protease activity.
[d]Purified courtesy of Dr. E. Regoeczi, Department of Pathology, McMaster University, Hamilton, Ontario, Canada.

addition to binding of all the necessary components of complement by antibody-coated sheep erythrocytes, a number of further steps are required before hemoglobin is released. An erythrocyte in this state has been isolated and designated E* (Mayer and Levine, 1954; Kabat and Mayer, 1961). A nucleated cell in this state has also been isolated and termed T* (Boyle *et al.,* 1976b,c,d). The isolation of this intermediate has provided an ideal tool with which to study the terminal stages of killing of a nucleated cell by antibody and complement.

With this intermediate, it was found that 3',5' cAMP blocked the transformation of T* to dead cells and that prolonged incubation at 37°C with the cyclic nucleotide caused a reversion of the cells from the potentially lethal state to a nondamaged form (Boyle *et al.,* 1976c). In addition, a diverse range of compounds with reported effects on cell membrane mobility or permeability (i.e., histamine, dimethylsulfoxide, NaF, EDTA, and cytochalasin B) have been found to block the transformation of T* to dead cells. However, prolonged incubation with these agents did not nullify the T* state (Boyle *et al.,* 1976d).

All the studies cited indicate that cellular events under metabolic control modulate the susceptibility of the cell to killing by complement. Since the action of C takes place on or in the cell membrane, it is postulated that the intracellular events, affected by the inhibitors, and cAMP most likely control membrane integrity. It is the task of future studies to elucidate the mechanisms whereby intracellular events govern cell surface properties and ultimately furnish explanations for the basis of the resistance of nucleated cells to immune injury.

4. Summary

The susceptibility of nucleated cells to the killing action of antibody plus C does not depend solely on antigen expression, class of antibody, or activation and fixation of C. While each of these points is important, other factors, such as (1) location of antigen relative to C binding sites, (2) sufficient number of cell surface areas susceptible to C action, (3) repair of C damaged area, (4) inactivation of cell-bound C components by the cell, and (5) other as yet undefined physical properties of the cell membrane, must also be considered.

ACKNOWLEDGMENT

We thank Ms. Nancy Branch for her expert help in preparing this manuscript.

References

Amos, D. B., Cohen, I., and Klein, W. J., 1970, Mechanism of immunological enhancement, *Transplant. Proc.* 2:68–75.

Baker, A. R., Borsos, T., and Colten, H. R., 1971, Cytotoxic action of antiserum and complement. Quantitation with a colony inhibition method, *Immunology* 101:33–43.

Basch, R. S., 1974, Effect of antigen density and non-complement fixing antibody on cytolysis by alloantisera, *J. Immunol.* 113:554–562.

Bickis, I. J., Quastel, J. H., and Vas, S. I., 1959, Effect of Ehrlich ascites antisera on the biochemical activities of Ehrlich ascites carcinoma cells *in vitro, Cancer Res.* 19:602–607.

Borsos, T., 1971, Immunoglobulin classes and complement-fixing activity, in: *Progress in Immunology,* pp. 841–848, Academic Press, New York.

Borsos, T., and Rapp, H. J., 1965a, Hemolysin titration bases on fixation of the activated first component of complement: evidence that one molecule of hemolysin suffices to sensitize an erythrocyte, *J. Immunol.* **95**:559–566.

Borsos, T., and Rapp, H. J., 1965b, Complement fixation on cell surfaces by 19S and 7S antibodies, *Science* **150**:505–506.

Borsos, T., Rapp, H. J., and Colten, H. R., 1970, Immune hemolysis and the functional properties of the second (C2) and fourth (C4) components of complement. I. Functional differences among C4 sites on cell surfaces, *J. Immunol.* **105**:1439–1446.

Borsos, T., Richardson, A. K., Ohanian, S. H., and Leonard, E. J., 1973, Immunochemical detection of tumor-specific and embryonic antigens of diethylnitrosamine-induced guinea pig tumors, *J. Nat. Cancer Inst.* **51**:1955–1960.

Boyle, M. D. P., Ohanian, S. H., and Borsos, T., 1975, Lysis of tumor cells by antibody and complement. III. Lack of correlation between antigen movement and cell lysis, *J. Immunol.* **115**:473–475.

Boyle, M. D. P., Ohanian, S. H., and Borsos, T., 1976a, Lysis of tumor cells by antibody and complement. VI. Enhanced killing of enzyme pretreated tumor cells, *J. Immunol.* **116**:661–668.

Boyle, M. D. P., Ohanian, S. H., and Borsos, T., 1976b, Studies on the terminal stages of antibody-complement mediated killing of a tumor cell. I. Evidence for the existence of an intermediate, T*, *J. Immunol.* **116**:1272–1275.

Boyle, M. D. P., Ohanian, S. H., and Borsos, T., 1976c, Studies on the terminal stages of antibody-complement mediated killing of a tumor cell. II. Inhibition of transformation of T* to dead cells by 3'5' cAMP, *J. Immunol.* **116**:1276–1279.

Boyle, M. D. P., Ohanian, S. H., and Borsos, T., 1976d, Studies on the terminal stages of antibody-complement mediated killing of a tumor cell. III. Effect of membrane active agents, *J. Immunol.* **117**:106–109.

Chang, S., 1967, Measurement of complement in patients with bone sarcoma, *Jpn J. Exp. Med.* **37**:97–106.

Chang, S., Stockert, E., Boyse, E. A., Hammerling, U., and Old, L. J., 1971, Spontaneous release of cytotoxic alloantibody from viable cells sensitized in excess antibody, *Immunology* **21**:829–838.

Cikes, M., 1970a, Antigenic expression of a murine lymphoma during growth in vivo, *Nature* **225**:645–646.

Cikes, M., 1970b, Relationship between growth rate, cell volume, cell cycle kinetics, and antigenic properties of cultured murine lymphoma cells, *J. Nat. Cancer Inst.* **45**:979–988.

Cikes, M., and Friberg, S., 1971, Expression of H-2 and Moloney leukemia virus-determined cell-surface antigens in synchronized cultures of a mouse cell line, *Proc. Nat. Acad. Sci. U.S.A.* **68**:566–569.

Cikes, M., and Klein, G., 1972a, Effect of inhibitors of protein and nucleic acid synthesis on expression of H-2 and Moloney leukemia virus-determined cell-surface antigens on cultured murine lumphoma cells, *J. Nat. Cancer Inst.* **48**:509–515.

Cikes, M., and Klein, G., 1972b, Quantitative studies of antigen exppression in cultured murine lymphoma cells. I. Cell surface antigens in "asynchronous" cultures, *J. Nat. Cancer Inst.* **49**:1599–1606.

Cikes, M., Friberg, S., and Klein, G., 1972, Quantitative studies of antigen expression in cultured murine lymphoma cells. II. Cell-surface antigens in synchronized cultures, *J. Nat. Cancer Inst.* **49**:1607–1611.

Cohen, S., 1968, The requirement for the association of two adjacent rabbit γG-antibody molecules in the fixation of complement by immune complexes, *J. Immunol.* **100**:407–413.

Cooper, N. R., Polley, M. J., and Oldstone, M. B. A., 1974, Failure of terminal complement components to induce lysis of Moloney virus transformed lymphocytes, *J. Immunol.* **112**:866–868.

Cunniff, R. V., and Stollar, B. D., 1968, Properties of 19S antibodies in complement fixation. I. Temperature dependence and a role of antigen structure, *J. Immunol.* **100**:7–14.

Dauphinee, M. J., Talal, N., and Witz, I. P., 1974, Generation of non-complement-fixing, blocking factors by lysosomal extract treatment of cytotoxic anti-tumor antibodies, *J. Immunol.* **113**:948–953.

Ellem, K. A. O., 1957, Studies on the mechanism of the cytotoxic action of antisera, *Aust. J. Sci.* **20**:116–117.

Ellem, K. A. O., 1958, Some aspects of the ascites tumor cell response to a heterologous antiserum, *Cancer Res.* **18**:1179–1185.

Evans, C. H., Ohanian, S. H., and Cooney, A. M., 1975, Tumor-specific and Forssman antigens of guinea-pig hepatoma cells: comparison of tumor cells grown *in vivo* and *in vitro, Int. J. Cancer* **15**:512–521.

Fass, L., and Herberman, R. B., 1969, A cytotoxic antiglobulin technique for assay of antibodies to histocompatibility antigens, *J. Immunol.* **102**:140–144.

Ferrone, S., Cooper, N. R., Pellegrino, M. A., and Reisfeld, R. A., 1971, The lymphocytotoxic reaction: the mechanism of rabbit complement action, *J. Immunol.* **107**:939–947.

Ferrone, S., Del Villano, B., Pellegrino, M. A., Lerner, R. A., and Reisfeld, R. A., 1972, Expression of HL-A antigens on the surface of cultured lymphoid cells: effects of inhibitors of protein and nucleic acid synthesis, *Tissue Antigens* **2**:447–453.

Ferrone, S., Cooper, N. R., Pellegrino, M. A., and Reisfeld, R. A., 1973, Interaction of histocompatibility (HL-A) antibodies and complement with synchronized human lymphoid cells in continuous culture, *J. Exp. Med.* **137**:55–68.

Ferrone, S., Pellegrino, M. A., Dierich, M. P., and Reisfeld, R. A., 1974, Effect of inhibitors of macromolecular synthesis on HL-A antibody mediated lysis of cultured fibroblasts, *Tissue Antigens* **4**:275–282.

Fish, F., Witz, I. P., and Klein, G., 1974, Tumor bound immunoglobulins. The fate of immunoglobulin disappearing from the surface of coated tumor cells, *Clin. Exp. Immunol.* **16**:355–365.

Flax, M. H., 1956, The action of anti-Ehrlich ascites tumor antibody, *Cancer Res.* **16**:774–783.

Frank, M. M., Rapp, H. J., and Borsos, T., 1965, Mechanism of the damage-producing steps of immune haemolysis, in: *Ciba Found. Symp., Complement* (G. E. W. Wolstenholme and J. Knight, eds.), pp. 120–126, J. & A. Churchill, London.

Friberg, S., 1972, Comparison of an immunoresistant and an immunosusceptible ascites subline from murine tumor TA3. II. Immunosensitivity and antibody-binding capacity in vitro and immunogenecity in allogeneic mice, *J. Nat. Cancer Inst.* **48**:1477–1489.

Goldberg, B., and Green, H., 1959, The cytotoxic action of immune gamma globulin and complement on Krebs ascites tumor cells. I. Ultrastructural studies, *J. Exp. Med.* **109**:505–510.

Gorer, P. A., and O'Gorman, P., 1956, The cytotoxic activity of isoantibodies in mice, *Transplant. Bull.* **3**:142–143.

Götze, D., Pellegrino, M. A., Ferrone, S., and Reisfeld, R. A., 1972, Expression of H-2 antigens during growth of cultured tumor cells, *Immunol. Commun.* **1**:533–544.

Green, H., and Goldberg, B., 1960, The action of antibody and complement on mammalian cells, *Ann. N.Y. Acad. Sci.* **87**:352–362.

Green, H., Barrow, P., and Goldberg, B., 1959, Effect of antibody and complement on permeability control in ascites tumor cells and erythrocytes, *J. Exp. Med.* **110**:699–713.

Harboe, M., 1964, Interaction between I^{131} trace-labelled cold agglutinin, complement and red cells, *Br. J. Haemat.* **10**:339–346.

Harboe, M., Müller-Eberhard, H., Fudenberg, H., Polley, M. J., and Mollison, P. L., 1963, Identification of components of complement participating in the antiglobulin reaction, *Immunology* **6**:412–420.

Haughton, G., and McGehee, M. P., 1969, Cytolysis of mouse lymph node cells by alloantibody: a comparison of guinea pig and rabbit complements, *Immunology* **16**:447–461.

Henney, C. S., and Ishizaka, K., 1968, Heterogeneity in antibodies specific for aggregated human γG-globulin, J. Immunol. **101**:79–91.

Hoyer, L. W., Borsos, T., Rapp, H. J., and Vannier, W. E., 1968, Heterogeneity of rabbit IgM antibody as detected by C'1a fixation, *J. Exp. Med.* **127**:589–603.

Humphrey, J. H., and Dourmashkin, R. R., 1965, Electron microscope studies of immune cell lysis, in: *Ciba Found. Symp., Complement* (G. E. W. Wolstenholme and J. Knight, eds.), pp. 175–186, J. & A. Churchill, London.

Humphrey, J. H., and Dourmashkin, R. R., 1969, The lesions in cell membranes caused by complement, *Adv. Immunol.* **11**:75–116.

Ishizaka, K., Ishizaka, T., Borsos, T., and Rapp, H. J., 1966, C'1 fixation by human isoagglutinins: fixation of C'1 by γG and γM but not by γA antibody, *J. Immunol.* **97**:716–726.

Ishizaka, T., Tada, T., and Ishizaka, K., 1968, Fixation of C' and C'1a by rabbit γG and γM antibodies with particulate and soluble antigens, *J. Immunol.* **100**:1145–1153.

Kabat, E. A., and Mayer, M. M., 1961, *Experimental Immunochemistry,* p. 176, Charles C. Thomas, Springfield, Illinois.

Kalfayan, B., and Kidd, J. G., 1953, Structural changes produced in Brown-Pearce carcinoma cells by means of a specific antibody and complement, *J. Exp. Med.* **97**:145–163.

Keisari, Y., and Witz, I. P., 1973, Degradation of immunoglobulins by lysosomal enzymes of tumors. I. Demonstration of the phenomenon using mouse tumors, *Immunochemistry* **10**:565–570.

Latta, H., and Kutsakis, A., 1957, Cytotoxic effects of specific antiserum and 17-hydroxycorticosterone on cells in tissue culture, *Lab. Invest.* **6**:12–17.

Lerner, R. A., Oldstone, M. B. A., and Cooper, N. R., 1971, Cell cycle-dependent immune lysis of Moloney virus-transformed lymphocytes: presence or viral antigens, accessibility to antibody, and complement activation, *Proc. Nat. Acad. Sci. U.S.A.* **68**:2584–2588.

Levy, N. L., Amos, D. B., Solovieff, G. V., and dos Reis, A. P., 1972, *In vitro* methods for assessment of antibody mediated tumor immunity, *Nat. Cancer Inst. Monogr.* **35**:5–11.

Linscott, W. D., 1970, An antigen density effect on the hemolytic efficiency of complement, *J. Immunol.* **104**:1307–1309.

Mayer, M. M., 1961, Development of the one-hit theory of immune hemolysis, in: *Immunochemical Approaches to Problems in Microbiology* (M. Heidelberger and O. J. Plescia, eds.), p. 268, Rutgers University Press, New Brunswick, New Jersey.

Mayer, M. M., 1972, Mechanism of cytolysis by complement, *Proc. Nat. Acad. Sci. U.S.A.* **69**:2954–2958.

Mayer, M. M., and Levine, L. J., 1954, Kinetics of immune hemolysis. III. Description of a terminal process which follows the Ca^{++} and Mg^{++} reaction steps in the action of complement on sheep erythrocytes, *J. Immunol.* **72**:511–515.

Miller, D. G., and Hsu, T. C., 1956, The action of cytotoxic antisera on the HeLa strain of human carcinoma, *Cancer Res.* **16**:306–312.

Mittal, K. K., Ferrone, S., Mickey, M. R., Pellegrino, M. A., Reisfeld, R. A., and Terasaki, P. I., 1973, Serological characterization of natural anti-human lymphocytotoxic antibodies in mammalian sera, *Transplantation* **16**:287–294.

Moller, E., 1963, Quantitative studies on the differentiation of isoantigens in newborn mice, *Transplantation* **1**:165–173.

Moller, E., and Moller, G., 1962, Quantitative studies of sensitivity of normal and neoplastic cells to the cytotoxic action of isoantibodies, *J. Exp. Med.* **115**:527–553.

Müller-Eberhard, H. J., 1968, Chemistry and reaction mechanisms of complement, *Adv. Immunol.* **8**:1–80.

Ohanian, S. H., and Borsos, T., 1975, Lysis of tumor cells by antibody and complement. II. Lack of correlation between amount of C4 and C3 fixed and cell lysis, *J. Immunol.* **114**:1292–1295.

Ohanian, S. H., Borsos, T., and Rapp, H. J., 1973, Lysis of tumor cells by antibody and complement. I. Lack of correlation between antigen content and lytic susceptibility, *J. Nat. Cancer Inst.* **50**:1313–1320.

Opferkuch, W., Rapp, H. J., Colten, H. R., and Borsos, T., 1971, Immune hemolysis and the functional properties of the second (C2) and fourth (C4) components of complement. II. Clustering of effective $\overline{C42}$ complexes at individual hemolytic sites, *J. Immunol.* **106**:407–413.

Pasternak, C. A., Warmsley, A. M. H., and Thomas, D. B., 1971, Structural alterations in the surface membrane during the cell cycle, *J. Cell Biol.* **50**:562–564.

Pellegrino, M. A., Ferrone, S., Cooper, N. R., Dierich, M. P., and Reisfeld, R. A., 1974, Variation in susceptibility of a human lymphoid cell line to immune lysis during the cell cycle. Lack of correlation with antigen density and complement binding, *J. Exp. Med.* **140**:578–590.

Plotz, P. H., Colten, H. R., and Talal, N., 1968, Mouse macroglobulin antibody to sheep erythrocytes: A non-complement-fixing type, *J. Immunol.* **100**:752–755.

Ran, M., Fish, R., Witz, I. P., and Klein, G., 1974, Tumor bound immunoglobulins. The *in vitro* disappearance of immunoglobulin from the surface of coated tumor cells, and some properties of released components, *Clin. Exp. Immunol.* **16**:335–353.

Rapp, H. J., and Borsos, T., 1970, *Molecular Basis of Complement Action,* Appleton-Century-Crofts, New York.

Rapp, H. J., Churchill, W. H., Jr., Kronman, B. S., Rolley, R. T., Hammond, W. G., and Borsos, T., 1968, Antigenicity of a new diethylnitrosamine-induced transplantable guinea pig hepatoma: pathology and formation of ascites variant, *J. Nat. Cancer Inst.* **41**:1–11.

Rosse, W., 1968, Fixation of the first component of complement (C'1a) by human antibodies, *J. Clin. Invest.* **47**:2430–2445.

Schlesinger, M., 1965, Immune lysis of thymus and spleen cells of embryonic and neonatal mice, *J. Immunol.* **94**:358–364.

Segerling, M., Ohanian, S. H., and Borsos, T., 1974, Effect of metabolic inhibitors on killing of tumor cells by antibody and complement, *J. Nat. Cancer Inst.* **53**:1411–1413.

Segerling, M., Ohanian, S. H., and Borsos, T., 1975a, Chemotherapeutic drugs increase killing of tumor cells by antibody and complement, *Science* **188**:55–57.

Segerling, M., Ohanian, S. H., and Borsos, T., 1975b, Enhancing effect by metabolic inhibitors on the killing of tumor cells by antibody and complement, *Cancer Res.* **35**:3195–3203.

Segerling, M., Ohanian, S. H., and Borsos, T., 1975c, Effect of metabolic inhibitors on the ability of tumor cells to express antigen and bind complement components C4 and C3, *Cancer Res.* **35**:3204–3208.

Segerling, M., Ohanian, S. H., and Borsos, T., 1976, The persistence of immunoglobulin, C4 and C3 bound to guinea pig tumor cells, *J. Nat. Cancer Inst.* **57**:145–150.

Shin, H. S., and Mayer, M. M., 1968, The third component of guinea pig complement system. II. Kinetic studies of the reaction of EAC′42a with guinea pig C3. Enzymatic nature of C′3 consumption, multiphasic character of fixation, and hemolytic titration of C′3, *Biochemistry* **7**:2997–3002.

Shipley, W. U., 1971, Immune cytolysis in relation to the growth cycle of Chinese hamster cells, *Cancer Res.* **31**:925–929.

Smith, J. K., and Becker, E. L., 1968, Serum complement and the enzymatic degradation of erythrocyte phospholipid, *J. Immunol.* **100**:459–474.

Thompson, J. J., and Hoffmann, L. G., 1974, Cooperative binding of a complement component to antigen–antibody complexes. I. Complexes containing rabbit IgG antibody, *Immunochemistry* **11**:431–445.

Winn, H. J., 1960, The immune response and the homograft reaction, *Nat. Cancer Inst. Monogr.* **2**:113–138.

Zbar, B., Bernstein, I. D., and Rapp, H. J., 1971, Suppression of tumor growth at the site of infection with living bacillus Calmette-Guerin, *J. Nat. Cancer Inst.* **46**:831–839.

7

Serum Bactericidal Activity and Complement

LOUIS H. MUSCHEL and JACK S. C. FONG

1. General Considerations

1.1. Interaction between Complement and Bacterial Cell Membranes

The bactericidal reaction provided the first demonstration of the existence and cooperative effect of a thermostable substance, which is peculiar to immune serum, and a thermolabile substance, which is present in both normal and fresh immune serum. This discovery by Bordet (1895) that the killing of *Vibrio cholerae* by serum was mediated by antibody and complement (C) represents a very significant landmark in the history of serology and immunochemistry.

The immune bactericidal reaction depends, then, upon the activity of the C system against antibody-sensitized bacteria. In addition to the gram-negative enteric bacteria and cholera organisms, which have been widely used in studies of the immune bactericidal reaction, other susceptible bacteria include *Treponema pallidum*, constituting the basis of the treponemal immobilization test for the detection of antibodies against the treponemes that cause syphilis (Nelson and Mayer, 1949), leptospirae (Johnson and Muschel, 1966), hemophilus (Dingle *et al.*, 1938), gonococcus (Glynn and Ward, 1970), meningococcus (Goldschneider *et al.*, 1969), pseudomonas (Muschel *et al.*, 1969a), and others. Predictably, the mycoplasma group, which possesses the simplest level of organization of the cell surface in bacteria, is also sensitive to the C system (Gale and Kenny, 1970).

LOUIS H. MUSCHEL • Research Department, American Cancer Society, New York, New York.
JACK S. C. FONG • Department of Pediatrics, McGill University, Montreal, Quebec, Canada.

LOUIS H. MUSCHEL
AND JACK S. C. FONG

Red cells are also destroyed by a similar mechanism, and this discovery too was largely the work of Bordet. In addition, protozoa (Anziano *et al.,* 1972) and even the nucleated cells of mammals are susceptible to attack by the C system (Green *et al.,* 1959). The vulnerability of many different cell types, however, may not be too unexpected. Investigations of the chemical composition of cell membranes isolated from various sources, including animal cells, fungi, and bacteria, have established a great deal of similarity in over-all composition. Biomembranes generally contain 20–30% lipid, 50–70% protein, and relatively small amounts of polysaccharide (Salton, 1968). All membranes are not susceptible, however, to the complements of all species. Rabbit C, for example, will not immobilize or kill *T. pallidum* sensitized by rabbit antibody, although it will function in the standard hemolytic system with sheep red cells sensitized by rabbit antibody (Müller and Segerling, 1970). On the other hand, cow C is ineffective in the standard hemolytic system with rabbit antiserum against sheep red cells, but will exert a potent bactericidal effect against *Salmonella typhi* sensitized with rabbit antibody (Muschel and Treffers, 1956b). Yet cow C reacts with sheep red cells sensitized by rabbit antibody to form an intermediate that may be lysed by EDTA-treated guinea pig serum (Fong *et al.,* 1971). The inactivity of whole rabbit or cow C in these experimental situations, therefore, would appear not to be dependent upon the species of antibody or class of antibody within a species. More likely, the late-acting C components, presumably enzymes, of some species, or the products of their activity, are incapable of reacting with substrates of certain membranes.

The chemical nature of the C lesion is not known, and it is difficult to summarize all the findings and hypotheses (Dourmashkin *et al.,* 1972; Humphrey and Dourmashkin, 1969). One attractive possibility is that one of the serum lipids is enzymatically altered and then inserted into the lipid layer of the cell membrane. This suggestion is compatible with the wide range of C substrates. Experimental evidence in favor of this concept is the finding that cell walls of *Escherichia coli* treated with active C have a higher proportion of unsaturated fatty acids than do walls treated with heated C. Fatty acids with a higher degree of unsaturation conceivably may facilitate the rearrangement of lipids in cell membranes (Dourmashkin *et al.,* 1972).

1.2. Metabolic Changes in Bacteria Induced by the Immune Bactericidal Reaction

Metabolic events occurring during the immune bactericidal activity have recently been studied by Melching and Vas (1971). In a complex medium, total RNA accumulation begins to decrease after 15 min, levels off until 30 min, and then declines markedly compared to control cultures with heated serum. The effect on DNA synthesis does not become evident until after 25 min. Protein synthesis is affected later in the reaction than either RNA or DNA synthesis. When the reaction was carried out in a simple medium with glucose as an energy source, then the pattern of results was similar to that obtained in the complex medium except that the cells were affected earlier with more drastic results. These findings are not necessarily incompatible with previous results by Amano *et al.* (1956), which indicated that one of the early effects of the bactericidal reaction was a loss in the ability to synthesize adaptive enzymes. Although interpreted as an effect upon protein synthesis, it is likely that transcription of the induced messengers was primarily affected.

1.3. The Metabolic State of a Culture and Its Sensitivity to Complement

Earlier studies (Maaløe, 1948) had indicated the importance of the medium in which organisms are grown or in which the reaction is conducted. Growth in diluted broth resulted in *Salmonella typhimurium* with low resistance as compared to that of bacteria grown in full broth that more nearly approached *in vivo* conditions, or in diluted broth to which glucose or other simple nitrogen-free compounds were added. More recent work (Melching and Vas, 1971) has also indicated less killing of *E. coli* by serum when the cells were grown in a complex medium. Moreover, with different energy sources, it was found that glycerol- and acetate-grown cells were less susceptible than cells grown with glucose or succinate as an energy source. The authors postulated that the ability of cells to carry on rapid membrane lipid synthesis may be involved because both acetate and glycerol are important precursors in lipid biosynthesis.

The availability of nutrients undoubtedly influences the metabolic states of bacteria, and it had been assumed, on the basis of limited experimental work, that the metabolic state of a culture influenced its susceptibility to C (Muschel, 1960b). Enhanced metabolic activity was found to render bacteria more susceptible to C. In this respect, the bactericidal action of C was erroneously assumed to mimic the action of penicillin. The finding that rod-shaped cells killed by ultraviolet light were lysed or converted to spheroplasts by the concerted action of the C system and lysozyme indicated that the surfaces of cells incapable of division were sensitive to C (Muschel *et al.*, 1959). Further analysis of this question by Crombie (1969) showed, moreover, that the primary factor in determining an organism's susceptibility to C was its size. With *S. typhi* 0901, mid-log- and mid-stationary-phase organisms were the largest and smallest, respectively, with surface area decreasing by a factor of 3 from the log to the stationary phase. With an excess of antibody, no differences in the sensitivity of log- and stationary-phase bacteria were noted. When antibody was limiting, however, with an equal number of organisms, the smaller stationary cells were at least three times more sensitive than log-phase cells. With an equal mass of log- and stationary-phase cells having approximately equal surface areas, however, the serum amount required to kill 50% of the stationary-phase cells was approximately equal to that amount required for the 50% endpoint against the log culture. Thus, the differential sensitivity of log-phase and stationary-phase cells may be explained simply on the basis of their differences in size.

Of particular interest in the interactions that may occur between a host's humoral and cellular defense systems are studies of serum resistance of bacteria following their intracellular residence. Increased serum resistance has been found with *Brucella abortus*, harvested from mononuclear phagocytes of the guinea pig (Stinebring *et al.*, 1960) and with *E. coli* from the peritoneal cells of the mouse (McElree *et al.*, 1966). Unfortunately, the mechanisms responsible for these observations have not been thoroughly investigated.

LOUIS H. MUSCHEL
AND JACK S. C. FONG

2. Methodology

2.1. Different Procedures Available for Assaying the Bactericidal Reaction

The standard method for estimating the number of bacteria, or other antimicrobial agents, surviving the action of serum is the plate count. Obviously, any method suitable for the determination of the viable number of organisms in culture may be applied to the immune bactericidal reaction. A photometric growth-assay procedure, similar to that being used for the determination of antibiotic activity, circumvents the more tedious plate-count methods and yields results reproducible to about 10% (Muschel and Treffers, 1956a). Using this method, the number of organisms surviving the bactericidal reaction, which may be below readable density, is subcultured. While still in log phase, the growth is stopped and the optical densities attained are related to the number of organisms subcultured. As currently used, the photometric assay requires a relatively large inoculum (about 10^7 organisms) of the test culture so that a readable density may be obtained in a reasonable length of time. However, within certain limits, the sensitivity of the bactericidal reaction for the detection of antibody varies inversely with the size of the test inoculum, and the photometric assay may be too insensitive for some purposes. For greater sensitivity and convenience in estimating the number of surviving bacteria, a modification of the plate-count procedure, using a very small number (100) of test organisms, has been adopted by various workers (Landy *et al.,* 1969). Tetrazolium reduction has also been used as an index of the number of organisms surviving the immune bactericidal reaction (Nagington, 1956). This method also allows a sharp reduction in the number of test organisms. Bactericidal antibody may be titrated with any of these methods by using different amounts of a test serum with an excess of added C (serum absorbed with heat-killed cells of the test organism of 0°C to remove normal antibody). Though obviously of limited application, such titrations constitute one of the most precise and sensitive methods for the measurement of antibody (Kabat, 1961). None of these procedures distinguishes actual lysis of the cell from any reaction that merely inhibits cell multiplication. The bactericidal reaction requires only antibody and C, whereas the rapid lysis of the killed cells, with the possible exception of cells of *V. cholerae,* also requires the enzyme lysozyme (Crombie and Muschel, 1967). For the estimation of immune bacteriolysis, a method based on the photometric determination of released nucleic acid has been developed (Amano *et al.,* 1958). Another procedure depends on the conversion of bacterial cells to spheroplasts. Cells that would ordinarily lyse are converted to spheroplasts when the reaction is conducted in the presence of a stabilizing medium containing 25% sucrose and 5% magnesium sulfate. The reaction is then stopped by the addition of formaldehyde, and the number of spheroplasts is determined by direct microscopic count (Crombie and Muschel, 1967). This technique demonstrated that C-killed cells of different organisms showed marked variation in their lysozyme sensitivity. The subsequent conversion of spheroplasts to ghosts has also been described as well as a kinetic analysis of the transformation of the rod-shaped organisms to spheroplasts and ghosts (Davis *et al.,* 1966).

2.2. Possible Use of the Bactericidal Reaction as an Indicator System for Complement Fixation

Complement-fixation reactions for the serological diagnosis of various microbial infections, including the Wassermann test, invariably use an indicator system consisting of sensitized erythrocytes. However, gram-negative bacteria, which are easily preserved and cultivated in the laboratory, may offer distinct advantages over sheep cells in some situations. Such procedures using bacteria have not been developed.

2.3. Detection and Assay of Antibody, Antigen, and Complement by the Bactericidal Reaction

Apart from its use as an indicator system in complement-fixation reactions, the bactericidal reaction conceivably could be useful in serological diagnosis as a method for the detection of antibody against different microbes. Extensive use of the bactericidal reaction in the public health or clinical laboratory has been largely restricted to the treponemal immobilization test. Because of the remarkable sensitivity of the bactericidal reaction in detection of antibody, it is quite likely that it would be valuable in the diagnosis of certain infections. For example, in an unpublished case of shigellosis acquired in the laboratory, an easily demonstrable rise in *Shigella* bactericidal antibody was obtained despite that apparent lack of response with the agglutination test.

The precision that may be achieved with the photometric growth assay method for the detection of human bactericidal *S. typhosa* anti-O antibody is illustrated in Figure 1. Also noteworthy is the well-marked increase in slope following immunization (Muschel and Treffers, 1956c).

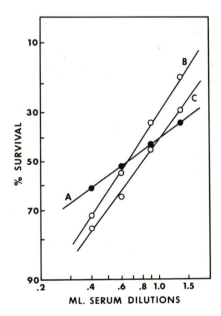

Figure 1. Bactericidal activity of human serum obtained before and after immunization with T. A. B. vaccine. (A) Preimmunization sample used at 1:12 dilution; (B) 7th day after last injection used at 1:120 dilution; (C) 11th day used at 1:120 dilution. Guinea pig C and *Salmonella typhosa* strain 0901 used for all sera. Log normal coordinates.

LOUIS H. MUSCHEL
AND JACK S. C. FONG

In addition to the detection of antibody, the immune bactericidal reaction, as well as other serological reactions, may be used for the detection of antigens with the aid of standard antisera. Recently, the immune bactericidal reaction was successfully applied to the classification of typing of the gonococci (Glynn and Howard, 1970). These results suggested that the antigens of the gonococci involved in the bactericidal reaction are lipopolysaccharides of several distinct specificities. Using rabbit antisera against 10 strains and normal human sera, 60 strains of the gonococci were classified into four main groups.

3. Immune Hemolysis: An Analogous Process

The killing of sensitized bacteria by C represents a process that is analogous to the lysis of sensitized red cells. Both immune hemolysis and the immune bactericidal reaction require the entire sequence of reactions of the C system (Goldman *et al.*, 1969), both have a requirement for divalent cations (Muschel and Treffers, 1956b), and both result in similar lesions in the respective cell membranes (Bladen *et al.*, 1966; Humphrey and Dourmashkin, 1969). Recently, however, the serum of a strain of guinea pigs presumably completely lacking in C4 was found to kill *E. coli* to a limited extent (Root *et al.*, 1972). This result may be interpreted nicely in accord with an alternative pathway for activation of the late-acting C components in which the endotoxin of the surface of the bacterial cells forms an intermediate complex on brief incubation with serum that comprises several guinea pig serum proteins, including C3. This complex then acts directly on C3 in a manner similar to sensitized sheep red cells with C1,4,2a (Marcus *et al.*, 1971). Crucial to support of this interpretation is the proof that natural antibody, C1, C4, and C2, are not required. However, whether it occurs by inapparent immunization or by normal physiological maturation, natural antibody of marked specificity is invariably present in the sera of the higher vertebrates, including even the serum of the colostrum-free piglet (Webb and Muschel, 1968). Thus, the contribution of the alternate pathway in the bactericidal reaction in normal animals may be slight.

In addition, the stoichiometric relation between antibody and C in the bactericidal reaction paralleled, quite closely, the corresponding data for hemolytic reactions (Muschel and Treffers, 1956b). On the other hand, the apparent differences between the immune bactericidal reaction and immune lysis of red cells may arise from the presence of a bacterial cell wall and its endotoxic constituents. It is well established that immune red cell lysis may occur from the combination of antibody with adsorbed surface antigens, which need not be integral components of those cells, and the resulting activation of the C system. Similarly with bacteria, antibody against substances such as albumin and globulin, which have been conjugated to the cell surface, may sensitize the organisms for the bactericidal reaction mediated by C (Adler, 1952; Rowley and Turner, 1968). The efficiency of this sensitization was found to be inversely proportional to the dimension of the conjugated molecules (Rowley and Turner, 1968). These observations suggest that the antigen–antibody reaction serves merely to concentrate C at a susceptible structure. It may be postulated that antigens of the cell wall or capsules of gram-negative bacteria may react like an adsorbed substance on the cell membrane of red cells.

4. Insensitivity of Gram-Positive Organisms and Mycobacteria

143

SERUM
BACTERICIDAL
ACTIVITY AND
COMPLEMENT

The insusceptibility of gram-positive bacteria to the C system may be related to the thickness of the cell wall of these organisms (15–80 mμm) compared to the relatively thin cell walls of gram-negative species, which range from 7.5–10 mμm. The presumably susceptible inner plasma membrane of gram-positive bacteria may be inaccessible or too far removed from the surface antigens of the cell wall, which constitute the locus of the antigen–antibody complexes that activate C. In accord with this view, protoplasts of gram-positive cells such as *Bacillus subtilis* were found to be very susceptible to the C system (Muschel and Jackson, 1966b). In addition, treatment of *Staphylococcus albus, Listeria monocytogenes,* or C resistant strains of *S. typhimurium* with tris, veronal buffers, low concentrations of EDTA, or ethanolamine rendered those organisms sensitive to killing by C (Reynolds and Rowley, 1969). These treatments, by their sequestration of metal ions in the cell-wall polysaccharides, may weaken their attachment to the underlying structures and allow the approach of antibody and C to the universally susceptible membranes (Reynolds and Pruul, 1971b).

Studies have not been performed to explain the resistance of mycobacteria to C. Possibly the lipid-rich thick wall is responsible by virtue of its size and/or probable anticomplementary activity of its lipid.

5. Anatomy of the Gram-Negative Bacterial Cell: Its Relationship to the Cell's Complement and Lysozyme Sensitivity

Because of the relatively narrow cell wall of the gram-negative bacteria, the locus of the antigen–antibody complex on the surface of the organism that activated C was believed to be sufficiently close to the inner cell membrane to permit destruction of the latter. The complexity of the cell wall of gram-negative bacteria, however, and the distance between their outer and inner membranes probably precludes this simple explanation. The gram-negative bacterial cell wall comprises an inner rigid peptidoglycan layer, which can be depolymerized by lysozyme, and a more flexible lipoprotein–lipopolysaccharide component, which overlaps the peptidoglycan and protects it from the action of lysozyme, possibly by impeding penetration of the enzyme into the wall. Gram-negative bacteria may be made sensitive to lysozyme by certain pretreatments, such as EDTA, which appear to act by disrupting the outer wall complex. Moreover, treatment of *E. coli* and other gram-negative bacteria with EDTA, which does not alter the growth rate of the organism or affect its viability, resulted in increased permeability of these organisms to actinomycin D and other substances. Together with other evidence, this finding has led to the suggestion that gram-negative bacteria may possess two membranes separated by the rigid peptidoglycan layer, and that both these membranes may function in permeability control (Salton, 1967). Because of the close association of the outer membrane to the surface antigens of the cell and because of the tremendous loss in the effectiveness of C when it is separated from its target by a distance equal only to that of a bovine serum albumin molecule, the suggestion was made that the outer membrane containing the antigenic lipopolysaccharide is the ultimate substrate for the C enzymes (Muschel and Gustafson, 1968). Possibly the polysaccharide of the molecule, which determines its antigenic specificity, reacts with antibody and the resulting immune complex activates C, resulting in an attack upon the lipid moiety. Moreover, the concept that the outer membrane is the immediate target of C is nicely in accord with the observation that untreated gram-negative bacteria are refractory to the action of lysozyme (Glynn, 1969), but when killed by C, lysozyme sensitivity is acquired, reflecting a loss of permeability control by the external barrier (Inoue *et al.*, 1959; Muschel *et al.*, 1959).

When C killed cells are exposed to lysozyme, the cells may be lysed or, in a protective milieu consisting of hypertonic sucrose and added magnesium ion, converted to rounded forms (spheroplasts), resulting from the degradation of the rigid peptidoglycan layer (Table 1). Rough organisms, such as *E. coli* B, are lysed by normal serum alone; a similar effect upon smooth forms, such as *S. typhi*, requires, in addition to normal serum as a C source, antiserum and lysozyme. Analysis of these reactions showed, for the rough strains, that normal serum served as an adequate source of antibody, C, and lysozyme; for the smooth strains, higher levels of antibody and lysozyme were needed (Table 1). Lysozyme, widely distributed in the fluids and tissues of the body, may play a significant role in host defenses not only against gram-positive bacteria upon which it exerts direct lytic action, but also as an adjunct to the complement system against gram-negative organisms.

These spheroplasts, formed by the synergistic activity of C and lysozyme, are stabilized by low concentrations of magnesium ion (Table 1), which seems to be uniquely effective in membrane stabilization. Moreover, magnesium ion protects *Aerobacter aerogenes* and other gram-negative organisms against the lethal effect of chilling. It is also interesting to note that under certain experimental conditions, the injury sustained by gram-negative organisms as a result of the action of C may be repaired by magnesium ion in concentrations from 0.03 M to 0.11 M. Many other substances tested, including anticomplementary substances, such as heparin and citrate, proteins, heated guinea pig serum, and salts of many other metals, were incapable of reversing the bactericidal action of C (Muschel and Jackson, 1966a). Thus, the bactericidal action of C, which requires a small concentration of magnesium ion, may be partially reversed by the addition of larger amounts of that ion.

6. Antigenic Targets of the Bactericidal Reaction

The antigenic targets of the bactericidal reaction against *S. typhi* have been studied (Muschel *et al.*, 1958; Nagington, 1956), and the results obtained are presumably applicable to all or most other *Salmonella* and *E. coli* strains. The Vi antigen of *S. typhi* and the other K antigens of *E. coli* (Muschel, 1960a) are associated with a strain's resistance to normal serum. The discovery that the Vi antigenic content of *S. typhi* was decreased by growing the organisms at temperatures above or below 37°C (Nicolle *et al.*, 1953) provided a way to demonstrate the significance of the Vi antigen. It was shown that *S. typhi* cultured at temperatures of either 18°C or 41.5°C lost most of its Vi antigen and became increasingly sensitive to serum bactericidal action. Similar results have been obtained with other Vi containing organisms (Osawa and Muschel, 1964a) and with *E. coli* (Glynn and Howard, 1970). Recultivation of these organisms at 37°C resulted in a return to serum resistance. Thus, the abnormal temperature effects a phenotypic change in the organism that is not transmissible.

TABLE 1. Formation of Protoplasts of *Salmonella typhosa* H901 by Serum Components

Experimental conditions	Test tube[a] (ml)		Control tubes[a] (ml)		
			Nonmotile rods	Ghosts	Protoplasts
Broth culture	0.1	0.1	0.1	0.1	0.1
S. typhosa anti-O[b]	0.1	0	0.1	0.1	0.1
Absorbed normal guinea pig serum[c]	0.5	0.5	0.5	0.5	0.5
Lysozyme (1 mg/ml)	0.1	0.1	0	0.1	0.1
10% MgSO$_4$ · 7H$_2$O	0.1	0.1	0.1	0	0.1
50% sucrose	0.1	0.1	0.1	0.1	0
Normal saline	0	0.5	0.1	0.1	0.1
Microscopic observation	Protoplasts	Motile rods	Motile rods, few clumps	Nonmotile rods	Ghosts	Protoplasts

[a]60 min. at 37°C prior to microscopic observation.
[b]1:1000 dilution in normal saline.
[c]Absorbed with washed, heat-killed cells of *S. typhosa* H901.

This loss of serum resistance when the organisms are cultured at elevated temperatures is obviously significant in considerations of the role of fever in host resistance. The elevated temperature of the fever may injure the parasite directly or activate defense reactions within the host. Conceivably, both mechanisms may operate in certain situations. In treponemal infections, it is not known whether the therapeutic effect of fever results mainly from the treponemicidal action of the higher temperatures or from possible antigenic changes induced by the fever that render the treponemas more susceptible to the C system. The latter possibility would seem to deserve serious consideration.

In addition to the K antigens, the presence of O antigen has been held to be associated with an organism's resistance to normal serum (Michael and Landy, 1961; Reynolds and Pruul, 1971a). With strains possessing both antigens, however, the difficult task of assessing the relative contribution of the separate antigens and of their interaction has not been thoroughly investigated.

An interesting finding regarding the O and Vi antigens as targets for the immune bactericidal reaction is the difference in the dose responses of anti-Vi and anti-O in the bactericidal reaction and also in protection tests *in vivo* (Muschel and Treffers, 1956c; Osawa and Muschel, 1964b). These results, showing that the Vi antibody gives a greater slope, provides some theoretical basis for understanding the great efficiency of the Vi antibody in mouse protection against challenge with virulent *S. typhi* organisms containing maximum amounts of both O and Vi antigens.

Generally, anti-H is not a bactericidal antibody (Osawa and Muschel, 1964b). Anti-H is also lacking in opsonic activity and mouse protection. Probably the H antigen determinants are insufficiently close to the vital substrates of the C system enzymes.

Since the presence of certain antigens on the surface of *Salmonella* and other organisms may be the consequence of lysogenization with particular phage types (Robbins and Uchida, 1962) and since, as we have seen, antigenic structures may influence susceptibility to the C system, it is not unexpected that lysogeny may change the sensitivity of certain organisms to C (Muschel *et al.*, 1968). Depending on the particular host and virus, lysogeny may result in increased serum resistance, no detectable change, or decreased serum resistance. Since the virulence of members of the Enterobacteriaceae has been associated with serum resistance in many studies (Roantree and Pappas, 1960; Rowley, 1954), the lysogenic state assumes critical significance in the host–parasite relationship. Similarly, the most dramatic effect of lysogeny involves the capacity of *Corynebacterium diptheriae* to produce toxin only as a result of infection with a suitable bacteriophage. Disease potential may be closely associated, therefore, not only with a bacterial agent, but also with the virus with which it is infected.

7. Sensitivity Differences between Rough and Smooth Strains

One of the distinguishing features between smooth and rough variants of the gram-negative bacteria is the relatively greater susceptibility of the latter to the bactericidal action of normal serum (Kauffman, 1950). Although this difference between smooth and rough forms has been well known for many years and repeatedly confirmed (Rowley, 1968), it has never been adequately explained nor is it possible to do so at this time. Nonetheless, certain exceptions to this generalization have been recently noted: the greater resistance of the rough organism, *S. typhi* Mrs. S., to normal serum compared with the smooth 0901 strain *S. typhi,* and the greater sensitivity of *Salmonella newington* compared with *Salmonella anatum,* although the latter organism is relatively rougher as determined by growth in broth (Muschel and Larsen, 1970). *S. anatum,* with the O factors 3,10, is converted to *S. newington* by infection with phage epsilon-15, resulting in the replacement of factor 10 by factor 15.

Resistance or susceptibility to normal serum may not necessarily be equated with an organism's reaction to the C system; antibody is required for the bactericidal reaction, and it may be present in limiting amounts in normal serum (Muschel and Larsen, 1970). For example, in the standard photometric growth-assay procedure, guinea pig serum alone gave a titer of 3.5 against smooth strain 20-A-10 of *V. cholerae,* reflecting the marked resistance of smooth *V. cholerae* strains to normal serum. In the presence of antiserum, the guinea pig serum titer was increased about thirtyfold, indicating that when adequately sensitized, *V. cholerae* is an organism with marked sensitivity to C. Similarly, normal guinea pig serum had a titer of 2.9 against a smooth strain of *E. coli* of serotype 0111-B4 and a titer of 15.0 against that strain's rough mutant, J-5. When homologous antiserum was used for sensitization, guinea pig serum titers, reflecting C titers, were quite comparable against the two organisms. Thus the marked difference in resistance of the two organisms to normal serum may be attributed to a lack of antibody against strain 0111-B4 in normal serum and not to that organism's resistance to C. Since the core polysaccharide of *Salmonella* and some *E. coli* serotypes are present in relatively large numbers of organisms, compared to the limited distribution of the specific determinants in strains similar to 0111-B4, the results suggest that antibody to the O-specific region of *E. coli* and other smooth organisms is often relatively lacking in normal sera. Thus, the additional work that is needed to adequately determine the basis of an organism's sensitivity to the C system must be performed with adequately sensitized organisms.

8. Antibody Source

8.1. Normal Serum and Immune Serum

The demonstration that antibody and C are both required for the bactericidal reaction is quite simple. An amount of normal untreated serum, which itself exerts no demonstrable effect against a particular organism, may produce a potent bactericidal effect when the cells of that organism are sensitized with an extremely small volume of heat-inactivated antiserum. Antibodies capable of complement fixation should be capable of functioning in the bactericidal reaction. Thus, both gamma M and gamma G antibodies, in conjunction with C, have been found to kill gram-negative bacteria, and gamma M is at least 20 times more effective than gamma G on a molar basis (Michael and Rosen, 1963; Robbins *et al.,* 1965). The report that gamma A antibody in colostrum caused lysis of *E. coli* in the presence of C and lysozyme (Adinolfi *et al.,* 1966) is compatible with more recent findings that gamma A can activate C via the alternate pathway.

Certain gram-negative enteric bacteria (Muschel, 1960b) and *T. pallidum* (Müller and Segerling, 1970) may, however, be killed by normal untreated serum itself. The specificity of this bactericidal reaction, mediated by normal serum, has been often questioned because the earlier experimental findings were in disagreement. The results that indicated a lack of specificity may be attributed to a variety of causes: an excessive loss of C during absorption procedures designed to determine the specificity of the reaction; the use of gram-positive bacteria that are killed by the beta lysins of serum, which function independently of antibody and C; and imprecise methods of assay. More recent findings have indicated a marked degree of specificity. When a sample of normal serum was absorbed with cells of one gram-negative organism without significant loss of C, then that serum's bactericidal activity against the organism whose cells were used for the absorption was lost. There was, however, little or no loss of activity against serologically unrelated organisms (Mackie and Finkelstein, 1932; Muschel, 1960a). Inhibition experiments with purified lipopolysaccharides have also confirmed the marked specificity of the normal bactericidal antibodies (Michael *et al.,* 1962). These relatively simple experiments have indicated that normal or natural antibody may sensitize the organism for its destruction by C.

Undoubtedly, the origin of certain of the natural antibodies is inapparent immunization. Whether normal physiological maturation can contribute to their formation is not entirely clear and probably is unanswerable experimentally, since it is not certain what abnormalities other than the relative absence of immunoglobulin formation may occur in an animal shielded from antigenic stimuli (Boyden, 1966; Hook *et al.,* 1966). In any event, the bactericidal reaction provides one of the simplest and most sensitive methods for the detection and study of the normal antibodies.

8.2. Bactericidal Activity without Antibody

In the apparent absence of normal antibody, certain experimental findings led to the conclusion that a nonspecific substance, called *properdin,* in conjunction with C, was responsible for certain of the biological activities of normal serum, including the destruction of certain gram-negative bacteria. Studies showing the marked specificity of the bactericidal reaction of normal serum refuted this contention and indicated that antibody represented an absolute requirement for the reaction (Osawa and Muschel, 1960). Since only a single molecule of antibody may be required for the killing of a bacterial cell, the immune bactericidal reaction represents possibly the most sensitive method available for the detection of certain antibodies. It has been demonstrated that only one gamma M molecule or two gamma G molecules are required for the immune lysis of red cells (Borsos and Rapp, 1965), and it is quite conceivable that certain gram-negative bacteria may be similarly sensitive.

A more startling proposal of great interest was made by Sterzl *et al.* (1965), who suggested that C alone might be responsible for the killing of gram-negative bacteria. The experimental basis for this concept was the finding that serum of the precolostral piglet, lacking in detectable immunoglobulin, was capable of gram-negative bactericidal activity. However, even with such sera, extensive absorption indicated that a specific sensitizing substance was required (Webb and Muschel, 1968).

With the recent documentation of C activation through an alternate pathway in which C3 is activated without the intervention of C1,4,2, a direct role of C-mediated-bactericidal activity, possibly in the absence of antibody, was indirectly suggested by experimental data of Götze and Müller-Eberhard (1971). These investigators showed an enhancement of *E. coli* survival when the serum sample was depleted of its C3 proactivator, an essential substance for the alternate pathway. However, restoration of activity by addition of the proactivator was not attempted. The situation is further confused by enhanced hemolytic activity with proactivator depleted serum.

When serum from C4 deficient guinea pigs was studied, a prolonged latent period and slow rate of bactericidal action against two rough strains of *E. coli* were observed. Such a defect could be corrected by the addition of purified C4 (Root *et al.,* 1972). These experiments also suggested that the alternate pathway of C activation might play a significant role in C-mediated-bactericidal activity, since it is well established that the interaction of endotoxins (LPS) of gram-negative bacteria with guinea pig serum leads to a marked depletion of C3 through C9 with little or no detectable loss of C1, C4, and C2. LPS may react, however, with natural antibodies to gram-negative bacteria, resulting in very efficient utilization of C1, C4, and C2, while depleting large quantities of the C3 complex (Snyderman *et al.,* 1971). Whether or not antibody represents an absolute requirement has not been determined (Gewurz, 1972). Moreover, a recent study using red cells coated with LPS indicated that a gamma-2 globulin containing natural antibody was required for the C mediated lysis of these cells (Phillips *et al.,* 1972).

While the relative contribution of the two pathways of C activation to bactericidal action has not been precisely determined, two points deserve to be mentioned. First, the classical terminal C components (C3–C9) function as the common pathway for both modes of C activation. Second, at least *in vitro,* the classical pathway involving antibody, which is almost invariably present in animals, and the entire C sequence provides an easily demonstrable, potent bactericidal reaction. The alternate pathway is relatively inefficient, and the extent of its contribution to the bactericidal activity against serum-sensitive forms is not yet available. Moreover, in the absence of antibody, the alternate pathway is apparently incapable of effecting the destruction of those organisms that are resistant to normal serum, such as the smooth forms of *V. cholerae.* Yet these forms are readily killed by antiserum and C.

8.3. Inhibition of the Bactericidal Reaction by an Excess of Antibody (Neisser-Wechsberg Phenomenon)

An interesting and paradoxical phenomenon, first described by Neisser and Wechsberg (1901), involves the inhibition of the immune bactericidal reaction by an excess of antiserum. Experimental procedures designed to elucidate the mechanism of this prozone phenomenon have indicated that with heat-inactivated antiserum, the prozone results from an excess of both specific antibody and nonspecific anticomplementary activity (Muschel *et al.,* 1969b). Nonspecific anticomplementary activity represents a major contribution to the prozone, since the effect was relatively slight with unheated antiserum or with the removal of serum substances unrelated to antibody. The inhibition of bactericidal activity by excess antiserum may be overcome, however, by an excess of the third C component factors (C3–C9), suggesting that the excess of antiserum interfered with the activation or function of the components acting at one of the late steps in the C sequence. Since rabbit antisera against bacteria show elevated levels of immunoconglutinin and since immunoconglutinin may exert an anticomplementary effect, it seemed possible that the nonspecific anticomplementary effect of antisera might be associated with immunoconglutinin. Removal of detectable amounts of immunoconglutinin from a rabbit antiserum resulted, however, in no significant effect upon the prozone reaction in tests with the homologous organism (Muschel et al., 1969b). In other experimental situations, immunoconglutinin may enhance the bactericidal reaction. The sera of rabbits in whom immunoconglutinin production was stimuated by the injection of kaolin coated with fresh serum showed enhanced bactericidal activity against several different bacteria (Mittal and Ingram, 1969). This result may be attributed to enhanced activation of C via an additional immune complex.

9. Complement Source

The lowest known vertebrate forms to have demonstrated adaptive immunity are the lampreys and primitive fishes (Finstad and Good, 1966). In all these forms, with the possible exception of hagfishes, a hemolytic system or components of a hemolytic system were found (Gewurz et al., 1966a). The serum of the chondrostean paddlefish (Polyodon spathula) demonstrated evidence of a conventional C system, including bactericidal activity. Among the elasmobranchs, the primitive shark Heterodontus gave slight but definite bactericidal activity against E. coli. The higher fish, represented by the carp, showed bactericidal activity against three rough strains of Enterobacteriaceae but not against eight smooth strains, thereby resembling mammalian serum in its activity spectrum (Muschel et al., 1964). Chicken serum is also bactericidal against gram-negative organisms (Collins, 1967).

Among mammals, normal sera of the human, guinea pig, horse, cow, and rabbit are effective bactericidal agents. Serum of the mouse is lacking in bactericidal action (Muschel and Muto, 1956), and that of certain hamsters is extremely weak. In the case of the mouse, the lack of activity may be associated with extreme lability of the second component or with the presence of an inhibitor of the second C component. Normal antibody of the mouse, in conjunction with C of other species, however, is capable of vigorous bactericidal action. With the exception of the mouse, there is little or no correlation between the hemolytic and bactericidal activity of C. This observation is not too unexpected, since the relative activity of C of different mammals will vary even when red cells of different species are used (Rice and Boulanger, 1952).

10. Interactions of the Immune Bactericidal Reaction

10.1. Antibiotics

There are several observations suggesting that when the immune bactericidal reaction or antibiotic has separate therapeutic or in vitro effects, then the combination may have additive value. In some cases, the combined effect may be greater than the effects of the individual components, which suggests a synergism, such as that reported, for example, with penicillin (Miller and Foster, 1944). On the other hand, sublethal doses of chloramphenicol have been reported to inhibit the immune bactericidal reaction (Michael and Braun, 1959).

With the use of a very precise assay method, the only effect observed with chloramphenicol or polymyxin and the immune bactericidal reaction was that of joint but independent actions (Muschel *et al.,* 1969a; Treffers and Muschel, 1954). Other tests with a variety of antibiotics, including the tetracyclines and penicillin, have indicated essentially similar results (Muschel, unpublished). Neither a synergism nor an antagonism was observed. Moreover, mutants of *S. typhi,* selected for increased resistance to chloramphenicol, were comparable to the parental strain in their susceptibility to the antibody C system (Treffers and Muschel, 1954).

Very few correlations have been made between the serum susceptibility of organisms and their antibiotic sensitivity. Different strains of *Pseudomonas aeruginosa,* all of which had approximately equal sensitivity to polymyxin, were extremely variable in their serum resistance (Muschel *et al.,* 1969a). *Paracolobactrum ballerup,* an organism that is refractory to C when grown at 37°C, became at least 50 times more sensitive to normal rabbit serum when that organism was cultivated at 43°C (Osawa and Muschel, 1964a). This altered reactivity, also demonstrated with the Ty2 strain of *S. typhi,* has been attributed to the loss of the Vi antigen. When cultured at the higher temperature, the sensitivity of *P. ballerup* to penicillin was increased at least fourfold, but with relatively slight changes in chloramphenicol sensitivity. However, *S. typhi* Ty2 became less sensitive to the action of both antibiotics when grown at temperatures above 37°C. These observations of a preliminary nature are obviously significant in considerations of the role of fever in host resistance.

10.2. Ethylenediaminetetraacetate

Various agents that partially remove or disrupt the structural organization of the LPS layer of smooth gram-negative bacteria might be expected to increase the C sensitivity of such treated cells. This has been found to be the case with EDTA (Muschel and Gustafson, 1968) and tris plus EDTA (Reynolds and Pruul, 1971b; Reynolds and Rowley, 1969). In addition, Feingold has found that cells grown in the presence of diphenylamine, which inhibits the synthesis of LPS, also became more serum sensitive (Cho *et al.,* 1967; Feingold, 1969). He has made the interesting suggestion that since the LPS is unique to the bacterial cell wall, one might find new drugs for the therapy of gram-negative infections. Such agents, which might have little effect on viability *in vitro,* could convert bacteria to a state of greater sensitivity to C-mediated reactions.

11. Role of the Immune Bactericidal Reaction in Gram-Negative Bacterial Infections

The final question involves the role of the immune bactericidal reaction in the defense of the host against gram-negative organisms. It is inconceivable that such a powerful and complicated mechanism, involving at least a dozen different proteins and ionic cofactors, afford no protection or survival value. An accurate assessment of its contributions to host defenses, however, has been difficult, if not impossible, primarily because of the lack of adequate controls. Normal antibody and C are almost invariably present, although naturally occurring C deficiencies in animals and humans have been studied. Moreover, the C system also contributes significantly to the activity of phagocytes. It is still doubtful, for example, whether the antibodies in typhoid fever act mainly by promotion of opsonization or by sensitization of the organism to the bactericidal action of C.

There is a great deal of indirect evidence implicating serum bactericidal activity in host defense mechanisms. Resistance to serum may be an important determinant of mouse virulence with gram-negative organisms as tested by intraperitoneal challenge (Rowley, 1954), in rabbits by intravenous challenge (Roantree and Pappas, 1960), and in human infections with *E. coli* (Muschel, 1960a). Moreover, organisms resistant to serum are more apt to be isolated from blood, whereas sensitive strains are particularly prone to occur in urine or stool (Fierer *et al.,* 1972; Roantree and Rantz, 1960). Susceptibility to meningococcal disease is related to a selective deficiency of antibody to the offending organism, and it is measured by the bactericidal activity of serum (Goldschneider *et al.,* 1969). Finally, field studies have demonstrated that the relative immunity of a population to cholera after administration of killed whole-cell antigen may be estimated by the vibriocidal antibody level (Mosley *et al.,* 1968).

The existence of a strain of guinea pigs lacking one or more of the components of the C3 complex was reported several decades ago (Hyde, 1923; Moore, 1919). The deficiency was carried as a single Mendelian recessive character. Although the strain died out in time, these guinea pigs survived in the laboratory, but were more liable than controls to experimental challenge and to adverse environmental conditions. More recently, the good health of C4 deficient guinea pigs under standard maintenance conditions has been noteworthy. As we indicated previously, however, the sera of these animals are not completely lacking in bactericidal activity. With C5 deficient mice, as might be expected, *in vivo* killing of *E. coli* is greatly impaired (Glynn and Medhurst, 1967).

Several strains of C6-deficient rabbits have been discovered and maintained (Lachmann, 1970). The quantitative absence of C6 in these animals renders them functionally deficient in C6–9. These rabbits are incapable of mounting a vigorous inflammatory response together with a subsequent increased susceptibility to infection and decreased ability for detoxification (Fong and Good, 1975).

In man, complement deficiency of early components Clr, C4, and C2 is not always accompanied by massive increases in susceptibility to infection (de Bracco *et al.,* 1974; Hauptmann *et al.,* 1974). Of these, extensive studies have been made of one apparently healthy individual with essential hypocomplementemia due to a deficiency of C2 (Gewurz *et al.,* 1966b). Hemolytic activity of this serum with maximally sensitized cells was extremely low, and its bactericidal titer was also low when tested with antiserum-sensitized organisms. However, near-normal titers were observed in tests of the serum's bactericidal activity against unsensitized bacteria. The reason for this apparently contradictory finding may be that the low C level was not the limiting factor in killing bacteria at normal antibody levels. Generally, in those experimental procedures in which test sera are not diluted to an appreciable extent and, therefore, are more nearly comparable to undiluted plasma *in vivo,* the C2 available in the hypocomplementemic individual was adequate. This study emphasizes the need for caution in drawing conclusions from deficiencies that are not absolute. Alternatively, the finding in the bactericidal activity of C2 deficient serum can also be explained in light of the two pathways of complement activation. It was shown that IgG natural antibodies activated the complement system mainly through the alternate pathway, whereas the interaction between immune IgG antibodies and the complement system followed the classical pattern (Bjornson and Michael, 1974). The late complement components C3–9 are positioned as the common pathway for both the classical- and the alternate-pathway activation of the complement system. These late components are expected to play a key role in bactericidal activities. Indeed, a patient with frequent gram-negative infection associated with abnormalities of C3 was reported (Alper *et al.,* 1970). His serum was devoid of bactericidal activity for smooth gram-negative bacilli and incapable of enhancement of phagocytosis of antibody-sensitized type II pneumococci. The infections encountered in this patient included pneumonia, β-hemolytic streptococcal septicemia, and meningococcal septicemia. Moreover, since the absolute deficiency of C4 in apparently healthy guinea pigs is associated with an intact alternate pathway for the activation of C, it has been inferred, on the basis of these and other observations, that the activation of C3, which is crucial for phagocytosis, plays a key role in resistance to bacterial infection.

Though C5 deficiency in mice is not associated with a major survival disadvantage under conditions of ideal husbandry in the laboratory, a dysfunction of C5 in human patients is accompanied by devastating morbidities and mortalities (Nilsson *et al.,* 1974). Both immunochemical and hemolytic assays revealed normal quantities of C5 in these patients, but a dysfunction of C5 dependent opsonization of yeast particles could be demonstrated. Such a deficit could be corrected by a small amount of purified C5 or normal human serum. These patients responded clinically to the administration of fresh plasma (Jacobs and Miller, 1972). Further, a patient lacking in C5 was shown to have many infections and to develop lupus erythematosus as well. Finally, Shin *et al.* demonstrated that challenge of C5 deficient mice with varying numbers of pneumococci revealed a rather increased susceptibility to infection by this organism.

Patients deficient in C6 or C7 were at first reported to be enjoying good health (Wellek and Opferkuch, 1975; Leddy *et al.,* 1974). While the membranolytic function of the C system is capable of killing bacteria, it is not the only mechanism for hosts' defense against bacterial invasion. Indeed, opsonizing and chemotactic activities of the C system may play a more important role in individuals with normal phagocytosis capabilities. On the basis of observations on C deficiency states in animals and patients, one may reasonably conclude that, despite the lack of one or more of the late- or early-acting components of C and consequently of hemolytic or bactericidal activity, the phagocytic mechanism may suffice for protection of the host against many microbial assaults. As information concerning patients with complement and C component deficiencies increases, evidence of enhanced susceptibility to certain infections and poorly understood increased frequency of apparently immunologically based diseases, such as lupus erythematosus and arthritis, has appeared (see Chapter 13). Further studies are necessary to ascertain to what degree these illnesses associated with C and C component deficiency are functions of defective bactericidal and cytolytic activities attributable to the C abnormalities.

12. Summary

LOUIS H. MUSCHEL
AND JACK S. C. FONG

Just as red cells sensitized with antibody are lysed by complement, gram-negative bacteria, spirochetes, many protozoa, and other organisms sensitized by antibody may be killed by the complement system. In a remarkable synergism between naturally occurring substances, gram-negative bacteria killed by complement are lysed by the enzyme lysozyme acting on a mucopeptide substrate exposed by the action of complement on the bacterial cell wall. Since protoplasts of gram-positive bacteria are sensitive to complement, the resistance of their whole cells probably results from the relatively large distance of the surface antigens of the cell, which constitute the locus of the antigen–antibody complexes that activate complement, from the susceptible plasma membrane.

This potent bacteriolytic mechanism, however, has not always been considered an important determinant of resistance to gram-negative bacteria. With commonly occurring "normal" antibody, it may play a significant part in the very early stages of infection. Its precise role is difficult to assess because phagocytosis may also depend on the activation of complement at the bacterial cell surface. The limited evidence currently available suggests that phagocytic activity mediated by complement may play a more important role in individuals with normal phagocytic capabilities.

References

Adinolfi, M., Glynn, A. A., Lindsay, M., and Milne, C. M., 1966, Serological properties of gamma A antibodies to *Escherichia coli* present in human colostrum, *Immunology* **10**:517–526.

Adler, F. L., 1952, Bactericidal action mediated by antibodies specific for heterologous antigens absorbed to bacterial cells, *Proc. Soc. Exp. Biol. Med.1* **79**:590–593.

Alper, C. A., Abramson, N., Johnston, R. B., Jandl, J. N., and Rosen, F. S., 1970, Increased susceptibility to infection associated with abnormalities of complement-mediated functions and of the third component of complement (C3), *N. Engl. J. Med.* **282**:349–354.

Amano, T., Inoue, K., and Tanigawa, Y., 1956, Studies on the immune bacteriolysis X. The influence of immune bacteriolysis upon the adaptive enzyme formation and on phage reproduction in the cells of *Escherichia coli* B, *Med. J. Osaka Univ.* **6**:1027–1034.

Amano, T., Fujikawa, K., Morioka, T., Miyana, A., and Ichikawa, S., 1958. Quantitative studies on immune bacteriolysis. I. A new method of quantitative estimation, *Biken J.* **1**:13–25.

Anziano, D. F., Dalmasso, A. P., Lelchuk, R., and Vasquez, C., 1972, Role of complement in immune lysis of *Trypanosoma cruzi*, *Infect. Immun.* **6**:860–864.

Bjornson, A. B., and Michael, J. G., 1974, Factors in human serum promoting phagocytosis of *Pseudomonas aeruginosa*. I. Interaction of opsonins with the bacterium, *J. Infect. Dis.* **130**:S119–S126.

Bladen, H. A., Evans, R. T., and Mergenhagen, S. E., 1966, Lesion in *Escherichia coli* membranes after action of antibody and complement, *J. Bacteriol.* **91**:2377–2381.

Bordet, J., 1895, Les leucocytes et les propriétés du serum chez les vaccines, *Ann. Inst. Pasteur* **9**:462–506.

Borsos, T., and Rapp, H. J., 1965, Complement fixation on cell surfaces by 19S and 7S antibodies, *Science* **150**:505–506.

Boyden, S. V., 1966, Natural antibodies and the immune response, *Adv. Immunol.* **5**:1–24.

Bracco, M. M. E. de, Windhorst, D., Stroud, R. M., and Moncada, B., 1974, The autosomal recessive mode of inheritance of Clr deficiency in a large Puerto Rican family, *Clin. Exp. Immunol.* **16**:183–188.

Cho, K. Y., Corpe, W. A., and Salton, M. R. J., 1967, Effect of diphenylamine on the fatty acid composition of some bacterial lipids, *Biochem. J.* **93**:26c–28c.

Collins, F. M., 1967, Serum mediated killing of three Group D Salmonellas, *J. Gen. Microbiol.* **46**:247–253.

Crombie, L., 1969, The influence of the growth phase of gram negative bacteria on their sensitivity to the antibody–complement lysozyme system, Thesis, University of Minnesota.

Crombie, L., and Muschel, L. H., 1967, Quantitative studies on spheroplast formation by the complement system and lysozyme on gram negative bacteria, *Proc. Soc. Exp. Biol. Med.* **124**:1029–1033.

Davis, S. O., Gemsa, D., and Wedgwood, R. J., 1966, Kinetics of the transformation of gram-negative rods to spheroplasts and ghosts by serum, *J. Immunol.* **96**:570–577.

Dingle, J. H., Fothergill, L. D., and Chandler, C. A., 1938, Studies on *Haemophilus influenzae*. III. The failure of complement of some animal species, notably the guinea pig, to activate the bactericidal function of sera of certain other species, *J. Immunol.* **34**:357–391.

Dourmashkin, R. B. Hesketh, R., Humphrey, J. R., Medhurst, F., and Payne, S. N., 1972, Electron microscopic studies of the lesions in cell membranes caused by complement, in: *Biological Activities of Complement* (D. G. Ingram, ed.), pp. 89–95, S. Karger, Basel.

Feingold, O. S., 1969, The serum bactericidal reaction. *IV.* Phenotypic conversion of *Escherichia coli* from serum resistance to serum sensitivity by diphenylamine, *J. Infect. Dis.* **120**:437–444.

Fierer, J., Finley, F., and Braude, A. I., 1972, A plaque assay in agar for detection of gram-negative bacilli sensitive to complement, *J. Immunol.* **109**:1156–1158.

Finstad, J., and Good, R. A., 1966, Phylogenetic studies of adaptive immune responses in the lower vertebrates, in: *Phylogeny of Immunity* (R. T. Smith, P. A. Miescher, and R. A. Good, eds.), pp. 173–189, University of Florida Press, Gainesville.

Fong, J. S. C., and Good, R. A., 1975, Congenital and experimentally induced complement deficiency in rabbits, in: *Immunodeficiency in Man and Animals* (R. A. Good, J. Finstad, and N. Paul, eds.), 2nd International Workshop, Sinauer Assoc., Sunderland, Mass.

Fong, J. S. C., Muschel, L. H., and Good, R. A., 1971, Kinetics of bovine complement. I. Formation of a lytic intermediate, *J. Immunol.* **107**:28–33.

Gale, J. L., and Kenny, G. E., 1970, Complement dependent killing of *Mycoplasma pneumoniae* by antibody: kinetics of the reaction, *J. Immunol.* **104**:1175–1183.

Gewurz, H., 1972, Alternate pathways to activation of the complement system, in: *Biological Activities of Complement* (D. G. Ingram, ed.), pp. 56–88, S. Karger, Basel.

Gewurz, H., Finstad, J., Muschel, L. H., and Good, R. A., 1966a, Phylogenetic inquiry into the origins of the complement system, in: *Phylogeny of Immunity* (R. T. Smith, P. A. Miescher, and R. A. Good, eds.), pp. 105–117, University of Florida Press, Gainesville.

Gewurz, H., Pickering, R. G. J., Muschel, L. H., Mergenhagen, S. E., and Good, R. A., 1966b, Complement dependent biological functions in complement deficiency in man, *Lancet* **ii**:356–360.

Glynn, A. A., 1969, The complement lysozyme sequence in immune bacteriolysis, *Immunology* **16**:463–472.

Glynn, A. A., and Howard, C. J., 1970, The sensitivity to complement of strains of *Escherichia coli* related to their K antigens, *Immunology* **18**:331–346.

Glynn, A. A., and Medhurst, F. A., 1967, Possible extracellular and intracellular bactericidal actions of mouse complement, *Nature (London)* **213**:608–610.

Glynn, A. A., and Ward, M. E., 1970, Nature and heterogeneity of the antigens of *Neisseria gonorrhoeae* involved in the serum bactericidal reaction, *Infect. Immun.* **2**:162–168.

Goldman, J. N., Ruddy, S., Austen, K. F., and Feingold, D. S., 1969, The serum bactericidal reaction. III. Antibody and complement requirements for killing a rough *Escherichia coli*, *J. Immunol.* **102**:1379–1387.

Goldschneider, I., Gotschlich, E. C., and Artenstein, M. S., 1969, Human immunity to the meningococcus. I. The role of humoral antibodies, *J. Exp. Med.* **129**:1307–1326.

Götze, O., and Müller-Eberhard, H. J., 1971, The C3-activator system an alternate pathway of complement activation, *J. Exp. Med.* **134**:90s–108s.

Green, H., Fleischer, R. A., Barrow, P., and Goldberg, B., 1959, The cytotoxic action of immune gamma globulin and complement on Krebs ascites tumor cells. II. Chemical studies, *J. Exp. Med.* **109**:511–521.

Hauptmann, G., Grosshans, E., Heid, E., Mayer, S., and Basset, A., 1974, Acute lupus erythematosus with total absence of the C4 fraction of complement, *Nouv. Presse Med.* **3**:881–882.

Hook, W. A., Toussaint, A. J., Simonton, L. A., and Muschel, L. H., 1966, Appearance of natural antibodies in young rabbits, *Nature (London)* **210**:543–544.

Humphrey, J. H., and Dourmashkin, R. R., 1969, The lesions in cell membranes caused by complement, *Adv. Immunol.* **11**:75–115.

Hyde, R., 1923, Complement deficient guinea pig serum, *J. Immunol.* **8**:267–286.

Inoue, K., Tanigawa, Y., Takubo, M., Satani, J., and Amano, T., 1959, Quantitative studies on immune bacteriolysis. II. The role of lysozyme in immune bacteriolysis, *Biken J.* **2**:1–20.

Jacobs, J. C., and Miller, M. E., 1972, Fatal familial Leiner's disease: a deficiency of the opsonic activity of serum complement, *Pediatrics* **49**:225–232.

Johnson, R. C., and Muschel, L. H., 1966, Antileptospiral activity of serum. I. Normal and immune serum, *J. Bacteriol.* **91**:1403–1409.

Kabat, E. A., 1961, Quantities of antibody detectable by various immunological procedures, in: *Experimental Immunochemistry* (E. A. Kabat and M. Mayer, eds.), p. 299, Charles C Thomas, Springfield, Illinois.

Kauffmann, F., 1950, *The Diagnosis of Salmonella Types,* p. 19, Charles C Thomas, Springfield, Illinois.

Lachmann, P. J., 1970, C6-deficiency in rabbits, in: *Protides of Biological Fluids* (H. Peeters, ed.), Vol. 17, Pergamon Press, Oxford.

Landy, M., Sanderson, R. P., and Jackson, A. L., 1969, Humoral and cellular aspects of the immune response to the somatic antigen of *Salmonella enteriditis, J. Exp. Med.* **122**:483–504.

Leddy, J. P., Frank, M. M., Gaither, T., Baum, J., and Klemperer, M. R., 1974, Hereditary deficiency of the sixth component of complement in man. I. Immunochemical, biologic, and family studies, *J. Clin. Invest.* **53**:544–553.

Maaløe, O., 1948, Pathogenic–apathogenic transformation of *Salmonella typhimurium, Acta Pathol. Microbiol scand.* **25**:414–430.

Mackie, J. T., and Finkelstein, M. H., 1932, The bactericidins of normal serum; characters, occurrence in various animals and the susceptibility of different bacteria to their action. *J. Hyg.* **52**:1–24.

Marcus, R. L., Shin, H. S., and Mayer, M. M., 1971, An alternate complement pathway: C-3 cleaving, activity not due to $\overline{C4,2a}$, on endotoxic lipopolysaccharide after treatment with guinea pig serum; relation to properdin, *Proc. Nat. Acad. Sci. U.S.A.* **68**:1351–1354.

McElree, H., Pitcher, J., and Arnivinn, J., 1966, Transiently acquired serum resistance by cell grown *Escherichia coli, J. Infect. Dis.* **116**:231–237.

Melching, L., and Vas, S. I., 1971, Effects of serum components on gram-negative bacteria during bactericidal reactions, *Infect. Immun.* **3**:107–115.

Michael, J. G., and Braun. W., 1959, Modification of bactericidal effects of human serum, *Proc. Soc. Exp. Biol. Med.* **102**:487–490.

Michael, J. G., and Landy, M., 1961, Endotoxic properties of gram-negative bacteria and their susceptibility to the lethal action of normal serum, *J. Infect. Dis.* **108**:90–94.

Michael, J. G., and Rosen, F. S., 1963, Association of "natural" antibodies to gram-negative bacteria with the gamma 1-macro-globulins, *J. Exp. Med.* **118**:619–626.

Michael, J. G., Whitby, J. L., and Landy, M., 1962, Studies on natural antibodies to gram-negative bacteria, *J. Exp. Med.* **115**:131–146.

Miller, C. P., and Foster, A. Z., 1944, Studies on action of penicillin: bactericidal action of penicillin on meningococcus in vitro, *Proc. Soc. Exp. Biol. Med.* **56**:205–208.

Mittal, K. R., and Ingram, D. G., 1969, Bactericidal activity of rabbit serum containing immunoconglutinin, *Immunology* **17**:677–684.

Moore, H. D., 1919, Complementary and opsonic functions in their relation to immunity. A study of the serum of guinea pigs naturally deficient in complement, *J. Immunol.* **4**:425–441.

Mosley, W. H., Benenson, A. S., and Barui, A., 1968, A serological survey for cholera antibodies in the cholera vaccine field trial population in rural East Pakistan. 2. A comparison of antibody titers in immunized and control populations and the relationship of antibody titer to cholera case rate, *Bull. WHO* **38**:335–346.

Müller, F., and Segerling, M., 1970, Comparative studies on the haemolytic and *Treponema pallidum* immobilizing complement activity in the serum of different species, *Immunology* **18**:13–18.

Muschel, L. H., 1960a, Bactericidal activity of normal serum against bacterial cultures. II. Activity against *Escherichia coli* strains, *Proc. Soc. Exp. Biol. Med.* **103**:632–636.

Muschel, L. H., 1960b, Serum Bactericidal actions, *Ann. N. Y. Acad. Sci.* **88**:1265–1272.

Muschel, L. H., and Gustafson, L., 1968, Antibiotic, detergent, and complement sensitivity of *Salmonella typhi* after ethylendiaminetetraacetic acid treatment, *J. Bacteriol.* **95**:2010–2013.

Muschel, L. H., and Jackson, J. E., 1966a, Reversal of the bactericidal reaction of serum by magnesium ion, *J. Bacteriol.* **91**:1399–1402.

Muschel, L. H., and Jackson, J. E., 1966b, The reactivity of serum against protoplasts and spheroplasts, *J. Immunol.* **97**:46–51.

Muschel, L. H., and Larsen, L. L., 1970, The sensitivity of smooth and rough gram-negative bacteria to the immune bactericidal reaction, *Proc. Soc. Exp. Biol. Med.* **133**:345–348.

Muschel, L. H., and Muto, T., 1956, Bactericidal reaction of mouse serum, *Science* **123**:62–64.

Muschel, L. H., and Treffers, H. P., 1956a, Quantitative studies on the bactericidal actions of serum and complement. I. A rapid photometric growth assay for bactericidal activity, *J. Immunol.* **76**:1–10.

Muschel, L. H., and Treffers, H. P., 1956b, Quantitative studies on the bactericidal actions of serum and complement. II. Some implications for the mechanism of the bactericidal reaction, *J. Immunol.* **76**:11–19.

Muschel, L. H., and Treffers, H. P., 1956c, Quantitative studies on the bactericidal actions of serum and complement. III. Observations on sera obtained after T. A. B. vaccination or during typhoid fever, *J. Immunol.* **76**:20–27.

Muschel, L. H., Chamberlin, R. H., and Osawa, E., 1958, Bactericidal activity of normal serum against bacterial cultures. I. Activity against *Salmonella typhi* strains, *Proc. Soc. Exp. Biol. Med.* **97**:376–382.

Muschel, L. H., Carey, W. F., and Baron, L. S., 1959, Formation of bactericidal protoplasts by serum components, *J. Immunol.* **82**:38–42.

Muschel, L. H., Jackson, J. E., and Gewurz, H., 1964, Phylogenic evolution of complement, *Fed. Proc. Fed. Amer. Soc. Exp. Biol.* **23**:505.

Muschel, L. H., Ahl, L. A., and Baron, L. S., 1968, Effect of lysogeny on serum sensitivity, *J. Bacteriol.* **96**:1912–1914.

Muschel, L. H., Ahl, A., and Fisher, W. W., 1969a, Sensitivity of *Pseudomonas aeruginosa* to normal serum and to polymyxin, *J. Bacteriol.* **98**:453–457.

Muschel, L. H., Gustafson, L., and Larsen, L. J., 1969b, Reexamination of the Neisser-Wechsberg (antibody prozone) phenomenon, *Immunology* **17**:525–533.

Nagington, J., 1956, The bactericidal action of typhoid antibody, *Br. J. Exp. Pathol.* **37**:385–396.

Neisser, M., and Wechsberg, F., 1901, Ueber die Wirkungsart bactericider Sera, *Muench. Med. Wochenschr.* **48**:697–700.

Nelson, R. A., and Mayer, M. M., 1949, Immobilization of *Treponema pallidum* in syphilitic infection, *J. Exp. Med.* **89**:369–393.

Nicolle, P., Jude, A., and Diverneau, G., 1953, Antigènes extravant l'action de certains bacteriophages, *Ann. Inst. Pasteur* **84**:27–50.

Nilsson, U. R., Miller, M. E., and Wyman, S., 1974, A functional serum of individuals with a familial opsonic defect, *J. Immunol.* **112**:1164–1176.

Osawa, E., and Muschel, L. H., 1960, The bactericidal action of serum and the properdin system, *J. Immunol.* **84**:203–212.

Osawa, E., and Muschel, L. H., 1964a, Studies relating to the serum resistance of certain gram-negative bacteria, *J. Exp. Med.* **119**:41–51.

Osawa, E., and Muschel, L. H., 1964b, The bactericidal actions of O and Vi antibodies against *Salmonella typhosa*, *J. Immunol.* **92**:281–285.

Phillips, J. K., Snyderman, R., and Mergenhagen, S. E., 1972, Activation of complement by endotoxin: a role for gamma 2 globulin, C1,C4 and C2 in the consumption of terminal complement components by endotoxin-coated erythrocytes, *J. Immunol.* **109**:334–341.

Pickering, R. J., Naff, G. B., Stroud, R. M., Good, R. A., and Gewurz, H., 1970, Deficiency of Clr in human serum: effects on the structure and function of macromolecular Cl, *J. Exp. Med.* **131**:803–815.

Reynolds, B. L., and Pruul, H., 1971a, Protective role of smooth lipopolysaccharide in the serum bactericidal reaction, *Infec. Immun.* **4**:764–771.

Reynolds, B. L., and Pruul, H., 1971b, Sensitization of complement-resistant smooth gram-negative bacterial strains, *Infect. Immun.* **3**:365–372.

Reynolds, B. L., and Rowley, D., 1969, Sensitization of complement resistant bacterial strains, *Nature London* **221**:1259–1261.

Rice, C. E., and Boulanger, P., 1952, Interchangeability of complement components of different animal species; in hemolysis of rabbit erythrocytes sensitized with sheep activity. *J. Immunol.* **68**:197–205.

Roantree, R. J., and Pappas, M. C., 1960, The survival of strains of enteric bacilli in the blood stream as related to their sensitivity to the bactericidal effect of serum, *J. Clin. Invest.* **39**:82–88.

Roantree, R. J., and Rantz, L. A., 1960, A study of the relationship of the normal bactericidal activity of the human serum to bacterial infection, *J. Clin. Invest.* **39**:72–81.

Robbins, P. W., and Uchida, T., 1962, Determinants of specificity in *Salmonella:* changes in antigenic structure mediated by bacteriophage, *Fed. Proc. Fed. Amer. Soc. Exp. Biol.* **21**:702–710.

Robbins, J. B., Kenny, K., and Suter, E., 1965, The isolation and biologic activities of rabbit gamma M and gamma G anti-*Salmonella typhimurium, J. Exp. Med.* **122**:385–402.

Root, R. K., Ellman, L., and Frank, M., 1972, Bactericidal and opsonic properties of C4-deficient guinea pig serum, *J. Immunol.* **109**:477–486.

Rowley, O., 1954, The virulence of strains of *Bacterium coli* for mice. *Br. J. Exp. Pathol.* **35**:528–538.

Rowley, O., 1968, Sensitivity of rough gram negative bacteria to the bactericidal action of serum, *J. Bacteriol.* **95**:1647–1650.

Rowley, O., and Turner, K. J., 1968, Passive sensitization of *Salmonella adelaide* to the bactericidal action of antibody and complement, *Nature London* **217**:657–658.

Salton, M. R. J., 1967, Structure and function of bacterial cell membranes, *Annu. Rev. Microbiol.* **21**:417–442.

Salton, M. R. J., 1968, Lytic agents, cell permeability, and monolayer penetrability, *J. Gen. Physiol.* **52**:227–252.

Snyderman, R., Gewurz, H., Mergenhagen, S., and Jensen, J., 1971, Effects of C4 depletion on the utilization of the terminal components of guinea pig complement by endotoxin, *Nature London New Biol.* **231**:152–154.

Sterzl, J., Mandel, L., Miler, I., and Riha, I., 1965, Development of immune reactions in the absence or presence of an antigenic stimulus, in: *Molecular and Cellular Basis of Antibody Formation* (J. Sterzl, ed.), pp. 351–370, Academic Press, New York.

Stinebring, W. R., Braun, W., and Pomales-Lebron, A., 1960, Modified serum resistance following intracellular residence, *Ann. N. Y. Acad. Sci.* **88**:1230–1236.

Treffers, H. P., and Muschel, L. H., 1954, The combined actions of chloramphenicol and of bactericidal antibody plus complement on Salmonella typhosa, *J. Exp. Med.* **99**:155–165.

Webb, P. M., and Muschel, L. H., 1968, Bactericidal antibody studies in maternal serum, colostrum, and newborn serum of the pig, *Can. J. Microbiol.* **14**:545–550.

Wellek, B., and Opferkuch, W., 1975, A case of deficiency of the seventh component of complement in man, *Clin. Exp. Immunol.* **19**:223–235.

8

Biologic Aspects of Leukocyte Chemotaxis

RALPH SNYDERMAN and MARILYN PIKE

1. Introduction

To protect a host against microbial invasion and the development of neoplasms, the immune system must discriminate self from nonself and then efficiently localize and eliminate material recognized as nonself. The process of localizing, degrading, and eliminating nonself can be termed an *immune effector function* and is largely mediated by the accumulation of wandering phagocytic cells, such as polymorphonuclear leukocytes (PMNs) and macrophages. One process that could result in the local accumulation of immune effector cells is chemotaxis, the unidirectional migration of cells along a concentration gradient of a chemoattractant substance. During the past decade, it has clearly been shown that the interaction of lymphocytes or immunoglobulins with antigens can result in the production or release of biologically active products that are capable of enhancing vascular permeability and attracting leukocytes. The production of chemotactic gradients as well as the ability of wandering cells to respond normally to such gradients appears to be critical for immunologically mediated host defense. Dysfunctions of leukocyte chemotaxis may render an individual more susceptible to infectious, inflammatory, and perhaps neoplastic diseases. In this chapter, we will review methodology for quantifying chemotaxis, describe factors that are chemotactic for polymorphonuclear leukocytes, and discuss recent observations of abnormalities of human leukocyte chemotaxis and their relationship to human disease states.

2. Methods for Quantifying Leukocyte Chemotaxis *in Vitro*

An early observation of directed leukocyte migration was made by Leber (1888), who injected inflammatory stimuli into rabbit corneas and noted the migra-

RALPH SNYDERMAN • Division of Rheumatic and Genetic Diseases, Duke University Medical Center, Durham, North Carolina. MARILYN PIKE • Department of Medicine, Duke University Medical Center, Durham, North Carolina.

RALPH SNYDERMAN
AND MARILYN PIKE

tion of inflammatory cells toward the site of injection. Various other techniques for quantifying leukocyte migration have evolved since these early experiments and have clearly shown that leukocytes are capable of migrating unidirectionally along chemical gradients of an attractant substance (chemotaxis). One method that allows the direct visualization and measurement of cell movement is time-lapse cinematography of cells migrating on glass slides. Techniques such as these, however, are laborious, only semiquantitative, and allow sampling of only a few cells at a time. The development by Boyden (1962) of an *in vitro* method for studying polymorphonuclear leukocyte chemotaxis has permitted major advances in our understanding of the mechanisms of inflammatory-cell accumulation. The Boyden technique has been modified and expanded to allow measurement of macrophage, basophil, neutrophil, and eosinophil migration *in vitro* (Ward *et al.*, 1965, 1969; Keller and Sorkin, 1965, 1969; Kay, 1970; Snyderman *et al.*, 1968, 1970, 1971b, 1972b; Kay and Austen, 1972; Boetcher and Leonard, 1973; Stroud *et al.*, 1974; Wilkinson, 1974). This technique measures leukocyte migration through porous filters that are used to separate a chemotaxis chamber into an upper and a lower compartment (Figure 1). A suspension of leukocytes is placed in the upper compartment of the chamber and the material being tested for chemotactic activity is placed in the lower compartment. The chambers containing leukocytes and chemotactic factor or control medium are incubated at 37°C for varying times, depending on the cell type being studied and the filter employed. Following incubation, the chambers are

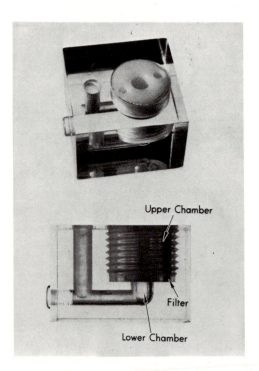

Figure 1. Chemotaxis chamber. A standardized cell suspension (0.4 ml) is placed in the upper compartment of the chamber and is separated from the chemotactic stimulant (0.85 ml) or medium alone in the lower compartment by a polycarbonate or nitrocellulose filter. From Snyderman *et al.* (1975d).

emptied, the filters are removed and stained, and the number of cells that migrated through the filter are quantitated microscopically, using an eyepiece grid. A widely used filter in chemotaxis studies is the nitrocellulose filter, which is approximately 150 μm thick and is available in several pore sizes, ranging from 0.4 to 8.0 μm. Chemotaxis can be scored by measuring the total number of cells per microscopic field that have migrated completely through the filter (Figure 2). Chemotaxis can

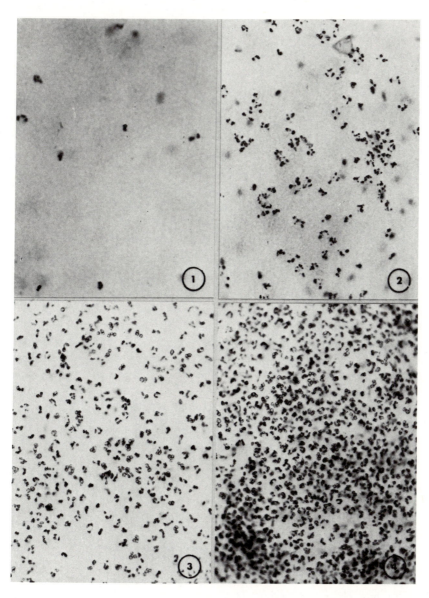

Figure 2. Neutrophil response to chemotactic factor generated by increasing doses of *V. alcalescens* endotoxin incubated in guinea pig serum: (1) serum alone; (2) serum plus 0.05 μg endotoxin; (3) serum plus 0.5 μg endotoxin; (4) serum plus 5.0 μg endotoxin. From Snyderman *et al.* (1968).

also be quantified by measuring the depth into the filter to which the leading front of cells has migrated (Zigmond and Hirsh, 1973). The nitrocellulose filter has also been used in a neutrophil chemotaxis radioassay employing chrominum-51 (Gallin *et al.,* 1973; Goetzl and Austen, 1972). In this assay, neutrophils labeled with chromium-51 are placed in the upper compartment of the chemotaxis chamber, which is separated from the chemotactic stimulant by two 5-μm nitrocellulose filters. The number of cells traversing the upper filter and migrating into the lower filter is proportional to the radioactivity incorporated into that filter. Jungi (1975) recently described a modified chemotaxis assay using a closed chamber that can be turned upside down during the incubation period. Then the leukocytes that are inside the filter when the chamber is turned migrate upward and are retained on the filter by gravity. This method eliminates any loss of cells due to their falling off the filter.

The other type of filter that has been used successfully in the Boyden chamber is the polycarbonate filter (Nuclepore®) (Horwitz and Garrett, 1971; Snyderman *et al.,* 1972b). This type of filter is 15 μm thick and is available in pore sizes ranging from 1 to 10 μm in diameter. For the study of macrophage migration, the 5-μm pore size is commonly used. This type of filter allows measurement of only those cells that have migrated to the lower surface. The polycarbonate filter is better than the nitrocellulose filter in the macrophage assay because the required incubation time is far less.

3. Chemotactic Factors

The accumulation of immune effector cells at sites of inflammation is mediated by a series of interrelated processes, initiated by the recognition of foreign substances or neoplastically transformed cells as nonself. An important consequence of the interaction of immune recognition components with antigenic materials is the production and/or release of chemotactic factors. These substances may be produced as the result of activation of certain enzyme cascade systems, or they may be synthesized and released by white blood cells, such as lymphocytes or mast cells. Chemotactic factors can be produced by direct cleavage of complement proteins by proteolytic enzymes released from cells and can also be produced by many types of bacteria. A summary of the chemotactic factors is presented in Table 1.

3.1. Chemotactic Factors Derived from the Complement System

It is now well established that the complement (C) system is an important immune effector and functions as a mediator of the acute inflammatory response. The role of C in mediating the local accumulation of PMNs and macrophages has become apparent during the last 13 years. Boyden (1962) demonstrated that immune complexes of antigen and antibody, while being potent inflammatory agents *in vivo,* were not directly chemotactic for neutrophils *in vitro.* If the immune complexes were incubated with serum, however, chemotactic activity was produced. The requirement for the production of this activity was suggested by the observation that prior heating of the serum (56°C for 30 min) prevented the formation of chemotactic activity. Ward *et al.* (1965, 1966) strengthened the contention that C was necessary for the production of neutrophil chemotactic activity by immune complexes in serum. With the use of partially purified C components, they reported activity associated with a macromolecular complex of activated C5, C6, and C7. Using bacterial endotoxin as a probe to determine the role of C in mediating leukotaxis, we demonstrated that, while not directly chemotactic for PMNs, endotoxin produced chemotactic activity when incubated with C-sufficient serum (Snyderman *et al.,* 1968). The fifth component of C was specifically required, and the great majority of chemotactic activity produced in serum treated with endotoxin was a product of about 15,000 daltons. The relatively low molecular weight of the chemotactic factor suggested that a cleavage product, rather than a macromolecular aggregate of C components, accounted for most of the activity produced upon C activation·in whole serum. Using highly purified guinea pic C components, Shin *et al.* (1968) showed that cleavage of C5 by the earlier-acting C components produced a 15,000-dalton product, termed C5a, that had chemotactic activity for PMNs. Human C5 cleaved by trypsin also produced chemotactic activity (Ward and Newman, 1969).

There is now substantial evidence for the biologic importance of C5a as a chemotactic factor for PMNs. The vast majority of chemotactic activity produced in serum upon its activation by immune complexes, aggregated gammaglobulins (Snyderman *et al.,* 1970), endotoxins (Snyderman *et al.,* 1968), staphylococcal protein A (Pike and Daniels, 1975), or cobra venom factor (Shin *et al.,* 1969) can be attributed to C5a. Human or mouse serum that is congenitally devoid of C5 is markedly deficient in producing chemotactic activity (Snyderman *et al.,*1971a, 1975d). Mice that are congenitally devoid of C5 also have a defective ability to

TABLE 1.   Chemotactic Factors[a]

Group	Factors
I. Humoral-derived factors	
(a) Complement system	C5a
	C3a
	C$\overline{567}$
(b) Clotting, kinin-forming, and fibrinolytic systems	Fibrinopeptide B
	Fibrin degradation products
	Kallikrein
	Plasminogen activator
II. Cellular-derived factors	
(a) Lymphocytes	LDCF
	Transfer factor
	PMN chemotactic factors
(b) Mast cells	ECF-A (eosinophil chemotactic factor of anaphylaxis)
	Histamine
III. Other sources	
	N-formyl-methionyl peptides
	Bacterial chemotactic factor
	Oxidized arachidonic acid
	Denatured proteins
	Collagen and collagen-derived peptides

[a]This list contains many, but not all, of the described chemotactic factors. See Wilkinson (1974) for a more comprehensive overview. The biological significance of most of these factors has not yet been documented.

mobilize PMNs in response to inflammatory agents *in vivo* (Synderman *et al.,* 1971a). In additon, C5a can be recovered from the synovial fluid of patients with inflammatory arthritidies, such as rheumatoid arthritis (Ward and Zvaifler, 1971). Moreover, the injection of highly purified C5a into the skin of animals results in a dramatic accumulation of polymorphonuclear leukocytes followed by the accumulation of macrophages (Jensen *et al.,* 1969). The inflammatory reaction in response to C5a injected *in vivo* appears quite similar to that produced by local antigen–antibody reactions (Arthus type).

Since large numbers of macrophages as well as PMNs are observed at sites of the injection of C5a *in vivo,* it became important to determine whether C5a was directly chemotactic for macrophages as well as for PMNs. Highly purified guinea pig C5, when cleaved with either the earlier-acting complement components or by trypsin (Snyderman *et al.,* 1971b), produced substantial amounts of chemotactic activity for guinea pig peritoneal macrophages. Polyacrylamide gel electrophoresis and molecular-sieve chromatography of cleaved C5 showed that the chemotactic activity for both PMNs and macrophages resided in the same or similar fragments of C5 (15,000 daltons) (Snyderman *et al.,* 1971b). Complement activated in the more physiologic milieu of whole serum also resulted in production of chemotactic activity for macrophages and human blood monocytes (Snyderman *et al.,* 1971b, Hausman *et al.,* 1972). Fractionation of serum treated with complement-activating agents demonstrated two peaks of chemotactic activity. One was a low-molecular-weight (ca. 15,000 daltons) heat-stable (30 min at 56°C) factor found only in activated serum. This activity was inhibited by incubation with monospecific antibody to C5 or C5a and had an elution profile similar to C5a. The other peak of chemotactic activity had a molecular weight of approximately 90,000 daltons and was present in both activated and unactivated serum. Human C5a derived from activated serum was chemotactic for human monocytes at concentrations as low as 3.3×10^{-9}M (Snyderman *et al.,* 1971b). The nature of the high-molecular-weight chemotactic activity present in both activated and untreated serum is still not identified, but its relationship to C5 has been shown. Fractionation of serum from C5 deficient and C5 normal mice indicates that the heavy molecular-weight peak of chemotactic activity is present in C5-sufficient mouse serum (Snyderman *et al.,* 1975d) but not in C5-deficient mouse serum.

Clearly, C5a is chemotactic for PMNs as well as mononuclear leukocytes, such as monocytes and macrophages. Thus, it can be assumed that prior accumulation of PMNs is not required for the accumulation of macrophages *in vivo,* since PMNs are not present in the mononuclear leukocyte preparations used *in vitro.* This is not to say that prior accumulation of PMNs does not enhance the subsequent accumulation of macrophages *in vivo.* It can be expected that the accumulation of PMNs with concomitant phagocytosis of foreign material would lead to the release of lysozomal enzymes that are capable of cleaving additional C5, thus producing higher local concentrations of C5a (Ward and Hill, 1970). The ability of intracellular proteolytic enzymes to cleave C5 and produce chemotactic fragments deserves emphasis. Neutrophils, macrophages, and parenchymal cells contain intracellular enzymes that can cleave C5 into fragments which contain chemotactic activity (Snyderman *et al.,* 1972a). The implication of these findings is that nonspecific tissue trauma as well as damage caused by cytopathic viruses can release enzymes that cleave C5 locally and thereby attract leukocytes to the area of tissue damage (Brier *et al.,* 1970).

In addition to the chemotactic activity associated with fragmentation of C5 and the activated macromolecular complex of C5, C6, and C7, C3 has also been reported to be a chemotactinogen. Taylor and Ward (1967) demonstrated that cleavage of human C3 by plasmin produced chemotactic activity for neutrophils. Bokisch *et al.* (1969) reported that the small-molecular-weight cleavage product of human C3, which had been cleaved by either trypsin or $C\overline{42}$, had chemotactic activity for neutrophils and was anaphylatoxic. Proteolytic enzymes derived from bacteria have also been reported to cleave C3 into fragments that are chemotactic for neutrophils (Chapitis *et al.,* 1971). While fragmentation products of C3 have been reported to be chemotactic for neutrophils *in vitro,* it must be emphasized that its relative activity as compared with C5a is substantially less. In addition, the injection of C3a into the skin of humans induces increased vascular permeability and neutrophil margination at capillary walls, but no chemotaxis of the neutrophils out of the vessel walls. Becker (1972) showed that C5a was a more potent activator of neutrophil esterases putatively involved in the chemotaxis response than was C3a.

In sum, the complement system appears to be an important mediator of leukocyte accumulation *in vivo.* Complement-derived chemotactic factors can be produced upon activation of the C system by either the classical or the alternative pathway (Sandberg *et al.,* 1972) by factors derived from the fibrinolytic systems, such as plasmin, and by proteolytic enzymes released from cells. Complement-mediated chemotaxis could then be expected to participate in inflammatory events in immune complex diseases, in virally induced cytopathic lesions, in nonspecific tissue trauma, and in areas of bacterial invasion. The relative importance of the various complement-derived chemotactic factors is still not certain; however, there are data that suggest that C5a is the major source of chemotactic activity supplied by the complement system. The evidence for this includes the fact that C5 deficient mice, which have normal quantities of C3, have a markedly defective accumulation of neutrophils *in vivo* when challenged with inflammatory agents, such as bacterial endotoxins (Snyderman *et al.,* 1971a). Moreover, rabbits that are congenitally devoid of C6 and thus unable to produce the trimolecular complex of C5, C6, and C7 produce normal amounts of chemotactic activity when their serum is activated *in vitro* (Stecher and Sorkin, 1969; Snyderman *et al.,* 1970). Finally, injection of C5a into the skin of animals as well as man produces substantial leukocyte accumulation, whereas injection of C3a produces increased vascular permeability and neutrophil margination but no neutrophil migration out of the vessel walls (Jensen *et al.,* 1969).

3.2. Chemotactic Factors Associated with the Kinin- and Clot-Forming Systems

The interrelationship between the biological activities of the complement, clotting, fibrinolytic, and kinin-forming systems has been well recognized (Ratnoff, 1969). For example, enzymes from one system have been shown to activate enzymes from other systems. In addition, naturally occurring inhibitors of one pathway may function as inhibitors of other pathways. It is of interest, therefore, to note that chemotactic activity has been attributed to products derived from the kinin-forming system as well as from fibrinolytic and clotting systems. Kaplan *et al.* (1972) have demonstrated that the conversion of prekallikrein to kallikrein by prekallikrein activator is associated with the production of chemotactic activity for neutrophils, and chemotactic activity produced during this reaction appears to be associated with kallikrein itself. In addition to being chemotactic for neutrophils, partially purified kallikrein is also chemotactic for human monocytes (Snyderman *et al.*, unpublished observations). The weight of the molecule associated with this activity is approximately 130,000 daltons.

Stecher and Sorkin (1972) have presented evidence that products derived from the fibrinolytic system are chemotactic for neutrophils. Following the conversion of fibrinogen to fibrin by prothrombin, the addition of plasmin to the fibrin clot produced chemotactic activity for neutrophils. However, neither plasmin nor fibrinogen alone was chemotactic. McKenzie *et al.* (1975) have also shown that products produced upon interaction of plasmin with human fibrinogen are chemotactic for human peripheral leukocytes. The digestion of human fibrinogen by plasmin resulted in the production of four fragments, one of which, termed *fragment* Y, with a molecular weight of approximately 30,000 daltons, was chemotactic. Additional chemotactic activity, with higher specific activity than fragment Y, was found in longer incubation–digestion mixtures and appeared to be attributable to low-molecular-weight peptides derived from fibrinogen. The interaction of thrombin with human fibrinogen also produces chemotactic activity, and this factor has been attributed to the release of fibrinopeptide B (McKenzie *et al.*, 1975). Thus, products derived from the kinin-forming system, fibrin-forming systems, and fibrinolytic pathways release materials that are chemotactic for leukocytes. Thus, it can be surmised that the release of these factors may attract leukocytes to areas of clot formation and might be important for the subsequent wound-healing processes.

3.3. Lymphocyte-Derived Chemotactic Factors

The observation that sensitized lymphocytes release biologically active effector molecules (lymphokines) after interaction with antigens *in vitro* or *in vivo* has contributed greatly to the understanding of how leukocytes accumulate at sites of delayed hypersensitivity. Factors produced by antigen-stimulated sensitized lymphocytes have been shown to be chemotactic for monocytes, macrophages, neutrophils, and lymphocytes (Ward *et al.*, 1969; Snyderman *et al.*, 1972b; Altman *et al.*, 1973; Wahl *et al.*, 1974). Ward *et al.* (1969) made the important observation that guinea pig lymphocytes, when stimulated with specific antigen, produced a chemotactic factor for homologous macrophages. This factor was reported to have a molecular weight of slightly less than 43,000 daltons and was shown to be separable from migration inhibitory factor (MIF) (Ward *et al.*, 1969). Supernatants of stimulated lymphocyte cultures have also been reported to be chemotactic for lymphocytes and neutrophils (Ward *et al.*, 1970). The neutrophil chemotactic factor could be distinguished from the macrophage chemotactic factor and the MIF by acrylamide gel electrophoresis. The chemotactic factor for lymphocytes has yet to be characterized. Boetcher and Leonard (1973) have shown that supernatants of human lymphocytes stimulated with PHA or PPD are also chemotactic for basophils.

The mechanisms of macrophage accumulation in human cellular immune inflammatory reactions have been studied in our laboratory (Snyderman *et al.*, 1972b; Altman *et al.*, 1973). Human peripheral blood leukocytes were isolated from individuals sensitive to tuberculoprotein (PPD). The incubation of these leukocytes with PPD or with the nonspecific mitogen phytohemagglutinin (PHA) resulted in the production of chemotactic activity for homologous and autologous monocytes. Kinetic studies of the production of a lymphocyte-derived chemotactic factor (LDCF) demonstrated that it is released prior to blastogenesis and that cell division is not necessary for its production (Altman *et al.*, 1973). This chemotactic activity has been shown to be released from stimulated lymphocyte cultures as early as 6 hr after introduction of antigen or mitogen *in vitro*. Characterization of this activity showed that it was due to a low-molecular-weight (ca. 12,500 daltons) factor, which was antigenically and isoelectrically distinct from the C5a fragment produced during activation of the complement system (Snyderman *et al.*, 1972b; Altman *et al.*, 1973, 1974a).

Several investigators have shown that chemotactic activity can be elaborated by bone marrow (B)–derived lymphocytes as well as by thymus-derived (T) lymphocytes. Mackler *et al.* (1974) and Altman *et al.* (1974a) have reported that human B lymphocytes, isolated after rosetting with sensitized sheep erythrocytes carrying the activated third component of complement (EAC3b), elaborated chemotactic activity when cultured with PHA or conconavalin A (Con A). Further studies by Wahl *et al.* (1974) have shown that polymeric B cell mitogens, including bacterial lipopolysaccharide and polymerized flagellin, can induce chemotactic lymphokine production by guinea pig splenic lymphocytes. Additionally, antigen–antibody complexes, aggregated gammaglobulin, anti-immunoglobulin, and antigen–antibody-complement complexes all served as adequate stimuli for mediator production by purified B lymphocytes in the absence of blastogenesis.

Activation of lymphocytes by antigen *in vitro* requires prior processing of these antigens by macrophages (Oppenheim *et al.*, 1968). Wahl *et al.* (1975) studied the macrophage requirement for chemotactic factor production by lymphocytes. Purified T cells depleted of macrophages did not produce LDCF when stimulated with specific antigens. Addition of macrophages to the lymphocyte cultures restored the ability of antigen-stimulated T lymphocytes to produce the chemotactic lymphokine. Purified B cells, however, produced chemotactic factor when cultured *in vitro* with a B cell mitogen in the absence of macrophages. These findings indicate a macrophage requirement for mediator production by T but not by B lymphocytes.

While recognition of the mediators produced by *in vitro* stimulation of lymphocytes has contributed toward our conceptual understanding of leukocyte accumulation in cellular immune reactions, the actual role played by these substances *in vivo* is as yet rudimentary. Cohen *et al.* (1973) detected the presence of a chemotactic factor for macrophages in skin sites of delayed hypersensitivity. A recently devised animal model has been employed in our laboratories to study the kinetics of inflammation in cell-mediated immune reactions *in vivo* (Postlethwaite and Snyderman, 1975). Specific antigens were introduced into the peritoneal cavities of immunized guinea pigs via indwelling, silicon–plastic catheters and fluid samples were removed at various times thereafter. Using these methods, we found that a macrophage chemotactic factor with a molecular weight of approximately 12,000 daltons was produced within 24 hr after the introduction of specific antigens into the peritoneal cavity. Concomitant with the appearance of this activity was the influx of macrophages. The majority of this activity could be attributed to a factor that could not be distinguished from the chemotactic activity produced by stimulated lymphocyte cultures (LDCF) *in vitro*. These data indicate that lymphokines are indeed produced *in vivo* during cellular immune reactions and that a chemotactic lympho-kine is responsible for the influx of macrophages to sites of delayed hypersensitivity.

3.4. Chemotactic Factors Produced by Bacteria

Culture filtrates of many bacteria grown *in vitro* are chemotactic for neutro-phils (Keller and Sorkin, 1967; Ward *et al.*, 1968). The greatest production of chemotactic activity occurs during the log phase of bacterial growth (Ward *et al.*, 1968). Several bacterial chemotactic factors have been described in different labora-tories and cannot be attributable to a single common entity. For example, Walker (1969) isolated from *Staphylococcus aureus* a neutrophil chemotactic factor that had a molecular weight above 10,000 daltons as indicated by its nondialyzability. On the other hand, Ward *et al.* (1968) found that chemotactic factors produced by a number of bacteria had a similar molecular weight of approximately 3600 daltons. Tempel *et al.* (1970) also found that chemotactic activities produced by three different types of bacteria that grow in the oral cavity have low molecular weight (less than 10,000 daltons). The exact chemical composition of chemotactic factors produced by bacteria is still unknown. Recent studies by Schiffmann *et al.* (1975), however, may shed some light on the nature of the bacterial chemotactic factors. These workers found that the chemotactic factors produced by bacteria in culture frequently had blocked end-terminal amino acid groups. They, moreover, showed that small formyl-methionyl peptides, analogous to those derived from the N-terminal regions of newly synthesized bacterial proteins, were chemotactic for guinea pig and rabbit leukocytes at concentrations as low as 10^{-9} M. We have recently shown that the formylated methionyl peptides are chemotactic for human monocytes and human neutrophils as well (Snyderman and Pike, unpublished observations). Nei-ther acylated peptides nor free methionine are active, thereby suggesting that formylation is specifically necessary for chemotactic activity. Since eukaryotic cells appear, for the most part, to initiate protein synthesis with nonacylated methionine, the chemotactic response of mammalian leukocytes to formylated amino acids may represent a simple recognition system that detects the presence of microbial agents. Additional products released by bacteria may also be chemotactic for neutrophils. Turner *et al.* (1975) have indicated that mild oxidation of arachidonic acid, which is present in many bacterial cell walls, results in the production of chemotactic activity for polymorphonuclear leukocytes.

Wilkinson *et al.* (1972, 1973) have identified macrophage-specific chemotactic activity produced by organisms belonging to the group *Corynebacterium parvum*. This activity is attributable to molecules that are nondialyzable and heat-stable at 60°C, but destroyed by boiling. The most striking feature about this factor is that its production by bacteria closely parallels the capacity of these bacteria to enhance carbon clearance by the infected hosts' reticuloendothelial system.

4. Defective Chemotaxis in Human Disease

The realization that defects in the immune system could result in the develop-ment of human disease has been recognized for the past 20 years. The earliest described defects in immunity were related to defective immune recognition function, i.e., deficient antibody synthesis or subnormal populations of lymphocytes. It is now becoming apparent, however, that abnormal immune function can also be due to defects in the effector limb of the immune system. Localization of leukocytes at sites of immune reactions requires recognition of foreign materials as nonself, the production of chemotactic factors, and the subsequent mobilization of effector cells in response to the factors produced. Defects in recognition, chemotactic factor production, or the response of leukocytes to chemotactic factors could all result in depressed immune reactions (Table 2). The following discussion will present, in brief, evidence that abnormalities in immune recognition function, chemotactic factor production, or chemotactic responsiveness of leukocytes can all be associated with abnormalities of the inflammatory response and certain human diseases.

4.1. Abnormalities of Host Recognition Factors

Complement-derived chemotactic factors are produced as a consequence of the interaction of antigen with immunoglobulins, IgM, IgG, and perhaps IgA. It can be postulated that individuals with agammaglobulinemia or hypogammaglobulinemia have depressed chemotactic factor production due to diminished activation of

TABLE 2.   Mechanism of Leukocyte Accumulation and Related Defects in Human Disease

Mechanism	Mediated by	Examples of defects

I. Recognition of nonself	Immunoglobulins
	Lymphocytes
	Macrophages
		(a) Defective recognition of nonself
		    Hypogammaglobulinemia
		    Lymphopenia

II. Activation of immune effector systems and production of chemotactic factors	Complement system
	Clotting system
	Kinin-forming system
	Lymphokines
		(a) Defective chemotactic factor production
		    Hypocomplementemias
		    Dysfunctional C5
		    Fletcher factor deficiency
		(b) Inhibitors of chemotactic factors
		    Glomerulonephritis
		    Hodgkin's disease
		    Cirrhosis
		    Anergic disease

III. Migration of leukocytes toward increasing gradients of chemotactic factors	PMNs
	Macrophages
	Monocytes
	Lymphocytes
		(a) Defective cellular chemotactic responses
		    Chronic mucocutaneous candidiasis
		    Chediak-Higashi syndrome
		    Lazy leukocyte syndrome
		(b) Inhibitors of the cellular chemotactic response
		    Rheumatoid arthritis
		    Hyper-IgE syndromes
		    Wiskott-Aldrich syndrome

IV. Ingestion and degradation of foreign materials	PMNs
	Macrophages
		(a) Defective degradation of foreign materials
		    Chediak-Higashi syndrome
		    Chronic granulomatous disease

the C system. This, indeed, was found to be the case by Steerman *et al.* (1971), who demonstrated the defective production of chemotactic activity by inflammatory stimuli in the serum of a patient with agammaglobulinemia.

4.2. Defective Chemotactic Factor Production

Deficiencies of the complement system may prevent normal activation of the C components responsible for chemotactic factor production. Gewurz *et al.* (1967) first demonstrated this phenomenon in individuals with deficiencies of C2. These patients manifested depressed neutrophil exudation *in vivo* and their serum was defective in generating chemotactic activity *in vitro*. This finding was confirmed by Gallin (1975), who showed that serum from patients deficient in C1r had decreased production of chemotactic activity. It is important to note that individuals with deficiencies of the early-acting C components (C1r or C2) have an increased incidence of inflammatory diseases, manifested clinically by a dermatomyositis or systemic lupus erythematosus-like syndrome (Day *et al.*, 1972; Ruddy *et al.*, 1972).

A familial dysfunction of the fifth component of complement has been described by Miller and Nilsson (1970), in which the individuals have increased susceptibility to bacterial infections. Serum from these patients generates less PMN chemotactic activity and supports less phagocytic activity than normal serum. Rosenfield and Leddy (1974) further demonstrated the importance of C5 as a chemotactinogen in humans. These investigators studied an individual with a complete absence of C5, who suffered from severe recurrent bacterial infections. The patient's serum had a marked inability to generate chemotactic activity when activated *in vitro*. Alper *et al.* (1970) described an individual with a congenital C3 deficiency caused by the hypercatabolism of this component due to a lack of C3b inactivator. Serum from this individual did not generate chemotactic activity when activated *in vitro*, perhaps because the activation of C3 is necessary for the cleavage of C5. Weiss *et al.* (1974) have demonstrated that serum from an individual with deficient plasma prekallikrein (Fletcher factor) produces diminished amounts of PMN chemotactic activity when incubated with kaolin. It is not known whether this individual suffered from susceptibility to infection.

Humoral inhibitors of chemotactic factors have been described in normal serum and in serum from individuals with certain diseases. Wilkinson *et al.* (1969) first demonstrated that certain serum fractions from normal subjects rendered chemotactic substances inactive. Berenberg and Ward (1973) and Till and Ward (1973, 1975) have recently described and characterized two distinct factors in serum that selectively inactivate the complement-derived and bacterial chemotactic factors.

The first suggestion that a humoral inhibitor of chemotactic factors might play a role in human disease was provided by Gewurz *et al.* (1967). These investigators demonstrated that the plasma from patients with acute and chronic glomerulonephritis contained a heat-labile (56°C for 30 min) inhibitor of chemotactic actitivy. It is interesting to note that this inhibitor disappeared from the plasma of patients treated by renal transplantation or nephrectomy. Ward and Berenberg (1974) recently described increased levels of a chemotactic factor inhibitor in the serum from patients with Hodgkin's disease. Serum from these patients had increased levels of inhibitory activity for C5a and bacterial chemotactic factors. It has not yet been reported if this inhibitory activity correlated with the stage of illness or the patient's immune responsiveness.

A serum inhibitor of the chemotactic activity of C3a, C5a, and kallikrein has been found in 12 of 16 patients with cutaneous anergy (Van Epps *et al.,* 1974). This inhibitor was a heat-stable, β-migrating substance, which had characteristics similar to immunoglobulin A.

4.3. Abnormalities of Chemotaxis of Unknown Etiology

The cellular and biochemical mechanisms by which leukocytes respond to chemotactic gradients are as yet unknown. It is known, however, that leukocyte chemotaxis is an energy-requiring process, which may depend on calcium fluxes with subsequent myofibril and myofilament formation as well as polymerization of actin (Gallin and Rosenthal, 1974). Defects in chemotaxis may, therefore, arise from anomalies in leukocyte membrane characteristics, biochemical processes required for energy, or contractile protein synthesis (Boxer *et al.,* 1974).

Several cellular deficiencies of neutrophil chemotaxis have been reported. Steerman *et al.* (1971) described a child with agammaglobulinemia and recurrent bacterial infections, who had a defect in chemotaxis and phagocytosis *in vivo* and *in vitro.* No inhibitor of chemotaxis could be detected in this patient's serum nor could the defect be reversed by incubating the patient's PMNs in normal plasma. This observation was confirmed by Gallin (1975), who studied two additional individuals with agammaglobulinemia and defective PMN chemotaxis. Abnormalities in PMN chemotaxis have also been reported in patients with Chediak-Higashi syndrome (Clark and Kimball, 1971; Wolf *et al.,* 1972).

Defects in neutrophil chemotaxis in which there is no detectable abnormality in phagocytosis or bactericidal activity have been described in patients with diabetes mellitus, with a disease termed *the lazy leukocyte syndrome,* and with a familial anomaly of neutrophil function. Mowat and Baum (1971b) have reported decreased PMN chemotaxis in patients with diabetes mellitus, which could be reversed by incubating the defective PMNs with glucose and insulin. The lazy leukocyte syndrome, as described by Miller *et al.* (1971), is a rare disease, characterized by severe peripheral neutropenia, recurrent bacterial infections, dermatitis, periodontitis, and impaired PMN chemotaxis and random motility. Children with this disease suffer from neutropenia, apparently because their cells lack the transport mechanism necessary for diapedesis, since normal numbers of PMNs are found in the bone marrow. The exact mechanism of the defect in this disease, be it structural or metabolic, is not known at this time. Miller *et al.* (1973) also described a familial PMN chemotactic defect in which individuals suffered from congenital icythyosis and recurrent infections with *Trichophyton rubrum.* This syndrome differs from the lazy leukocyte syndrome in that the familial anomaly is associated with neither defective random motility nor peripheral neutropenia.

The accumulation of macrophages at sites of inflammation is particularly important for host defense against viral, fungal, and mycobacterial infection. Since the development of the methodology for assaying human peripheral blood monocyte chemotaxis has only recently been described, our knowledge of monocyte chemotactic dysfunctions in human disease processes is rudimentary at present.

The first observation of an abnormality in monocyte chemotaxis was made in a

RALPH SNYDERMAN
AND MARILYN PIKE

child with recurrent mucocutaneous candidiasis and delayed cutaneous anergy to *Candida* antigen (Snyderman *et al.*, 1973). Immunologically, this patient had delayed cutaneous anergy to monilial as well as other ubiquitous antigens; she had normal lymphocyte transformation; and her lymphocytes produced MIF. In contrast to normal lymphocyte function, this patient's monocyte chemotactic responsiveness to C5a and LDCF ranged from 2–11% of normal when compared to age-matched controls. Nine months after initiation of transfer-factor therapy, the patient's monocyte chemotaxis had improved to approximately 80% of normal. In addition, after transfer-factor therapy and concomitant with the improvement of her monocyte chemotaxis, the patient's skin reaction to *Candida* became positive, and clinical improvement of her disease followed. Depressed monocyte chemotactic responsiveness in two additional patients with chronic mucocutaneous candidiasis was confirmed by Gallin (1975).

During the past 20 years, a considerable body of data has accumulated that suggests a central role for the immune system in protecting the host against the development and spread of neoplasms (Waldmann *et al.*, 1972). Using experimental animals, a number of investigators have shown that cellular immune reactions can destroy tumors and that the accumulation of macrophages is associated with tumor killing (Zbar *et al.*, 1970). It is therefore important to determine whether the ability of macrophages to respond to chemotactic stimuli and thus accumulate at sites of delayed hypersensitivity reactions is impaired in individuals with tumors.

Boetcher and Leonard (1974), Hausman *et al.* (1973), and our laboratory have studied monocyte chemotactic responsiveness *in vitro* in patients with neoplastic diseases and have found their responses to be depressed. Boetcher and Leonard (1974) have shown that of 44 patients with various types of cancer, 24 individuals had depressed monocyte chemotaxis. Hausman *et al.* (1973) have shown that 24 patients with renal cell carcinoma or carcinoma of the bladder had chemotactic responses that were approximately 30% below normal. We studied monocyte chemotactic responsiveness to a chemotactic lymphokine (LDCF) in 98 patients with cancer (Snyderman *et al.*, 1974, 1975b,c; Snyderman and Stahl, 1975; Snyderman and Mergenhagen, 1975). Of these patients, 45 had recurrent malignant melanoma and the rest had a variety of common neoplasms, including carcinoma of the lung, breast, colon, prostate, and kidney. None of the patients was undergoing chemotherapy. Approximately 50% of the patients with cancer had depressed monocyte chemotactic responsiveness with values below the 95th percentile of the responses of a large population of age-matched normals and hospitalized controls (Figure 3). The patients with recurrent malignant melanoma in this particular study were to be placed on BCG therapy (Seigler *et al.*, 1973). It was determined that none of the patients prior to admission to the protocol had evidence of distant metastases. Of patients with melanoma tested prior to receiving BCG, 45% had depressed chemotactic responses. The responses of the melanoma patients were determined following treatment with BCG. Immunization with BCG and subsequent intralesional injection of BCG enhanced the chemotactic responsiveness of all but two individuals who had depressed chemotaxis prior to therapy (Figure 4). Patients whose chemotaxis was normal prior to immunotherapy did not have enhanced responsiveness following BCG treatment. The possible prognostic significance of depressed monocyte chemotactic responsiveness is indicated by the finding that of 25 patients with depressed chemotaxis prior to immunotherapy, 9

(36%) died of their disease during the follow-up period, which ranged from 1 month to 2 years. In contrast, none of the 15 individuals whose chemotaxis was normal died during the same time period. These data further indicate that enhancement of monocyte chemotaxis by BCG is not necessarily accompanied by a better prognosis. An hypothesis that could reconcile the seemingly paradoxical observation that depressed chemotaxis is associated with poor prognosis in cancer patients and that enhancement of chemotaxis by BCG does not necessarily improve prognosis is that there is a heterogeneous population of monocytes. It can be speculated that certain monocytes are capable of participating in tumoricidal reactions while others are not. BCG immunization may bring into the circulation or enhance the chemotactic responsiveness of those cells that are not particularly suited for tumor killing. This hypothesis is consistent with the observation that systemic immunization with BCG does not enhance local tumor destruction; for BCG to destroy tumors, it must be injected directly into the tumor and produce a delayed hypersensitivity reaction at the tumor site.

A group of patients with either renal carcinoma or carcinoma of the breast were tested for monocyte chemotactic responsiveness both before and after surgical excision of the tumor. All 12 patients tested with depressed chemotaxis prior to removal of the tumor had enhancement of monocyte chemotactic responsiveness postoperatively (Table 3). Thus, these data indicate that the presence of a tumor itself might depress monocyte chemotactic responsiveness.

This hypothesis was tested by implanting tumors in mice and determining their effect on macrophage accumulation in response to an inflammatory stimulus *in*

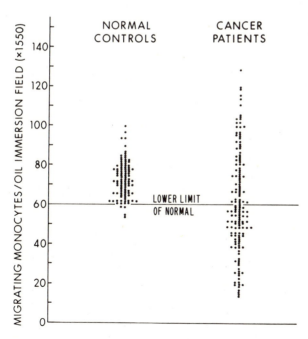

Figure 3. Monocyte chemotactic responsiveness of normal controls and patients with neoplastic disease. The lower limit of normal indicates the level below which only 5% of the normal responses fall. Approximately 54% of the cancer patients had chemotaxis values below this level.

vivo (Snyderman *et al.*, 1975a,c). The implantation of syngeneic tumor cells subcutaneously in the thigh resulted in the depression of macrophage migration into the peritoneal cavities of these animals in response to proteose peptone or phytohemaglutinin. By 5 days after tumor implantation, prior to the time the tumor was palpable, macrophage migration was depressed by as much as 60% compared to control animals implanted with syngeneic liver or spleen cells. While the mechanism by which tumors depress macrophage migration *in vivo* is not yet defined, lysates of several mouse tumors, but not of normal tissues, depressed mouse macrophage chemotactic responsiveness *in vitro* (Snyderman and Pike, 1976). The

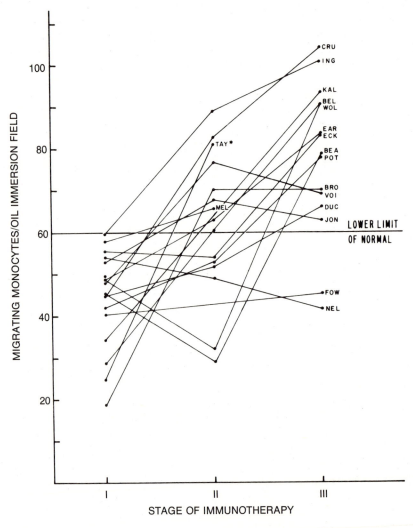

Figure 4. Effect of BCG immunotherapy on the monocyte chemotactic responsiveness of patients with malignant melanoma whose responses were depressed prior to therapy. Stage I: Before BCG administration; Stage II: 4 weeks after intradermal injection of BCG; Stage III: 4 weeks after inoculation of tumor nodules with BCG.

inhibitory activity derived from lysates of a BP8 sarcoma is dialyzable, heat stable (56°C × 30 min), and inhibits macrophage accumulation in response to inflammatory stimuli when injected *in vivo*. The hypothesis that neoplasms may have anti-inflammatory effects was suggested by Graham and Graham (1964), who reported prolonged skin homografts in mice treated with extracts from human cancer tissue. Fauve *et al.* (1974) further demonstrated that mouse neoplasms growing *in vitro* produce a low molecular-weight factor, which inhibits the accumulation of neutrophils at inflammatory sites *in vivo*. The biological importance of anti-inflammatory products produced by neoplasms remains to be determined, but these findings support the hypothesis that malignant neoplasms may prevent their own destruction by inhibiting the accumulation of cytotoxic cells at tumor sites.

Certain viral infections have recently been shown to depress monocyte chemotactic responsiveness *in vitro* and *in vivo*. In studies by Kleinerman *et al.* (1974), human peripheral blood monocytes were incubated *in vitro* with herpes simplex, influenza, vaccinia, polio, or REO viruses. Herpes simplex and influenza virus markedly decreased the *in vitro* chemotactic responsiveness of monocytes to LDCF. Infection with vaccinia, polio, or REO viruses had no effect on the chemotaxis of monocytes. Live virus was required for the depression of chemotaxis, but the effect was not caused by cell death. In order to determine whether the effect of viruses also occurred *in vivo*, mice were injected with influenza virus (Kleinerman *et al.*, 1976). By 6 days after infection, macrophage chemotaxis to inflammatory stimuli *in vivo* was depressed. Studies of human monocyte function in patients during a recent influenza epidemic demonstrated that infection by this virus produced a transient but dramatic depression of chemotaxis (Kleinerman *et al.*, 1975). Fifteen patients with serologically proved acute influenza infection were

TABLE 3. Effect of Tumor Removal on Monocyte Chemotactic Responsiveness

Patient	Neoplasm	Chemotactic response[a]	
		Pre-op	Post-op
G.W.	Renal adenocarcinoma	21.3 ± 4.2	83.3 ± 5.6
A.G.	Renal adenocarcinoma	20.9 ± 2.6	86.9 ± 7.6
T.W.	Renal adenocarcinoma	58.2 ± 2.9	74.3 ± 1.7
C.F.	Renal adenocarcinoma	57.6 ± 5.0	91.9 ± 5.2
M.B.	Breast carcinoma	49.2 ± 0.9	78.3 ± 1.3
C.M.	Breast carcinoma	25.9 ± 1.9	54.9 ± 3.6
V.P.	Breast carcinoma	37.6 ± 5.4	52.6 ± 5.0
M.P.	Breast carcinoma	32.6 ± 1.7	81.2 ± 0.7
M.S.	Breast carcinoma	48.2 ± 2.6	69.2 ± 1.9
M.W.	Breast carcinoma	32.9 ± 3.5	40.6 ± 9.4
M.W.	Breast carcinoma	46.6 ± 3.6	114.2 ± 3.9
A.W.	Breast carcinoma	51.9 ± 0.7	69.3 ± 3.6
	Mean ± 1 SEM:	40.6 ± 3.7	74.2 ± 5.5
		($P < 0.0005$)	
	Mean of 6 patient controls:	69.9 ± 10.3	70.9 ± 4.9
		($P > 0.2$)	
	Normal mean:	71.6 ± 8.2	

[a]Mean ± SEM of monocytes that have migrated in response to LDCF.

found to have depressed monocyte chemotactic responsiveness with values ranging from 30 to 70% of normal. The monocyte chemotactic responses of these patients returned to normal by 3 weeks after the acute illness. These findings indicate that a viral infection can transiently depress monocyte function *in vivo,* rendering the host more susceptible to microbial invasion or perhaps neoplastic transformation.

4.4. Humoral Inhibitors of Leukocyte Chemotactic Responsiveness

Hill and Quie (1974) have noted depressed PMN chemotactic responsiveness in patients with recurrent bacterial and fungal infections associated with increased circulating levels of immunoglobulin E. Since IgE mediated the release of histamine, the authors speculated that this substance was responsible for the chemotaxis defect and reported that histamine depressed PMN chemotactic responsiveness *in vitro*.

Depressed chemotaxis in patients with rheumatoid arthritis has been reported by Mowat and Baum (1971a). These investigators also demonstrated that normal cells incubated with rheumatoid-factor–immunoglobulin complexes have depressed chemotactic activity. It was speculated that such immune complexes could be responsible for the defect in patients with rheumatoid arthritis. A humoral inhibitor of monocyte chemotaxis has been demonstrated in patients with Wiskott-Aldrich syndrome (Altman *et al.,* 1974b). Immunologically, patients with this disease have depressed cellular immunity and defective antibody synthesis. Altman *et al.* (1974b) have studied cellular-immune effector function in six individuals with Wiskott-Aldrich syndrome and found their monocyte chemotaxis *in vitro* to be impaired. Incubation of normal monocytes in the plasma of these patients produced a depression of the chemotaxis of the normal cells, indicating the presence of a humoral inhibitor. An interesting observation made in this study was that the lymphocytes from patients with this disease produced excessive amounts of LDCF when cultured *in vitro* in the absence of antigens or mitogens. The authors reasoned that hyperproduction of LDCF *in vivo* by circulating lymphocytes could desensitize peripheral blood monocytes and hinder their chemotactic responsiveness to sites of delayed hypersensitivity.

5. Summary and Conclusions

The availability of new *in vitro* and *in vivo* techniques for quantitating leukocyte chemotaxis has allowed the definition of humoral and cellular-derived chemotactic factors as well as the role abnormal chemotaxis plays in certain human diseases. A cleavage product of the fifth component of complement, C5a, is highly chemotactic for leukocytes and may be an important mediator of their accumulation at local sites of humoral immune reactions. Chemotactic factors derived from the clotting, fibrinolytic, and kinin-forming systems may similarly attract leukocytes to areas of tissue injury or wound healing. Accumulation of macrophages at sites of delayed hypersensitivity appears to be mediated by a chemotactic lymphokine released by stimulated lymphocytes.

The inability of a host to rapidly mobilize leukocytes to sites of immunological reactions could result in the ineffective elimination of foreign substances and render the host more susceptible to infections and inflammatory or neoplastic diseases.

Most humans or experimental animals with neoplasms have defective monocyte chemotaxis, and there is increasing evidence that tumors themselves may exert an inhibitory effect on macrophage function. Within the next few years, further study of the relationship of depressed chemotaxis and disease may offer a clearer insight into the diagnosis and treatment of abnormal immune function.

ACKNOWLEDGMENT

Ralph Snyderman is a Howard Hughes Investigator.

References

Alper, C. A., Abramson, N., Johnston, R. B., Jr., Jandl, J. H., and Rosen, F. S., 1970, Increased susceptibility to infection associated with abnormalities of complement-mediated functions and of the third component of complement (C3), *N. Engl. J. Med.* **282**:349–354.

Altman, L. C., Snyderman, R., Oppenheim, J. J., and Mergenhagen, S. T., 1973, A human mononuclear leukocyte chemotactic factor: characterization, specificity and kinetics of production by homologous leukocytes, *J. Immunol.* **110**:801–810.

Altman, L. C., Mackler, B. F., and Chassey, B. M., 1974a, Physiochemical characterization of chemotactic lymphokines produced by human thymus derived (T) and bone marrow derived (B) lymphocytes, *J. Reticuloendothel. Soc.* **16**(Suppl.):15a.

Altman, L. C., Snyderman, R., and Blaese, R. M., 1974b, Abnormalities of chemotactic lymphokine synthesis and mononuclear leukocyte chemotaxis in Wiskott-Alrich syndrome, *J. Clin. Invest.* **54**:486–493.

Becker, E. L., 1972, The relationship of the chemotactic behavior of the complement-derived factors, C3a, C5a and C$\overline{567}$, and a bacterial chemotactic factor to their ability to activate the proesterase I of rabbit polymorphonuclear leukocytes, *J. Exp. Med.* **135**:376–387.

Berenberg, J. L., and Ward, P. A., 1973, Chemotactic factor inactivation in normal human serum, *J. Clin. Invest.* **52**:1200–1206.

Boetcher, D. A., and Leonard, E., 1973, Basophil chemotaxis: augmentation by a factor from stimulated lymphocyte cultures, *Immunol. Commun.* **2**:421–429.

Boetcher, D. A., and Leonard, E. J., 1974, Abnormal monocyte chemotactic response in cancer patients, *J. Nat. Cancer Inst.* **52**:1091–1099.

Bokisch, V. A., Müller-Eberhard, H. J., and Cochrane, C. G., 1969, Isolation of a fragment (C3a) of the third component of human complement containing anaphylatoxin and chemotactic activity and description of an anaphylatoxin inactivator of human serum, *J. Exp. Med.* **129**:1109–1130.

Boyden, S., 1962, The chemotactic effect of mixtures of antibody and antigen on polymorphonuclear leukocytes, *J. Exp. Med.* **115**:453–466.

Boxer, L. A., Hedley-Whyte, E. T., and Stossel, T. P., 1974, Neutrophil actin dysfunction and abnormal neutrophil behavior, *N. Engl. J. Med.* **291**:1093–1099.

Brier, A. M., Snyderman, R., Mergenhagen, S. E., and Notkins, A. L., 1970, Inflammation and *herpes simplex* virus; release of a chemotaxis-generating factor from infected cells, *Science* **170**:1104–1106.

Chapitis, J., Ward, P. A., and Lepow, I. H., 1971, Generation of chemotactic activity from human serum and purified components of complement by *Serratia* proteinase, *J. Immunol.* **107**:317 (abstract).

Clark, R. A., and Kimball, H. R., 1971, Defective granulocyte chemotaxis in the Chediak-Higashi syndrome, *J. Clin. Invest.* **50**:2645–2652.

Cohen, S., Ward, P. A., Toshida, T., and Burek, C. L., 1973, Biologic activity of extracts of delayed hypersensitivity skin reaction sites, *Cell Immunol.* **9**:363–376.

Day, N. K., Geiger, H., Stroud, R., DeBracco, M., Mancado, B., Windhorst, D., and Good, R. A., 1972, C1r deficiency: an inborn error associated with cutaneous anergy and renal disease, *J. Clin. Invest.* **51**:1102–1108.

Fauve, R. M., Hevin, B., Jacob, H., Gaillard, J. A., and Jacob, F., 1974, Anti-inflammatory effects of murine malignant cells, *Proc. Nat. Acad. Sci. U.S.A.* **71**:4052–4056.

Gallin, J. I., 1975, Abnormal chemotaxis: cellular and humoral components, in: *The Phagocytic Cell in Host Resistance* (J. A. Bellanti and D. H. Dayton, eds.) pp. 227–248, Raven Press, New York.

Gallin, J. I., and Rosenthal, A. A., 1974, Regulatory role of divalent cations in human granulocyte chemotaxis: evidence for an association between calcium exchanges and microtubule assembly, *J. Cell Biol.* **62**:594–609.

Gallin, J. I., Clark, R. A., and Kimball, H. R., 1973, Granulocyte chemotaxis. An improved *in vitro* assay employing ^{51}Cr labeled granulocytes, *J. Immunol.* **110**:233–240.

Gewurz, H. A., Page, A. R., Pickering, R. J., and Good, R. A., 1967, Complement activity and neutrophil exudation in man. Studies in patients with glomerulonephritis, essential hypocomplementemia and agammaglobulinemia, *Int. Arch. Allergy Appl. Immunol.* **32**:64–90.

Goetzl, E. J., and Austen, K. F., 1972, A neutrophil immobilizing factor derived from human leukocytes. I. Generation and partial characterization, *J. Exp. Med.* **136**:1564–1580.

Graham, J. B., and Graham, R. M., 1964, Tolerance agent in human cancer, *Surg. Gynecol. Obstet.* **118**:1217–1222.

Hausman, M. S., Snyderman, R., and Mergenhagen, S. E., 1972, Humoral mediators of chemotaxis of mononuclear leukocytes, *J. Inf. Dis.* **125**:595–602.

Hausman, M. S., Brosman, S., Snyderman, R., Mickey, M. R., and Fahey, J., 1973, Defective monocyte function in patients with genitourinary carcinoma, *Clin. Res.* **21**:646A.

Hill, H. R., and Quie, P. G., 1974, Raised serum IgE levels and defective neutrophil chemotaxis in three children with eczema and recurrent bacterial infections, *Lancet* **1**:183–187.

Horwitz, D. A., and Garrett, N. A., 1971, Use of leukocyte chemotaxis in vitro to assay mediators generated by immune reactions I. Quantification of mononuclear and polymorphonuclear leukocyte chemotaxis with polycarbonate (nucleopore) filters, *J. Immunol.* **106**:649–655.

Jensen, J., Snyderman, R., and Mergenhagen, S. E., 1969, Chemotactic activity: A property of guinea pig C5 anaphylatoxin, in: *Cellular and Humoral Mechanisms in Anaphylaxis and Allergy* (Third Int. Congress of Allergy and Anaphylaxis), pp. 265–278, S. Karger, Basel.

Jungi, T. W., 1975, Assay of chemotaxis by a reversible Boyden chamber eliminating cell detachment, *Int. Arch. Allergy Appl. Immunol.* **48**:341–352.

Kaplan, A. P., Kay, A. B., and Austen, K. F., 1972, A prealbumin activator of prekallikrein III. Appearance of chemotactic activity for human neutrophils by the conversion of prekallikrein to kallikrein, *J. Exp. Med.* **135**:81–97.

Kay, A. B., 1970, Studies on eosinophil leukocyte migration II. Factors specifically chemotactic for eosinophils and neutrophils generated from guinea pig serum by antigen antibody complexes, *Clin. Exp. Immunol.* **7**:723–737.

Kay, A. B., and Austen, K. F., 1972, Chemotaxis of human basophil leukocytes, *Clin. Exp. Immunol.* **11**:557–563.

Keller, H. U., and Sorkin, E., 1965, I. On the chemotactic and complement-fixing activity of gammaglobulins, *Immunology* **9**:241–248.

Keller, H. U., and Sorkin, E., 1967, Studies on chemotaxis V. On the chemotactic effect of bacteria, *Int. Arch. Allergy Appl. Immunol.* **31**:505–517.

Keller, H. U., and Sorkin, E., 1969, Studies on chemotaxis XIII. Differences in the chemotactic response of neutrophil and eosinophil polymorphonuclear leukocytes, *Int. Arch. Allergy Appl. Immunol.* **35**:279–290.

Kleinerman, E. S., Snyderman, R., and Daniels, C. A., 1974, Depression of human monocyte chemotaxis by *herpes simplex* and influenza virus, *J. Immunol.* **113**:1562–1567.

Kleinerman, E. S., Daniels, C. A., and Snyderman, R., 1975, Depression of human monocyte chemotaxis during acute influenza infection, *Lancet* **2**:1063–1065.

Kleinerman, E. S., Snyderman, R., and Daniels, C. A., 1976, Effect of virus infection on the inflammatory response: depression of macrophage accumulation in influenza infected mice, *Am. J. Path.*, in press.

Leber, T. 1888, Über die Entstehung der Entzündung und die Wirkung der entzündungerregenden Schädlichkeiten, *Fortschr. Med.* **4**:460–480.

Mackler, B. F., Altman, L. C., Rosenstreich, D. L., and Oppenheim, J. J., 1974, Induction of lymphokine production by EAC and of blastogenesis by soluble mitogens during human B cell activation, *Nature London* **249**:834–837.

McKenzie, R., Pepper, D. S., and Kay, A. B., 1975, The generation of chemotactic activity for human leukocytes by the action of plasmin on human fibrinogen, *Thrombosis Res.* **6**:1–8.

Miller, M. E., and Nilsson, U. F., 1970, A familial deficiency of the phagocytosis-enhancing activity of serum related to a dysfunction of the fifth component of complement (C5), *N. Engl. J. Med.* **282**:354–358.

Miller, M. E., Oski, F. A., and Harris, M. B., 1971, Lazy-leukocyte syndrome: a new disorder of neutrophil function, *Lancet* **1**:665–669.

Miller, M. E., Norman, M. G., Koblenzer, P. J., and Schonauer, T., 1973, A new familial defect of neutrophil movement, *J. Lab. Clin. Med.* **82**:1–8.

Mowat, A. G., and Baum, J., 1971a, Chemotaxis of polymorphonuclear leukocytes from patients with rheumatoid arthritis, *J. Clin. Invest.* **50**:2541–2549.

Mowat, A. G., and Baum, J., 1971b, Chemotaxis of polymorphonuclear leukocytes from patients with diabetes mellitus, *N. Engl. J. Med.* **284**:621–627.

Oppenheim, J. J., Levanthal, B. G., and Hersh, E. M., 1968, The transformation of column purified lymphocytes with nonspecific and specific antigenic stimuli, *J. Immunol.* **101**:262–270.

Pike, M. C., and Daniels, C. A., 1975, Production of C5a upon the interaction of staphylococcal protein A with human serum, *Fed. Proc. Fed. Amer. Soc. Exp. Biol.* **34**:853A.

Postlethwaite, A. E., and Snyderman, R., 1975, Characterization of chemotactic activity produced *in vivo* by a cell mediated immune reaction in the guinea pig, *J. Immunol.* **114**:274–278.

Ratnoff, O. D., 1969, Some relationships among hemostasis, fibrinolytic phenomena, immunity and the inflammatory response, *Adv. Immunol.* **10**:145–227.

Rosenfield, S. I., and Leddy, J. P., 1974, Hereditary deficiency of the fifth component of complement of man, *Clin. Res.* **22**:162A.

Ruddy, S., Gigli, I., and Austen, K. F., 1972, The complement system of man, *N. Engl. J. Med.* **287**:592–596.

Sandberg, A. L., Snyderman, R., Frank, M. M., and Osler, A. G., 1972, Production of chemotactic activity by guinea pig immunoglobulins following activation of the C3 complement shunt pathway, *J. Immunol.* **108**:1227–1231.

Schiffmann, E., Corcoran, B. A., and Wahl, S. M., 1975, *N*-Formyl methionyl peptides as chemo-attractants for leukocytes, *Proc. Nat. Acad. Sci. U.S.A.* **72**:1059–1062.

Seigler, H. F., Shingleton, W. W., Metzgar, R. S., Buckley, C. E., and Bergoe, P. M., 1973, Immunotherapy in patients with melanoma, *Ann. Surg.* **178**:352–359.

Shin, H. S., Snyderman, R., Friedman, E., Mellors, A., and Mayer, M. M., 1968, Chemotactic and anaphylatoxic fragment cleaved from the fifth component of guinea pig complement, *Science* **162**:361–363.

Shin, H. S., Gewurz, H., and Snyderman, R., 1969, Reaction of cobra venom factor with guinea pig complement and generation of an activity chemotactic for polymorphonuclear leukocytes, *Proc. Soc. Exp. Biol Med.* **131**:203–207.

Snyderman, R., and Mergenhagen, S. E., 1976, Chemotaxis of macrophages, in: *Immunobiology of the Macrophage* (D. S. Nelson, ed.), pp. 323–348, Academic Press, New York.

Snyderman, R., and Pike, M. C., 1976, An inhibitor of macrophage chemotaxis produced by neoplasms, *Science* **192**:370–372.

Snyderman, R., and Stahl, C., 1975, Defective immune effector function in patients with neoplastic and immune deficiency diseases, in: *The Phagocytic Cell in Host Resistance* (J. A. Bellanti and D. H. Dayton, eds.), pp. 267–281, Raven Press, New York.

Snyderman, R., Gewurz, H., and Mergenhagen, S. E., 1968, Interactions of the complement system with endotoxic lipopolysaccharide. Generation of a factor chemotactic for polymorphonuclear leukocytes, *J. Exp. Med.* **128**:259–275.

Snyderman, R., Phillips, J. K., and Mergenhagen, S. E., 1970, Polymorphonuclear leukocyte chemotactic activity in rabbit serum and guinea pig serum treated with immune complexes. Evidence for C5a as the major chemotactic factor, *Infect. Immun.* **1**:521–525.

Snyderman, R., Phillips, J. K., and Mergenhagen, S. E., 1971a, Biological activity of complement *in vivo*: role of C5 in the accumulation of polymorphonuclear leukocytes in inflammatory exudates, *J. Exp. Med.* **134**:1131–1143.

Snyderman, R., Shin, H. S., and Hausman, M. S., 1971b, A chemotactic factor for mononuclear leukocytes, *Proc. Soc. Exp. Biol. Med.* **138**:387–390.

Snyderman, R., Shin, H. S., and Dannenberg, A. M., 1972a, Macrophage proteinase and inflammation. The production of chemotactic activity from the fifth component of complement, *J. Immunol.* **109**:869–898.

Snyderman, R., Altman, L. C., Hausman, M. S., and Mergenhagen, S. E., 1972b, Human mononuclear leukocyte chemotaxis: a quantitative assay for mediators of humoral and cellular chemotactic factors, *J. Immunol.* **108**:857–860.

Snyderman, R., Altman, L. C., Frankel, A., and Blaese, R. M., 1973, Defective mononuclear leukocyte chemotaxis: a previously unrecognized immune dysfunction, *Ann. Intern. Med.* **78**:509–513.

Snyderman, R., Dickson, J., Meadows, L., and Pike, M. C., 1974, Defective mononuclear leukocyte chemotaxis in patients with cancer, *Clin. Res.* **22**:430A.

Snyderman, R., Blaylock, B., and Pike, M. C., 1975a, Depression of macrophage chemotaxis *in vivo* in tumor bearing mice, *Fed. Proc. Fed. Amer. Soc. Exp. Biol.* **34**:991A.

Snyderman, R., Pike, M. C., and Altman, L. C., 1975b, Abnormalities of leukocyte chemotaxis in human disease, *Ann. N. Y. Acad. Sci.* **256**:386–401.

Snyderman, R., Pike, M. C., Meadows, L., Wells, S., and Hemstreet, G., 1975c, Depression of monocyte chemotaxis by neoplasms, *Clin. Res.* **23**:297A.

Snyderman, R., Pike, M. C., McCarley, D., and Lang, L., 1975d, Quantification of mouse macrophage chemotaxis *in vitro:* role of C5 for the production of chemotactic activity, *Infect. Immun.* **11**:488–492.

Stecher, V. J., and Sorkin, E., 1969, Studies on chemotaxis. XII. Generation of chemotactic activity for polymorphonuclear leukocytes in sera with complement deficiencies, *Immunology* **16**:231–239.

Stecher, V. J., and Sorkin, E., 1972, The chemotactic activity of fibrin lysis products, *Int. Arch. Allergy Appl. Immunol.* **43**:879–886.

Steerman, R. L., Snyderman, R., Leiken, S. L., and Colten, H. R., 1971, Intrinsic defect of the polymorphonuclear leukocyte resulting in impaired chemotaxis and phagocytosis, *Clin. Exp. Immunol.* **9**:939–946.

Stroud, R. M., Shin, H. S., and Shelton, E., 1974, Complement components: assays, purification and ultrastructure methods, in: *Immune Responses at the Cellular Level* (T. Zacharia, ed.), pp. 161–211, Marcel Dekker, New York.

Taylor, F. B., and Ward, P. A., 1967, Generation of chemotactic activity in rabbit serum by plasminogen–streptokinase mixtures, *J. Exp. Med.* **126**:149–158.

Tempel, T. R., Snyderman, R., Jordan, H. V., and Mergenhagen, S. E., 1970, Factors from saliva and oral bacteria, chemotactic for polymorphonuclear leukocytes. Their possible role in gingival inflammation, *J. Periodontology* **41**:3/71–12/78.

Till, G., and Ward, P. A., 1973, The chemotactic factor inactivator in human serum, *J. Immunol.* **111**:299A.

Till, G., and Ward, P. A., 1975, Two distinct chemotactic factor inactivators in human serum, *J. Immunol.* **114**:843–847.

Turner, S., Campbell, J., and Lynn, W. S., 1975, Arachidonic acid, a precursor of polymorphonuclear leukocyte (PMN) chemotaxis, *Clin. Res.* **23**:54A.

Van Epps, D. C., Palmer, D. L., and Williams, R. C., Jr., 1974, Characterization of serum inhibitors of neutrophil chemotaxis associated with anergy, *J. Immunol.* **113**:189–200.

Wahl, S. M., Iverson, G. M., and Oppenheim, J. J., 1974, Induction of guinea pig B-cell lymphokine synthesis by mitogenic and non-mitogenic symbols to Fc, Ig and C3 receptors, *J. Exp. Med.* **140**:1631–1645.

Wahl, S. M., Wilton, J. M., Rosenstreich, D. L., and Oppenheim, J. J., 1975, The role of macrophages in the production of lymphokines by T and B lymphocytes, *J. Immunol.* **114**:1296–1301.

Waldmann, T. A., Strober, W., and Blaease, R. M., 1972, Immuno-deficiency disease and malignancy: various immunologic deficiencies of man and the role of immune processes in the control of malignant disease, *Ann. Intern. Med.* **77**:605–628.

Walker, W. S., Bartlet, R. L., and Kurtz, H. M., 1969, Isolation and partial characterization of a staphylococcal leukocyte cytotaxin, *J. Bacteriol.* **97**:1005–1008.

Ward, P. A., 1969, Chemotaxis of human eosinophils, *Amer. J. Pathol.* **54**:121–128.

Ward, P. A., and Berenberg, J. L., 1974, Defective regulation of inflammatory mediators in Hodgkin's disease. Supra-normal levels of chemotactic factor inactivator, *N. Engl. J. Med.* **290**:76–80.

Ward, P. A., and Hill, J. H., 1970, C5 chemotactic fragments produced by an enzyme in lysosomal granules of neutrophils, *J. Immunol.* **104**:535.

Ward, P. A., and Newman, L. J., 1969, A neutrophil chemotactic factor from human C5, *J. Immunol.* **102**:93–99.

Ward, P. A., and Zvaifler, N. J., 1971, Complement-derived leukotactic factors in inflammatory synovial fluids of humans, *J. Clin. Invest.* **50**:606–616.

Ward, P. A., Cochrane, C. G., and Müller-Eberhard, H. J., 1965, The role of serum complement in chemotaxis of leukocytes *in vitro, J. Exp. Med.* **122**:327–346.

Ward, P. A., Cochrane, C. G., and Müller-Eberhard, 1966, Further studies on the chemotactic factor of complement and its formation *in vivo, Immunology* **11**:141–153.

Ward, P. A., Lepow, I. H., and Newman, L. J., 1968, Bacterial factors chemotactic for polymorphonuclear leukocytes, *Amer. J. Pathol.* **52**:725–736.

Ward, P. A., Remold, H. G., and David, J. R., 1969, Leukotactic factors produced by sensitized lymphocytes, *Science* **163**:1079–1081.

Ward, P. A., Remold, H. G., and David, J. R., 1970, The production from antigen-stimulated lymphocytes of a leukotactic factor distinct from migration inhibitory factor, *Cell. Immunol.* **1**:162–174.

Weiss, A. S., Gallin, J. I., and Kaplan, A. P., 1974, Fletcher-factor deficiency. A diminished rate of Hageman factor activation caused by absence of pre-kallikrein with abnormalities of coagulation, fibrinolysis, chemotactic activity and kinin generation, *J. Clin. Invest.* **53**:622–633.

Wilkinson, P. C., 1974, Principles of the measurement of leukocyte chemotaxis using Boyden's method, in: *Chemotaxis and Inflammation* (P. C. Wilkinson, ed.), pp. 33–53, Churchill-Livingstone, Edinburgh.

Wilkinson, P. C., Borel, J. F., Stecher-Levin, V. J., and Sorkin, E., 1969, Macrophage and neutrophil-specific chemotactic factors in serum, *Nature (London)* **222**:244–250.

Wilkinson, P. C., O'Neill, G. J., Wapshaw, K. G., and Symon, D. N. K., 1972, Enhancement of macrophage chemotaxis by adjuvant-active bacteria, *Ann. Immunol.* **4**:119–130.

Wilkinson, P. C., O'Neill, G. J., and Wapshaw, K. G., 1973, Role of anaerobic cornyeforms in specific and non-specific immunological reactions II. Production of a chemotactic factor specific for macrophages, *Immunology* **24**:997–1006.

Wolf, S. M., Dale, D. C., Clark, R. A., Root, R. K., and Kimball, H. R., 1972, The Chediak-Higashi syndrome: studies of host defense, *Ann. Intern. Med.* **76**:293–306.

Zbar, B., Wepsic, H. T., Rapp, H. J., Stewart, L. C., and Borsos, T., 1970, Two-step mechanism of tumor graft rejection in syngeneic guinea pigs: II. Initiation of reaction by a cell fraction containing lymphocytes and neutrophils, *J. Nat. Cancer Inst.* **44**:701–717.

Zigmond, S. H., and Hirsch, J. G., 1973, Leukocyte locomotion and chemotaxis: new methods for evaluation and demonstration of cell derived chemotactic factor, *J. Exp. Med.* **137**:387–410.

9

Phylogenetics and Ontogenetics of the Complement Systems

MARK BALLOW

1. Introduction

The biological significance of the complement (C) systems, e.g., the classical and alternative C pathways, has recently become more fully appreciated with the recognition of a number of C deficiencies associated with disease in man and laboratory animals (see Chapters 11 and 13). Activation of the C system results in several important biological functions, including enhancement of phagocytosis, cell lysis, bactericidal activity, chemotactic factors, and anaphylatoxins, which lead to the augmentation of various effector host defense mechanisms in inflammation. Although much information is available on these C-dependent biological functions, a whole new concept is developing of the importance of the C system in specific immune responses in relation to cell–cell cooperation (Pepys, 1972), antigen focusing (Dukor *et al.*, 1970), and secondary signals (Dukor *et al.*, 1974). Although many questions remain to be answered, ontogenetic and phylogenetic studies of the C systems might help to determine the role of C in these new biological functions.

This review will examine the development (ontogeny) and the evolution (phylogeny) of the C systems and hopefully will provide new insights into the relationship between the emergence of the C system and the evolution of the cellular (T cell) and humoral (B cell) immune systems.

2. Ontogeny of the Human Complement System

2.1. Biosynthesis of Complement Components in the Human Fetus

The study of the C system during the stages of fetal development has been enhanced by the availability of several methodologies. *In vitro* cultures of fetal

MARK BALLOW • Department of Pediatrics, UConn Health Center, Farmington, Connecticut.

tissue, which are incubated in the presence of tissue-culture media containing ^{14}C- or ^{3}H-labeled amino acids, are used to study the synthesis of C components. The incorporation of these labeled amino acids into newly synthesized C proteins is studied by radioautography using monospecific antisera and immunoelectrophoresis. However, certain precautions in the interpretations of such immunoautoradiographs are necessary concerning specificity (Hochwald *et al.*, 1965). Ideally, such studies should be coupled with functional hemolytic assays, which are now possible, employing microtest systems and C cellular intermediates (Colten, 1972; Chapter 3).

In an early study of fetuses ranging in age from 9 to 24 weeks, Adinolfi and Gardner (1967) detected C3 and C4 in all sera of fetuses more than 14 weeks gestation by immunoelectrophoresis. In a subsequent study, these investigators (Adinolfi *et al.*, 1968) studied the production of C3 and C4 in tissue-culture fluids from fetuses at 10–20 weeks' gestation by radioautography. Both C3 and C4 were synthesized by liver fragments in 14-week-old fetuses. Functionally active C3 and C4 were demonstrated in two sera from fetuses at 18–20 weeks' gestation by the agglutination of red cell C intermediates with specific antisera.

Gitlin and Biasucci (1969) investigated the development of immunoglobulins, C3, C1-esterase inhibitor (C1-INH), and other serum proteins in human embryos and yolk-sac fetal tissues of 29 days' to 18 weeks' gestation with radioimmunoelectrophoresis by the incorporation of ^{14}C-labeled amino acids in fetal tissue cultures. The synthesis of C3 and C1-INH was demonstrated as early as 29 days' gestation. The serum concentrations of C3 increased from a low of 1.9 mg/100 ml at 5.5 weeks' gestation to a range of 58–167 mg/100 ml between 28 and 41 weeks' gestation. The serum concentrations of C1-INH at 6.5 weeks' gestation was 20% of the normal pooled adult reference sera and reached adult levels by 28 weeks' gestation.

Kohler (1973) studied the onset of synthesis of C components in the human fetus, 8–25 weeks' gestation, by culturing tissues in the presence of ^{14}C-labeled lysine and isoleucine amino acids, followed by immunoelectrophoresis and autoradiography. C5 synthesis was detected as early as 8 weeks' gestation; C3 and C4 production began at 11 weeks' gestation. Interestingly, C1q synthesis began at a later period in gestation, 14 weeks.

New advances in C research employing microtest systems and C intermediate cell components have made it possible to detect the *in vitro* synthesis and kinetics of biologically active C components. In an early study, Colten *et al.* (1968) presented evidence that the bowel epithelium from a 19-week-gestation human fetus was capable of producing hemolytically active C1 *in vitro*. Subsequently, Colten (1972) demonstrated that human liver was capable of synthesizing biologically active C2 and C4 as early as 8 weeks' gestation; C1-INH was detected at 11 weeks gestation in fetuses 11–17 weeks' gestation; and C3 was demonstrated at 14 weeks from fetuses at 14–18 weeks' gestation. *In vitro* production of these biologically active C components was temperature-dependent and reversibly inhibited by inhibitors of protein synthesis. These C components were also detectable immunochemically by radioimmunodiffusion assay of the tissue culture fluids. Recently, Colten (1973) demonstrated the synthesis of hemolytically active C5 from human fetuses at 9 weeks' gestation.

On the basis of the studies presented in the preceding paragraphs, the human fetus is capable of synthesizing the first five components of the C system in the first trimester of gestation. Further studies are necessary on the ontogeny of the

remaining C components, C6–9, and the C components of the properdin pathway in
the human fetus. These studies are now possible with the modern techniques of
microhemolytic assays and the availability of specific antisera. Such investigations
will provide information on the cell types that produce C proteins (see Chapter 3)
and the regulatory systems that influence C synthesis and secretion from these cells.

185

PHYLOGENETICS
AND ONTOGENETICS
OF THE
COMPLEMENT
SYSTEMS

2.2. Transplacental Passage of C Components

2.2.1. Genetic Polymorphism

Although the fetus is known to synthesize C proteins, placental transfer of C
components remains a possibility. Most of the fetal serum IgG late in gestation is
derived from placental transfer from the mother (Brambell, 1970). The differences
in phenotype between maternal and fetal plasma proteins have provided evidence
for the fetal synthesis rather than the placental transfer from mother to fetus for
several plasma proteins (Rausen *et at.,* 1961a, b). Propp and Alper (1968) examined
paired maternal and cord sera for C3 genetic polymorphism. Of 25 paired sera, 8
demonstrated allotypic differences for C3, providing evidence for the synthesis of
C3 by the fetus and the absence of placental passage from the mother to the fetus for
this C component. Bach *et al.* (1971) examined C4 polymorphism in paired maternal
and cord plasma with significant discordance in 9 of 52 pairs, indicating a lack of
transplacental passages for C4. Similar polymorphism and allotypic differences
between paired maternal and cord sera have been demonstrated for properdin factor
B (Alper *et al.,* 1972).

2.2.2. Serum Levels of C Components in Newborns from Families with Genetic C Deficiencies

Inherited genetic deficiencies of C components in the mother have been useful
in examining the question of fetal synthesis of C components vs. placental transfer.
A mother, heterozygous for C2 deficiency with half plasma levels of C2, gave birth
to a child with no detectable levels of C2 (Ruddy *et al.,* 1970). In a family with C1-
INH deficiency and hereditary angioedema, a child of a normal mother had no
demonstrable C1-INH (Ruddy *et al.,* unpublished data). Examination of maternal
and cord sera of other newly described genetic C deficiencies in man (see Chapter 5)
will provide an opportunity to study the synthesis and transplacental passage of
other C components.

2.3. Developmental Aspects of C Components in the Newborn

A number of studies are in good agreement that the concentrations of total
hemolytic C and C components in cord sera of full-term newborns are approximately half the levels in paired maternal sera. C levels are generally higher in
maternal serum than normal human reference sera. In an early study by Fischel and
Pearlman (1961), the ratio of newborn-to-maternal sera concentrations for total
hemolytic C was 0.5. In studies by Fireman *et al.* (1969) and Adinolfi (1970), the
mean ratio of total hemolytic C activity in cord sera of full-term infants to maternal
levels was 0.53 and 0.495, respectively. The analysis of other C components were
determined by immunochemical radial diffusion techniques in several studies

employing specific antisera. Newborns were found to be deficient in C1q, C3, C4, and C5 compared to paired maternal serum concentrations. The mean neonatal C3 concentration was 88.8 mg/100 ml compared to the mean maternal C3 level of 178.3 mg/100 ml in a study by Propp and Alper (1968). Kohler (1968) reported that the mean cord-to-maternal sera ratios for C1q, C3, C4, and C5 were 0.75, 0.56, 0.55, and 0.6, respectively. In close agreement, Fireman *et al.* (1969) showed that the ratios of the mean neonatal serum concentrations of C3, C4, and C5 to maternal levels were, respectively, 0.54, 0.56, and 0.61.

A correlation exists between the levels of C and the gestational age of the infant. Fireman *et al.* (1969) showed a general trend for the serum concentrations of CH50, C3, C4, and C5 to increase with the length of the gestation. In a study by Sawyer *et al.* (1971), the fetal–maternal ratios for C3, C4, and C1q determined immunochemically in infants below (low birth weight) and above 2000 g were significantly different: 0.35 to 0.71 for C3; 0.32 to 0.52 for C4; and 0.54 to 0.84 for C1q. A positive correlation was shown between the levels of C3, C4, and C1q, and

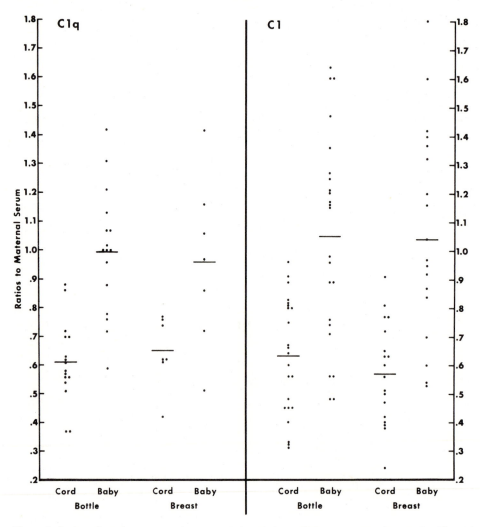

Figure 1. Ratios of cord to maternal sera, or baby (4 days of age) to maternal sera, for Clq and hemolytic Cl in bottle-fed and breast-fed groups. The bar in each group represents the mean.

the birth weight was analogous to the correlations found with the gestation age in the study by Fireman *et al.* (1969).

Quantitation of serum C components in cord or newborn sera by hemolytic assay has been reported in only a few studies. In an early study, Fischel and Pearlman (1961) showed that newborn sera were deficient in C1, C2, and C4; and C3 compared to paired maternal sera using the classical R reagents. Sawyer *et al.* (1971) reported that both hemolytic C2 and C4 were reduced in full-term newborn sera (newborn-to-maternal ratio for C2, 0.83, and for C4, 0.73).

Recently Ballow *et al.* (1974), employing cellular intermediate C components and a semimicro hemolytic method, assayed all nine C components in paired cord–maternal sera. The serum levels of C components in bottle-fed vs. breast-fed infants at 4 days of age were compared to examine the possibility of passive transfer of C components by the colostrum as seen in suckling piglets (Day *et al.*, 1969). The cord sera contained about half the maternal serum levels for C1q, hemolytic C1, C4, and C2 (Figures 1 and 2), ranging from ratios of 0.45 to 0.65. At 4 days of age, however,

187

PHYLOGENETICS
AND ONTOGENETICS
OF THE
COMPLEMENT
SYSTEMS

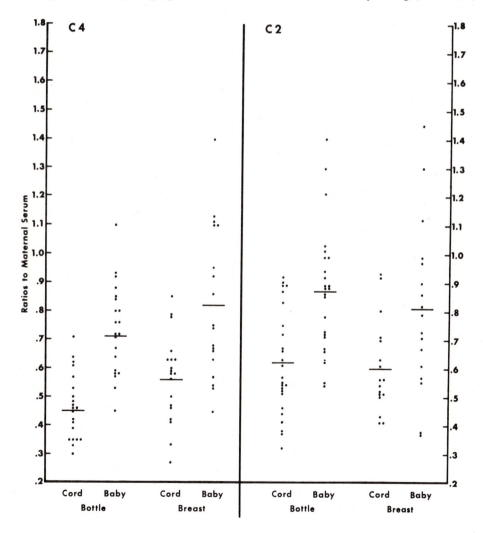

Figure 2. Distribution of ratios of cord or baby to maternal sera for C4 and C2.

a marked increase in serum levels of these C components occurred, approaching maternal concentrations. No differences were observed between the sera of breast-fed and bottle-fed infants. This study (Ballow *et al.*, 1974) was the first to examine all the late C components, C3–9. The cord sera contained approximately half the hemolytic activities for C3, C5, C6, and C7 as those present in the paired maternal sera (Figures 3 and 4). In contrast, a marked deficiency of hemolytic C8 and C9 was demonstrated at birth (Figure 5). The cord sera contained only 5–10% of the maternal levels of hemolytic C9. All C components increased significantly from birth to 4 days of age, except for C3, and again, no differences were seen between the bottle-fed and breast-fed groups. Although these investigations demonstrated the presence of substantial amounts of C3, C4, and Factor B, measured immuno-chemically in human colostrum at 24–72 hr after birth, no evidence was found for the passive transfer of either the early or late C components in the breast-fed infants.

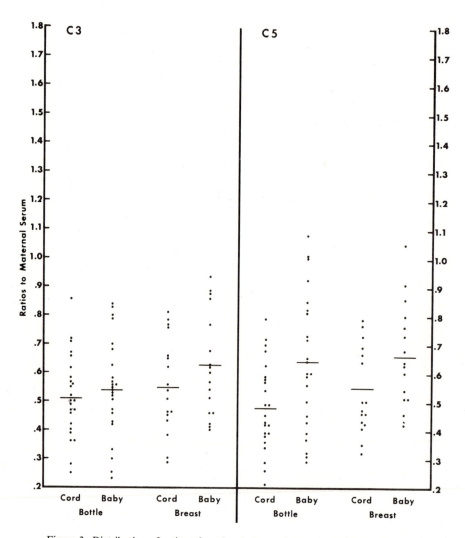

Figure 3. Distribution of ratios of cord or baby to maternal sera for C3 and C5.

Only a few studies have examined the levels of C components beyond the first week of life. Sawyer *et al.* (1971) followed the levels of C1q, C4, and C3 on three low-birth-weight (< 2500 g) infants from 7 to 34 days after birth. In general, the serum concentration of these C components either fell slightly or remained stable after birth. Gitlin and Biasucci (1969) found that the serum levels of C3 in three neonates remained stable or decreased very slightly over the first 2 weeks after birth. Fireman *et al.* (1969) measured, immunochemically, the levels of C3, C4, and C5 during the first 12 months of life. The concentrations of these C components gradually rose after birth to approach normal adult levels by 6 months of age. Other studies on the development of the C system beyond the immediate neonatal period are needed for the other C components.

Very little is known about the development of the C components of the alternate pathway (see Chapter 4). Properdin Factor B has been the only component of the alternate pathway measured in cord sera. In a study by Stossel *et al.*

189

PHYLOGENETICS
AND ONTOGENETICS
OF THE
COMPLEMENT
SYSTEMS

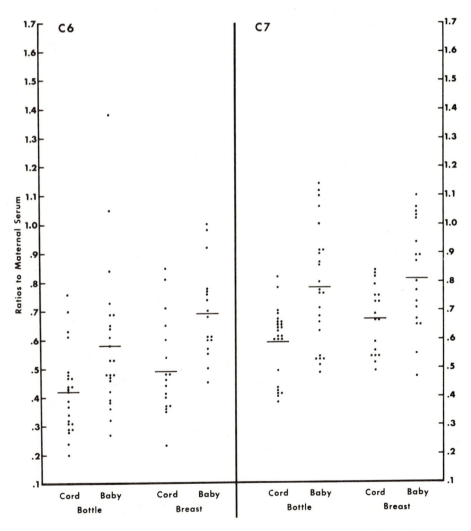

Figure 4. Distribution of ratios of cord or baby to maternal sera for C6 and C7.

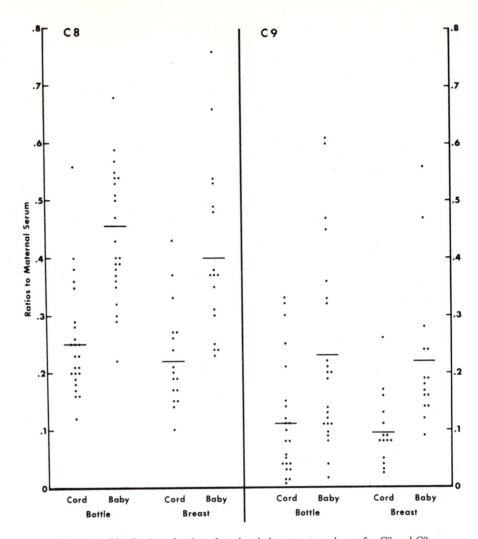

Figure 5. Distribution of ratios of cord or baby to maternal sera for C8 and C9.

(1973), cord sera had lower Factor B levels than the pooled adult reference sera. Of 40 cord sera associated with impaired opsonic activity, 6 had significantly lower levels of Factor B. In a study by Alper *et al.* (1972), the mean cord sera Factor B level was 12 mg/100 ml compared to a mean of 42 mg/100 ml for the paired maternal sera.

3. Ontogenetic Study of Complement in Animals

The study of the ontogeny of C in other animal species has, in general, revealed results similar to those for man. Of 24 fetal lambs examined by Rice and Silverstein (1964), none exhibited significant total hemolytic C activity earlier than 123 days' gestation (gestational period, 150 days). After birth, there was a progressive increase in total C activity during the first few weeks, but at 10 weeks of age, the

191

PHYLOGENETICS
AND ONTOGENETICS
OF THE
COMPLEMENT
SYSTEMS

total hemolytic C levels were still below adult levels. In the goat, total C activity was detected after 115 days' gestation (Adinolfi, 1972). C1 synthesis was present in sheep embryos of 39 weeks' gestation; the levels of C1 reached adult values 2 days after birth (Colten *et al.*, 1968). In bovine fetuses, total hemolytic C activity was detected in the latter part of the first trimester (Gewurz *et al.*, 1966).

Gewurz *et al.* (1966) showed in chickens that total hemolytic C activity was present between the 13th and the 18th day of the 21-day incubation period. In a recent study, Gabrielsen *et al.* (1973) followed the development of total C and hemolytic C1 in chickens. Both total C activity and C1 were detected on day 13 of egg incubation and rose slowly in the late prehatching period (total C, 20–30 CH50/ ml). On the day of hatching (day 21), levels increased sharply (total C, 90 CH50/ml) and continued to rise at a steady rate to day 19 posthatching (total C, 280 CH50/ml).

The Minnesota miniature piglets have been a useful animal to study the development of the C system, particularly because this animal has a multilayered, impermeable placenta, separating maternal and fetal blood proteins. Day *et al.* (1969) showed that as early as the 40th day of gestation (115–120 day gestational period), fetal sera contained measurable amounts of total hemolytic C, hemolytic C1, C2, and C3 terminal (C3t). Hemolytic C4 activity was first measurable at 77 days of gestation. A marked increase in C1, C4, and C2 activity occurred in the 3-day-old suckling piglet in contrast to the non-colostrum-fed piglet. Pig colostrum contained large amounts of C1q, hemolytic C1, C2, C4, and C3t. These observations suggested that C proteins were transferred to the newborn piglet via the colostrum.

C1q synthesis was detected early in gestation (day 48) from pig intestinal tissue cultures employing ^{14}C-labeled amino acids and radioautography with specific antisera (Day *et al.*, 1970c.) Geiger *et al.* (1972a) investigated the ontogenetic development in fetal piglets of the late C components and Factor B. The synthesis of hemolytic C8 was demonstrated in a 47-day-gestation piglet embryo from tissue cultures of the liver, lung, and midgut (Geiger *et al.*, 1972b). Hemolytic C5, C6, and C7 were measurable in very low titers in fetal sera early during gestation (60 days), but increased strikingly between 100–110 days' gestation to 10% of adult levels. C3 was measurable in very low titers in fetal pigs less than 100 days' gestation, but increased at 100–110 days' gestation to 30% of adult levels. C8 and C9 showed a steady increase during embryonic development and at the end of gestation were 20% and 33% of adult levels, respectively. All the late C components reached adult levels by the 12th day of life. In contrast to C3, C5, C6, and C7, the levels of Factor B, measured functionally, could be detected as early as the 47th day of gestation and increased markedly between the 80th and the 90th day of gestation. The development of Factor B in fetal piglet sera appeared to precede the development of C3 in this study.

4. Phylogeny of the C System

4.1. Limitations in Studying the Phylogeny of the C System

The study of the phylogeny of the C system has proved difficult because of the complexity of the C assay systems. Total hemolytic C activity has been assayed by the hemolysis of sensitized red cells with the test serum serving as the C source

(Mayer, 1961) or with the test serum as the source for both C and natural antibody using unsensitized red cells. Cobra venom factor (CVF) has been used to study the alternative C pathway (see Chapter 2) and the terminal C components, C3–9, by the indirect lysis of unsensitized erythrocytes (Ballow and Cochrane, 1969; Pickering *et al.*, 1969; Götze and Müller-Eberhard, 1971) or by the inhibition or depletion of C hemolytic activity (Day *et al.*, 1970a). Finally, individual C components are assayed by the lysis of C cellular intermediates using purified C components and sensitized red cells.

Guinea pig sera, the classic source for C, is not always the most efficient complement sera and depends on the antibody source and the target cells (Muir, 1911; Gigli and Austen, 1971). Furthermore, the titer of hemolytic activity is influenced by the number of red cells and the reaction volume of the assay. Another problem has been incompatibilities between C components of different species (Rice and Crowson, 1950; Gigli and Austen, 1971). Thus, the study of the phylogenetic development of C is impeded by the complex interactions in the lytic assay system among the target cell, the antibody source, and the C source.

4.2. Complement in Mammals

The chemical nature and the biological interaction of the nine components of the classical C system have been characterized in man (Müller-Eberhard, 1968) and in the guinea pig (Nelson *et al.*, 1966). In addition, serum protein inhibitors, which modulate the activation sequence and the biological activity of C reaction products, have been described (Gigli, 1974). Recently, much progress has been made in delineating a second system of serum proteins in man (Osler and Sandberg, 1973) involved in the activation of the terminal C sequence: the properdin or alternative C system. Components of the C system have been measured in other mammalian species, at least functionally, i.e., in rabbits (Nelson and Biro, 1968), dogs (Sargent *et al.*, 1970), rats (Miyakawa *et al.*, 1971; Ballow *et al.*, 1975), sheep (Rice and Silverstein, 1964), cows (Gewurz *et al.*, 1968; Fong *et al.*, 1971), pigs (Geiger *et al.*, 1972a), and cats (O'Neill *et al.*, 1976).

Recently, Schur *et al.* (1975) analyzed the antigenic properties and functional activities of C components in subhuman primates. Antibodies to human C components cross-reacted with the C components of apes, except for C1q. Antigenic cross-reactivity was variable in Old World monkeys. Functional analysis showed similar levels in man and primates. Thus, many of the C proteins of apes and Old World monkeys were homologous in function and antigenicity to the C proteins in man, indicating a close phylogenetic relationship between man and other primates.

4.3. Complement in Lower Vertebrates

4.3.1. Birds

It was known for many years that classic rabbit hemolysin was a poor activator of chicken complement (Noguchi and Bronfenbrenner, 1911). Nevertheless, avian sera do contain total hemolytic C activity if the antibody source is guinea pig hemolysin or the natural hemolysins in avian sera (Muir, 1911). Even though

193

PHYLOGENETICS
AND ONTOGENETICS
OF THE
COMPLEMENT
SYSTEMS

erythrocytes sensitized with rabbit hemolysin fail to activate avian C, immune complexes made from rabbit sera do consume chicken hemolytic C activity (Day *et al.,* 1970b). Serum C from a variety of vertebrate sources fail to interact with chicken antibodies (Gigli and Austen, 1971). These species' incompatibilities with avian C have hampered the delineation of C components in chicken sera, although Gabrielsen *et al.* (1973) have recently been able to titer chicken C1 with $EAC4_{hu}$.

4.3.2. Reptiles

The presence of hemolytic C activity in snake serum was demonstrated by Flexner and Noguchi in 1903. Studies by Bond and Sherwood (1939) showed that snake sera from 13 different species had natural hemolysins and C activity for human and sheep erythrocytes.

Day *et al.* (1970b) demonstrated hemolytic C activity in cobra and turtle sera using rabbit hemolysin. The lytic activity seemed to be analogous to the C system of higher vertebrates because it was heat labile, temperature dependent, potentiated by antibody, and inhibitable by EDTA. The C activity could be depleted by immune complexes, endotoxin lipopolysaccharides (LPS), and CVF. However, the CVF-induced passive lysis of unsensitized erythrocytes was not supported by cobra or turtle sera (Day *et al.,* 1970a), but if the passive lysis assay was performed in two steps, with frog sera supplying the terminal C components, then the reptilian sera were active in CVF-induced passive lysis of unsensitized erythrocytes. These studies suggest that reptilian sera contain not only C components analogous to the classical C system, but components of the alternative C pathway that can interact with CVF and LPS.

4.3.3. Amphibians

Hemolytic C in amphibian sera was first described by Cushing (1945). Legler and Evans (1966) examined the sera of three different orders of amphibians for the presence of hemolytic C activity. Each of the amphibian sera had natural hemolytic activity for a variety of different erythrocytes that could be potentiated by heterologous antibody. Amphibian C appeared to be comparable to mammalian C by a number of inactivation procedures: heat (45–48°C), EDTA, hydrazine, carrageenin (except *Rana pipiens,* leopard frog), and antigen–antibody precipitates (except *N. maculosus,* mud puppy). Day *et al.* (1970b) confirmed these findings in their studies of two amphibian species, leopard and bull frogs.

The anticomplementary activity of LPS and CVF in amphibian sera suggested the presence of the alternative C pathway (Day *et al.,* 1970a,b). The CVF-induced passive lysis of unsensitized red cells was greater in frog sera than in other vertebrate sera (Day *et al.,* 1970a). The hemolysis induced by CVF with frog serum was inhibited by known C inactivators as demonstrated in higher vertebrates. Using a two-step assay for CVF-induced passive lysis, Day *et al.* (1970a) showed that a divalent cation-dependent complex formed with CVF in frog sera and that this complex could initiate lysis by activation of the terminal components of frog C. CVF complexes formed with invertebrate hemolymph, but not guinea pig sera, induced the lysis of unsensitized erythrocytes with EDTA frog sera supplying the terminal C components. Thus these findings suggest that the sera of the amphibian group contain C components that are homologous to higher vertebrates of both the classic and alternative pathways, although species incompatibilities do exist.

4.3.4. Bony Fishes (Osteichthyes)

The bony fish represent the crucial evolutionary deviation between primitive lower vertebrates and phylogenetic pathways leading to the lungfish, the amphibians, and the higher vertebrates. Distinct from the primitive elasmobranchs are the chondrostean fish (paddlefish and sturgeon), which are believed to be the survivors of the primitive ray-finned fishes and today represent some of the most primitive bony fish. The holostean bowfin and garpike are also primitive fish, which are derived from the ancient ganoids and which represent evolutionary deviations that occurred phylogenetically proximal to the teleost deviations. The teleosts represent 95% of the fishes in the world today.

All members of the bony fish have natural hemolysins and hemolytic C activity. The C activity is temperature-dependent (optimal at 28°C) and could be potentiated with carbowax (Legler and Evans, 1967). Although classic rabbit hemolysins did not enhance hemolytic C activity, potentiation with other vertebrate hemolysins was possible depending on the source of serum (Legler and Evans, 1967; Gewurz et al., 1966). The lytic activity appeared to be analogous to the C system in higher vertebrates, since the hemolytic activity was blocked by EDTA (and restored by the addition of divalent cations), heat labile, and consumed by immune complexes and LPS (Day et al., 1970b).

No CVF-induced passive lysis activity or anticomplementary CVF effect was found in the sera of the carp (teleost) or paddle fish (chondrostean) by Day et al. (1970a). The reason was not explored further, but may indicate species incompatibilities or the lack of a protein of the alternative pathway analogous to properdin Factor B of mammalian serum which complexes with CVF. A two-step analysis of the CVF-induced passive lysis assay would be helpful in examining these possibilities.

4.3.5. Elasmobranchs (Chondrichthyes)

Legler and Evans (1967) demonstrated that sera from the lemon shark and nurse shark hemolyzed the erythrocytes of several species. High hemolytic titers were obtained with rabbit and sheep red cells with an optimal temperature range of 25–30°C. The hemolysis of sheep erythrocytes was potentiated by turtle antibody and carbowax. None of the elasmobranch sera were potentiated by classic rabbit hemolysin. In contrast, Day et al. (1970b) showed that rabbit antibody potentiated the C activity of the nurse shark, but not the C of the horned shark.

Hemolytic activity was found to be extremely labile to dilution, slow freezing, or storage at −20 and −70°C, but could be kept at 4°C for a period of 5 days (Legler and Evans, 1967). Inactivation of C activity occurred at lower temperatures than were seen with guinea pig sera (48–50°C), but other inactivation procedures, i.e., EDTA, carrageenin, and hydrazine; and recombination experiments (Legler and Evans, 1967) suggested a C system similar to that of higher vertebrates. Jensen

195

PHYLOGENETICS
AND ONTOGENETICS
OF THE
COMPLEMENT
SYSTEMS

(1969) isolated a factor from nurse shark serum, which inactivates the C4 in the sera of various mammalian species. The shark C4 inactivator may be analogous to human C1s, but a possible relationship awaits further analysis.

In the nurse shark, hemolytic C activity was consumed by *Escherichia coli* LPS (Day *et al.*, 1970b). Although the passive lysis-inducing activity of CVF was absent, CVF was anticomplementary for the serum of the nurse shark (Day *et al.*, 1970a). These observations of C activation by LPS and CVF indicates a system resembling the alternative C pathway of mammals may exist in the nurse shark and perhaps in other elasmobranchs.

4.3.6. Cyclostomes—Hagfish and Sea Lampreys (Agnatha)

The cyclostomes are an interesting phylogenetic class situated at an immunologic transitional position. The sea lamprey is the lowest known vertebrate form to demonstrate all components of an adaptive immune response. This primitive vertebrate has antibody production capacity, although poor; secondary responses; delayed hypersensitivity reaction; and both first- and second-set homograft rejection (Finstad and Good, 1966).

Gewurz *et al.* (1966) studied both the hagfish and the sea lamprey for the presence of C-like activity comparable to that of the C of higher vertebrates. The serum of lampreys has a "natural" hemolysin for rabbit red cells, which is potentiated by carbowax and increased at lower temperatures. However, unlike the known antibody C system in higher forms, the lysis was heat-stable, not blocked by EDTA, and not potentiated by presensitization of the erythrocytes. In addition, lamprey serum had no bactericidal activity against gram-negative bacteria. A "natural" agglutinin, active against rabbit and sheep red cells, could not be increased by immunization or removed by absorption and was incapable of sensitizing sheep or rabbit erythrocytes for lysis by guinea pig C. Thus, the studies of the sea lamprey disclosed no evidence for a classic hemolytic C system or sensitizing agglutinin antibody, but an alternative, modified, or primitive cytolytic system does seem to exist.

Efforts to demonstrate a hemolytic C system have failed in the hagfish. Recently, Day *et al.* (1970a) showed that hagfish serum interacted with CVF to induce the lysis of erythrocytes. However, a two-step analysis or the effects of C inhibitors on the CVF-induced passive lysis activity was not pursued to delineate further the presence of a primitive alternative C system analogous to the pathway in man.

4.4. Invertebrates

Day *et al.* (1970a) studied the hemolymph of three invertebrates, the *Limulus*, or horseshoe crab, the sipunculid worm, and the starfish. Both the hemolymph of the horseshoe crab and the sipunculid worm interacted with CVF to induce the lysis of red cells when incubated at 0°C for 18 hr. Preformed complexes of CVF–horseshoe crab serum and CVF–starfish serum induced the lysis of erythrocytes in the presence of EDTA–frog serum, suggesting that the hemolymph of both these invertebrates was capable of activating the terminal C components of frog serum.

The lysis was C-dependent, as shown by the use of known inhibitors of the C system. When CVF–frog serum complex was added to the different hemolymphs in EDTA, lysis was observed with the starfish hemolymph.

These studies suggested that the hemolymph of several invertebrate species has a factor that is capable of interacting with CVF analogous to properdin Factor B of the alternative C pathway in man. In addition, the hemolymph of the starfish and perhaps the sipunculid worm has a CVF-activatable system that induces the lysis of erythrocytes similar to the terminal C component system of higher vertebrates.

In a subsequent recent study of starfish hemolymph, Day *et al.* (1972) isolated a factor that complexes with purified CVF in activating the terminal C system of the frog. The starfish hemolymph factor (HLF) has a low molecular weight (2000), and once it has been reacted with CVF, the HLF can be separated from the CVF by sucrose density gradient in an active form. This active form of HLF (HLFa) can cleave purified human C3 to release anaphylatoxin. These interesting studies allude to a primitive alternative C pathway in which a factor isolated from invertebrate hemolymph, analogous to Factor B in man, is capable of activating a lytic system.

5. Humoral Immunity, Cellular Immunity, and Complement in Phylogenetic Perspective

5.1. Origin of the Classical Hemolytic C System

Fossil records indicate that the now extinct ostracoderms are the earliest vertebrates on record existing some 400 million years ago. The cyclostomes, the lamprey and the hagfish, are believed to be the most primitive vertebrates in existence today and are the lowest known vertebrate forms to demonstrate an adaptive immune response (Hildemann, 1972b; Finstad and Good, 1966). Cellular immune competence with specific immunologic memory is present in the cyclostomes (Hildemann, 1972b and 1974). However, the B cell or humoral immune capacity is poorly developed in these primitive vertebrates, responding feebly to only one of ten antigens (Brucella) (Finstad and Good, 1966) and, with the production of IgM-type antibodies, only to potent xenogenic antigens (Hildemann, 1972b). The sera of cyclostomes have a lytic and agglutinating system that does not resemble C-like activity of higher vertebrates (Gewurz *et al.*, 1966). The very poor humoral immune system in this most primitive vertebrate form may account for this primitive cytotoxic system and may be related to the absence of a classic hemolytic complement system.

The progressive emergence of a more sophisticated immune capacity as well as the appearance of a hemolytic C system analogous to that of higher vertebrates appears to have evolved after the deviation leading to the modern cyclostomes. Complex adaptive immune responses can be traced to the morphological appearance of a discrete thymus and plasma cells (Table 1) (Good *et al.*, 1966). The primitive elasmobranchs have greater humoral and cellular immunologic vigor than the hagfish and the lamprey. The development of a definitive thymus and spleen perhaps correlates with the appearance of a hemolytic activity which is characteristic of a C-dependent antibody system (Day, 1970b; Gewurz *et al.*, 1966). With the emergence of plasma cells, the higher sharks and the chondrostean fish, i.e., paddlefish, are capable of vigorous antibody formation, although restricted to an

197

PHYLOGENETICS
AND ONTOGENETICS
OF THE
COMPLEMENT
SYSTEMS

IgM-like immunoglobulin (Marchalonis and Cone, 1973; Litman *et al.*, 1971) and exhibit a high degree of hemolytic activity comparable to the C system of higher vertebrates (Legler and Evans, 1967; Day *et al.*, 1970b). In contrast, the sting ray (*Dasyatis americana*) has an extremely low level of hemolytic activity (Legler and Evans, 1967) and no true plasma cells (Good *et al.*, 1966).

An evolutionary progression in both cellular and humoral immunity is evident with the bony fish, the Osteichthyes (Hildemann, 1972a, 1974). Serum hemolytic C activity is well established (Day *et al.*, 1970a,b; Gewurz *et al.*, 1966; Gigli and Austen, 1971). Immunoglobulin classes distinct from IgM-like molecules emerge at the phylogenetic level of the teleosts (Marchalonis and Cone, 1973; Litman *et al.*, 1971). Amphibians, reptiles, birds, and other higher vertebrates synthesize multiple classes of immunoglobulin, with plasma cells appearing in the lamina propria of the gut (Good *et al.*, 1966). True lymph nodes do not appear until mammals, but primitive lymph-node analogs are present in amphibians (Good *et al.*, 1966). Various T cell functions, such as proliferative responses to mitogens, MLC responses, graft vs. host reactions, T–B cell cooperation, and lymphokine production have been demonstrated in certain amphibians and reptiles (Marchalonis, 1974). Central lymphoid tissue of the tonsillar and bursal types apparently developed in the primitive reptiles, followed by the emergence of tonsillar and Peyer's patch lymphoid tissue in the higher reptiles and mammals and the bursa of Fabricius in the birds (Good *et al.*, 1966).

Nine components of the classical hemolytic C system have been recognized functionally in man (Müller-Eberhard, 1968) and the guinea pig (Nelson *et al.*, 1966). Although our knowledge of the hemolytic C component system in vertebrates lower than the mammal is less complete, present information supports the concept that a hemolytic C system similar to man developed with the higher sharks (elasmobranchs). It would appear from the data on the cyclostomes and the sting ray that the development of a classical hemolytic C system closely parallels the appearance of plasma cells and the capacity for a vigorous antibody response (see Table 1).

5.2. Origin of the Alternative C Pathway

Although a variety of agglutining, bactericidal, and lytic substances have been described in invertebrates, immunoglobulin-type antibodies have not been identified to date (Marchalonis and Cone, 1973). In contrast, cellular recognition beyond phagocytic mechanisms and cellular incompatibility reactions exist among certain advanced invertebrates (see Table 1) (Hildemann, 1974). Transplantation immunity with immunologic memory has been demonstrated in two phyla of advanced invertebrates, the annelid worms and the echinoderms.

In earthworms, both xenografts and allografts are slowly rejected after an initial period of healing (Cooper, 1971). Short-term memory is demonstrable in that accelerated rejection occurs if the second graft is placed soon after the initial rejection phenomenon. Cells (coelomocytes) from previously sensitized donor earthworms upon passive transfer are capable of provoking an accelerated reaction in naïve unimmunized host worms (Duprat, 1970; Cooper, 1970). Echinoderms, which possess a diversity of leukocytic cell types, including lymphocyte-like cells, exhibit specific allograft immunity with at least short-term memory (Hildemann and

TABLE 1. Evolution of the Immune and Complement Systems

Time millions of years (geologic period)	Development of the immune system [a]	Phylogeny	Development of the complement system [b]		
			Hemolytic activity CH50	C-depletion LPS/CVF	CVF-induced passive lysis
2 (Cenozoic) (Mesozoic)	T and B cell systems; Lymphokines; T–T/T–B collaboration; T suppressor cells	MAN — MAMMALIA — guinea pig	+	+/+	+
135	Bursa of Fabricius	AVES	+	+/+	+
(Paleozoic) 275	Tonsillar lymphoid tissue; Graft vs. host disease	REPTILIA — turtle	+	+/+	+[c]
		cobra	+	+/+	+[c]
325	Acute graft rejection; MLC, MIF production; Well-defined thymus and spleen; Primitive lymph nodes; Plasma cells in gut; Multiple immunoglobulin classes	AMPHIBIA — frog	+	+/+	+
340	Immunoglobulin class other than IgM (lungfish)	Crossopterygii — Dipnoi lungfish — Sarcopterygii	+	+/+	+
	Defined Hassell's corpuscles; Lymphocytes respond to PHA; Numerous plasma cells; Vigorous antibody formation	Teleostei — Holostei gar, bowfin — Chondrostei paddlefish — OSTEICHTHYES	+	+/–	–
360	?Hassell's corpuscles; Plasma cells	Elasmobranchii higher sharks, rays	+	+/+	–

199

PHYLOGENETICS
AND ONTOGENETICS
OF THE
COMPLEMENT
SYSTEMS

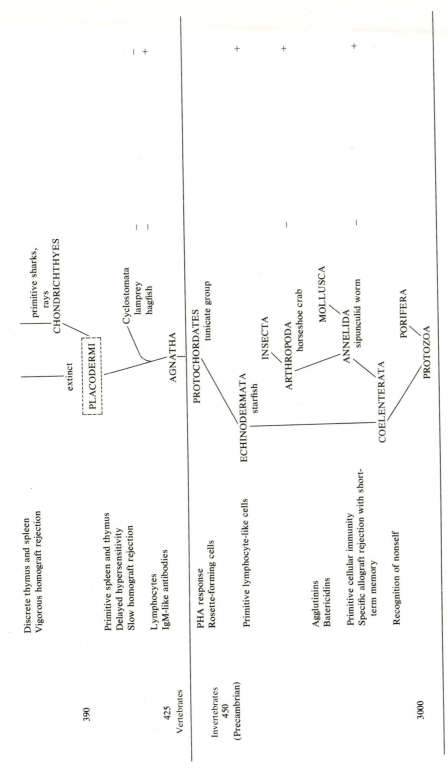

[a]From Good et al. (1966) and Hildemann (1972).
[b]From Day et al. (1970a,b).
[c]Frog and turtle sera will support the CVF-induced passive lysis of erythrocytes if it is performed in two steps.

Dix, 1972). Vertebrates are thought to have evolved from the tunicate group of protochordates (Berill, 1955). These invertebrates have differentiated leukocytes (Smith, 1970). Immunoincompatibility at the level of colony specificity has been demonstrated in a variety of colonial tunicates (Freeman, 1970). Preliminary experiments by Hildemann *et al.* (1974) have demonstrated the existence of transplantation immunity in the solitary tunicate. Other studies by these investigators have shown that the lymphocytes of the solitary tunicate *Ciona intestinalis* can form rosettes with sheep red blood cells (?T cell rosettes) (Hildemann and Reddy, 1973) and respond to the mitogen, PHA (Hildemann, 1974). Thus it appears that cellular immunocompetence similar to cell-mediated immunity in higher vertebrates evolved in the more advanced invertebrates long before the capacity to produce circulating immunoglobulin antibodies.

Although classical hemolytic C activity is not measurable in the sera of the most primitive of vertebrates, e.g., the cyclostomes, and in the hemolymph of invertebrates, lysis-inducing activity by CVF is present (Day *et al.,* 1970a). In addition, Day *et al.* (1972) have isolated a factor from starfish hemolymph that complexes with frog serum. Thus, the most primitive of vertebrates, the hagfish, and several invertebrate species have a system that is perhaps similar to the alternative C pathway and the terminal C sequence of man. The importance of this alternative C system in phylogeny remains to be further explored. However, this C system may enhance the existing primitive phagocytic and inflammatory defense mechanisms (Good and Papermaster, 1964; Hildemann, 1972b) in the absence of an adaptive immune response. Perhaps, as pointed out by Day (1970a), the alternative C pathway in man has really evolved from a primitive C pathway of the invertebrates. It is intriguing to observe the concomitant development of the alternative C system and cell-mediated immunity in the invertebrates (Table 1), particularly in view of the fact that cellular immunity evolved long before the capacity to elaborate circulating antibodies. Recently several investigators (Pepys, 1972; Dukor *et al.,* 1970, 1974) have initiated interest in the role of the C system in cellular immune responses. Phylogenetic studies of the relationship between cellular immunocompetence and the C system (the alternative pathway) may help delineate the mechanisms and pathophysiology of C proteins in the immune response.

6. Summary

The development (ontogeny) and the evolution (phylogeny) of the C systems were reviewed in this chapter. Modern techniques of microhemolytic assays, tissue culture, and immunoautoradiography have made possible the study of the C system during fetal development. The human fetus is capable of synthesizing the first five components (C1q to C5) of the C system as well as the C1-INH in the first trimester of gestation.

Studies of C3 and C4 genetic polymorphism and the serum levels of C2 and C1-INH in newborns of families with genetic C deficiencies have indicated that the placental transfer of C components does not occur. The levels of C are directly related to the gestational age of the infant. The concentrations of total hemolytic C and C components in cord sera of full-term newborns are approximately half the levels in paired maternal sera, except for C8 and C9, which are 5–10% of maternal levels. The concentrations of C components increase after birth to reach adult levels

201

PHYLOGENETICS
AND ONTOGENETICS
OF THE
COMPLEMENT
SYSTEMS

by 6 months of age. Although colostrum contains substantial amounts of C3, C4, and Factor B, no evidence was found for the passive transfer of these C components in breast-fed infants. Studies of the ontogeny of C in animal species have revealed similar findings as those in man.

The study of the phylogeny of the C system has proved difficult because of the complexities of the C assay systems and the incompatibilities between C components of different animal species. Hemolytic C activity has been demonstrated in mammals other than man down through phylogeny to the elasmobranchs (sharks). The sea lamprey, the lowest known vertebrate to have an adaptive immune response, does not appear to have a classical hemolytic C system similar to man. On the other hand, studies have indicated that the hemolymph of several invertebrate species contains a factor that is capable of interacting with CVF and activating a lytic system analogous to the alternative C pathway in man. The progressive emergence of a sophisticated immune capacity in phylogeny correlates with the appearance of a hemolytic C system that is dependent on antibody activation. The development of a classical hemolytic C system similar to man closely parallels the appearance of plasma cells in the higher sharks and the capability for a vigorous antibody response.

Although immunoglobulin-type antibodies have not been identified, certain advanced invertebrates, the annelid worms, and the echinoderms demonstrate cellular recognition and transplantation immunity similar to the cell-mediated immunity of higher vertebrates. Invertebrate hemolymph contains a CVF-activatable system suggesting a primitive alternative C pathway. The evolutionary development of this primitive C pathway, together with cellular immunocompetence, probably was of importance as the major defense mechanism in the invertebrate in the absence of a humoral adaptive immune response. Thus perhaps the alternative C pathway in man has emerged from a primitive C system of the invertebrates and represents the "primary" C system in evolutionary development.

References

Adinolfi, M., 1970, Levels of two components of complement (C'4 and C'3) in human fetal and newborn sera, *Dev. Med. Child Neurol.* **12**:306–308.

Adinolfi, M., 1972, Ontogeny of components of complement and lysozyme, in: *Ciba Found. Symp., Ontogeny of Acquired Immunity,* (R. Porter and J. Knight, eds.), pp. 65–85, Associates Scientific Publishers, Amsterdam.

Adinolfi, M., and Gardner, B., 1967, Synthesis of β1E and β1C components of complement in human foetuses, *Acta Paediatr. Scand.* **56**:450–554.

Adinolfi, M., Gardner, B., and Wood, C. B. S., 1968, Ontogenesis of Two Components of human complement: β1E and β1C-1A globulins, *Nature (London)* **219**:189–191.

Alper, C. A., Boenisch, T., and Watson, L., 1972, Genetic polymorphism in human glycine-rich-beta-glycoprotein, *J. Exp. Med.* **135**:68–80.

Bach, S., Ruddy, S., MacLaren, J. A., and Austen, K. F., 1971, Electrophoretic polymorphism of the fourth component of human complement (C4) in paired maternal and foetal plasmas, *Immunology* **21**:869–878.

Ballow, M., and Cochrane, C. A., 1969, Two anticomplementary factors in cobra venom: hemolysis of guinea pig erythrocytes by one of them, *J. Immunol.* **103**:944–952.

Ballow, M., Fang, F., Good, R. A., and Day, N. K., 1974, Developmental aspects of complement components in the newborn: the presence of complement components and C3 proactivator (Properdin Factor B) in human colostrum, *Clin. Exp. Immunol.* **18**:257–266.

Ballow, M., Good, R. A., and Day, N. K., 1975, Complement in graft versus host disease. I. Depletion of complement components during a systemic graft versus host reaction in the rat, *Proc. Soc. Exp. Biol. Med.* **148**:170–176.

Berill, N. J., 1955, *The Origin of Vertebrates,* Oxford University Press, New York.

Bond, G. C., and Sherwood, N. P., 1939, Serological studies of the reptilia. II. The hemolytic property of snake serum, *J. Immunol.* **36**:11–16.

Brambell, F. W. R., 1970, The transmission of antibodies in: *The Transmission of Passive Immunity from Mother to Young* (A. Neuberger and E. L. Tatum, eds.), pp. 242–250, North-Holland Publishing Company, Amsterdam und London.

Colten, H. R., 1972, Ontogeny of the human complement system: *In vitro* biosynthesis of individual complement components by fetal tissues, *J. Clin. Invest.* **51**:725–730.

Colten, H. R., 1973, Biosynthesis of the fifth component of complement (C5) by human fetal tissues, *Clin. Immunol. Immunopathol.* **1**:346–352.

Colten, H. R., Gordon, J. M., Borsos, T., and Rapp, H. J., 1968, Synthesis of the first component of human complement in vitro, *J. Exp. Med.* **128**:595–604.

Cooper, E. L., 1970, Transplantation immunity in helminths and annelids, *Transplant. Proc.* **3**:216–221.

Cooper, E. L., 1971, Phylogeny of transplantation immunity: graft rejection in earthworms, *Transplant. Proc.* **3**:214–216.

Cushing, J. E., Jr., 1945, A comparative study of complement. I. The specific inactivation of the components, *J. Immunol.* **50**:61–89.

Day, N. K. B., Pickering, R. J., Gewurz, H., and Good, R. A., 1969, Ontogenetic development of the complement system, *Immunology* **16**:319–326.

Day, N. K. B., Gewurz, H., Johannsen, R., Finstad, J., and Good, R. A., 1970a, Complement and complement-like activity in lower vertebrates and invertebrates, *J. Exp. Med.* **132**:941–950.

Day, N. K., Good, R. A., Finstad, J., Johannsen, R., Pickering, R. J., and Gewurz, H., 1970b, Interactions between endotoxic lipopolysaccharides and the complement system in the sera of lower vertebrates, *Proc. Soc. Exp. Biol. and Med.* **133**:1397–1401.

Day, N. K., Gewurz, H., Pickering, R. J., and Good, R. A., 1970c, Ontogenetic development of C1q synthesis in the piglet, *J. Immunol.* **104**:1316–1319.

Day, N., Geiger, H., Finstad, J., and Good, R. A., 1972, A starfish hemolymph factor which activates vertebrate complement in the presence of cobra venom factor, *J. Immunol.* **109**:164–167.

Dukor, P., Bianco, C., and Nussenzweig, V., 1970, Tissue localization of lymphocytes bearing a membrane receptor for antigen–antibody-complement complexes, *Proc. Nat. Acad. Sci. U.S.A.* **67**:990–997.

Dukor, P., Schumann, G., Gisler, R. J., Dierich, M., König, W., Hadding, U., and Bitter-Suermann, D., 1974, Complement-dependent B-cell activation by cobra venom factor and other mitogens?, *J. Exp. Med.* **139**:337–354.

Duprat, P. C., 1970, Specificity of allograft reaction in *Eisenia foetida, Transplant. Proc.* **2**:222–225.

Finstad, J., and Good, R. A., 1966, Phylogenetic studies of adaptive immune responses in the lower vertebrates, in: *Phylogeny of Immunity* (R. T. Smith, P. A. Miescher, and R. A. Good, eds.), pp. 173–188, University of Florida Press, Gainesville.

Fireman, P., Zuchowski, D. A., and Taylor, P. M., 1969, Development of human complement system, *J. Immunol.* **103**:25–31.

Fishel, C. W., and Pearlman, D. S., 1961, Complement components of paired mother-cord sera, *Soc. Exp. Biol. Med. Proc.* **107**:695–699.

Flexner, S., and Noguchi, H., 1903, Snake venom in relation to hemolysis, bacteriolysis, and toxicity, *J. Exp. Med.* **6**:277–301.

Fong, J. S. C., Muschel, L. H., and Good, R. A., 1971, Kinetics of bovine complement. I. Formation of a lytic intermediate, *J. Immunol.* **107**:28–33.

Freeman, G., 1970, Transplantation specificity in echinoderms and lower chordates, *Transplant. Proc.* **2**:236–239.

Gabrielsen, A. E., Pickering, R. J., Linna, T. J., and Good, R. A., 1973, Haemolysis in chicken serum. II. Ontogenetic development, *Immunology* **25**:179–184.

Gewurz, H., Finstad, J., Muschel, L. M., and Good, R. A., 1966, Phylogenetic inquiry into the origins of the complement system, in: *Phylogeny of Immunity* (R. T. Smith, P. A. Miescher, and R. A. Good, eds.) pp. 105–117, University of Florida Press, Gainesville.

Gewurz, H., Pickering, R. J., and Good, R. A., 1968, Complement and complement component activities in diseases associated with repeated infections and malignancy, *Int. Arch. Allergy* **33**:368–388.

Geiger, H., Day, N., and Good, R. A., 1972a, The ontogenetic development of the later complement components in fetal piglets, *J. Immunol.* **108**:1098–1104.

203

PHYLOGENETICS
AND ONTOGENETICS
OF THE
COMPLEMENT
SYSTEMS

Geiger, H., Day, N., and Good, R. A., 1972b, Ontogenetic development and synthesis of hemolytic C8 by piglet tissues, *J. Immunol.* **108**:1092–1097.

Gigli, I., 1974, Control mechanisms of the classical and alternate C sequences, *Transplant. Proc.* **6**:9–12.

Gigli, I., and Austen, K. F., 1971, Phylogeny and function of the complement system, *Annu. Rev. Microbiol.* **25**:309–332.

Gitlin, D., and Biasucci, A., 1969, Development of γG, γA, γM, β1C/β1A, C'1 esterase inhibitor, ceruloplasmin, transferrin, hemopexin, haptoglobin, fibrinogen, plasminogen, α^1-antitrypsin, oroscomucoid, B-lipoprotein, α^2-macroglobulin and prealbumin in the human conceptus, *J. Clin. Invest.* **48**:1433–1446.

Good, R. A., and Papermaster, B. W., 1964, Ontogeny and phylogeny of adaptive immunity, *Adv. Immunol.* **4**:1–115.

Good, R. A., Finstad, J., Pollara, B., and Gabrielsen, A. E., 1966, Morphologic studies on the evolution of the lymphoid tissues among the lower vertebrates, in: *Phylogeny of Immunity* (R. T. Smith, P. A. Miescher, and R. A. Good, eds.), pp. 149–170, University of Florida Press, Gainesville.

Götze, O., and Müller-Eberhard, H. J., 1971, The C3-activation system: an alternate pathway of complement activation, *J. Exp. Med.* **134**:90S–108S.

Hildemann, W. H., 1972a, Transplantation reactions of two species of osteichthyes (Teleostei) from South Pacific Coral Reefs, *Transplantation* **14**:261–267.

Hildemann, W. H., 1972b, Phylogeny of transplantation reactivity, in: *Transplantation Antigens* (B. D. Kahan and R. A. Reisfeld, eds.), pp. 3–73, Academic Press, New York.

Hildemann, W. H., 1974, Some new concepts in immunological phylogeny, *Nature London* **250**:116–120.

Hildemann, W. H., and Dix, T. G., 1972, Transplantation reactions of tropical Australian echinoderms, *Transplantation* **15**:624–633.

Hildemann, W. H., and Reddy, A. L., 1973, Phylogeny of immune responsiveness: marine invertebrates, *Fed. Proc. Fed. Amer. Soc. Exp. Biol.* **32**:2188–2194.

Hochwald, G. M., Thorbecke, G. J., and Asofsky, R., 1965, Sites of formation of immune globulins and of a component of C'3: I. A new technique for the demonstration of the synthesis of individual serum proteins by tissues in vitro, *J. Exp. Med.* **114**:459–470.

Jensen, J. A., 1969, A specific inactivator of mammalian C'4 isolated from nurse shark (*Ginglymstoma cirratum*), *J. Exp. Med.* **130**:217–241.

Kohler, P. F., 1968, Quantitative comparison of complement in the mother and newborn, *Fed. Proc. Fed. Amer. Soc. Exp. Biol.* **27**:491 (abstract).

Kohler, P. F., 1973, Maturation of the human complement system. I. Onset time and sites of fetal C1q, C4, C3, and C5 synthesis, *J. Clin. Invest.* **52**:671–677.

Legler, D. W., and Evans, E. E., 1966, Comparative immunology: hemolytic complement in amphibia, *Proc. Soc. Exp. Biol. Med.* **121**:1158–1162.

Legler, D. W., and Evans, E. E., 1967, Comparative immunology: hemolytic complement in elasmobranchs, *Proc. Soc. Exp. Biol. Med.* **124**:30–34.

Litman, G. W., Frommel, D., Chartrand, S., Finstad, J., and Good, R. A., 1971, Significance of heavy chain mass and antigenic relationship in immunoglobulin evolution, *Immunochemistry* **8**:345–349.

Marchalonis, J. J., 1974, Phylogenetic origin of antibodies and immune recognition, in: *Progress in Immunology II,* Vol. 2 (C. Brent and J. Holborow, eds.), pp. 249–259, North-Holland Publishing Co., Amsterdam.

Marchalonis, J. J., and Cone, R. W., 1973, The phylogenetic emergence of vertebrate immunity, *Aust. J. Exp. Med. Sci.* **51**:461–488.

Mayer, M. M., 1961, Complement and complement fixation, in: *Experimental Immunochemistry* (E. A. Kabat and M. M. Mayer, eds.), pp. 133–240, Charles C. Thomas, Springfield, Illinois.

Miyakawa, Y., Sekine, T., Shibata, S., and Nichioka, K., 1971, Studies on rat complement: a method for titration of rat C1, C2, C3, C4, as well as C5, and the effect of rabbit nephrotoxic serum on the first five components of complement in rat serum, *J. Immunol.* **106**:545–551.

Muir, R., 1911, Relationships between the complements and immune bodies of different animals; the mode of action of immune body, *J. Pathol. Bacteriol.* **16**:523–534.

Müller-Eberhard, H. J., 1968, Chemistry and reaction mechanisms of the complement system, *Adv. Immunol.* **8**:1–80.

Nelson, R. A., Jr., and Biro, C. E., 1968, Complement components of a hemolytically deficient strain of rabbits, *Immunology* **14**:525–540.

Nelson, R. A., Jensen, J., Gigli, I., and Tamura, R., 1966, Methods for the separation purification and measurements of the nine components of hemolytic complement in guinea pig serum, *Immunochemistry* **3**:111–135.

Noguchi, H., and Bronfenbrenner, J., 1911, The comparative merits of various complements and amboceptors in the serum diagnosis of syphilis, *J. Exp. Med.* **13**:78–91.

Osler, A. G., and Sandberg, A. C., 1973, Alternate complement pathway, *Prog. Allergy* **17**:51–92.

Pepys, M. B., 1972, Role of complement in induction of the allergic response, *Nature London New Biol.* **237**:157–159.

Pickering, R. J., Wolfson, M. R., Good, R. A., and Gewurz, H., 1969, Hemolysis induced by cobra venom factor activation of terminal complement (C') components in guinea pig serum (GPS), *Fed. Proc. Fed. Amer. Soc. Exp. Biol.* **28**:818.

Pillemer, L., Blum, L., Lepow, I. H., Todd, E. W., and Wardlaw, A. C., 1954, The properdin system and immunity. I. Demonstration and isolation of a new serum protein, properdin, and its role in immune phenomenon, *Pediatrics* **52**:134–136.

Propp, R. P., and Alper, C. A., 1968, C'3 synthesis in the human fetus and lack of transplacental passage, *Science* **162**:672–673.

Rausen, A. R., Gerald, P. S., and Diamond, L. K., 1961a, Haptoglobin patterns in cord blood serums, *Nature London* **191**:717.

Rausen, A. R., Gerald, P. S., and Diamond, L. K., 1961b, Genetical evidence for synthesis of transferrin in the foetus, *Nature London* **192**:182.

Rice, C. E., and Crowson, C. N., 1950, The interchangeability of the complement components of different animal species. II. In the hemolysis of sheep erythrocytes sensitized with rabbit amboceptor, *J. Immunol.* **65**:201–210.

Rice, C. E., and Silverstein, A. M., 1964, Haemolytic complement activity of sera of foetal and new-born lambs, *Can. J. Comp. Med. Vet. Sci.* **28**:34–37.

Ruddy, S., Kelmperer, M. R., Rosen, F. S., Austen, K. F., and Kumate, J., 1970, Hereditary deficiency of the second component of complement in man: correlation of C2 haemolytic activity with immunochemical measurements of C2 protein *Immunology* **18**:943–954.

Sargent, A. U., and Austen, K. F., 1970, The effective molecular titration of the components of dog complement, *Proc. Soc. Exp. Biol. Med.* **133**:1117–1122.

Sawyer, M. K., Forman, M. L., Kuplic, L. S., and Stiehm, E. R., 1971, Developmental aspects of the human complement system, *Biol. Neonate* **19**:148–162.

Schur, P. H., Connelly, A., and Jones, T. C., 1975, Phylogeny of complement components in non-human primates, *J. Immunol.* **114**:270–273.

Smith, M. J., 1970, The blood cells and tunic of the ascidian halocynthia aurantium (Pallas). I. Hematology, tunic morphology, and partition of cells between blood and tunic, *Biol. Bull.* **138**:354–378.

Stossel, T. P., Alper, C. A., and Rosen, F. S., 1973, Opsonic activity in the newborn: role of properdin, *Pediatrics* **52**:134–136.

10

The Chemistry and Biology of the Proteins of the Hageman Factor-Activated Pathways

RICHARD J. ULEVITCH and CHARLES G. COCHRANE

1. Introduction

The initiation of the intrinsic clotting system, the formation of bradykinin, and one pathway of plasminogen activation all require the activation of Hageman factor (factor XII). These pathways are shown schematically in Figure 1. Activation of Hageman factor, prekallikrein plasma thromboplastin antecedent (factor XI), and the plasminogen activator are all characterized by the conversion of a zymogen to an enzymatically active protease. This singular biochemical event, activation of zymogen, can produce rapid and diverse alterations in both humoral and cellular-based mediation systems.

The purposes of this review are to describe the biochemical and biological properties of the zymogen as well as the active molecule and to summarize some recent observations that have provided new concepts about the regulation of the activation of the Hageman factor activated pathways. This discussion will focus on the components of the Hageman factor activated pathways of man and will be limited to a review of recent investigation conducted with highly purified proteins. Previous reviews have documented earlier work in the field (Ratnoff, 1966; Austen, 1974; Cochrane *et al.*, 1973a).

RICHARD J. ULEVITCH and CHARLES G. COCHRANE • Department of Immunopathology, Scripps Clinic and Research Foundation, La Jolla, California.

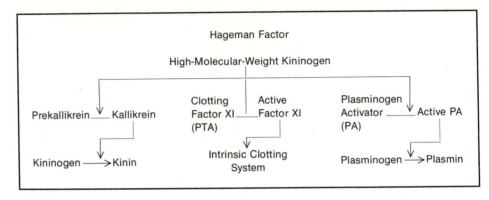

Figure 1. Hageman factor–activated pathways of kinin formation, coagulation, and fibrinolysis.

2. Biochemical Properties of the Components of the Hageman Factor-Activated Pathways

2.1. Hageman Factor

Hageman factor was discovered with the observation of a patient whose blood and plasma were observed to show a prolonged clotting time with defective activation of factor XI (Margolis, 1959). The defects were found to result from an absolute deficiency of the initial protein of the intrinsic system, named for the propositus bearing the defect (Ratnoff, 1966; Smink et al., 1967).

The purification of Hageman factor in the precursor form has been intensively pursued by several groups of investigators. Although active forms of the molecule were prepared in the early 1960s (Ratnoff and Davie, 1962), it was not until this decade that efforts to isolate precursor Hageman factor from human plasma were successful. Preparative methods from this laboratory (Revak et al., 1974), from Saito et al. (1974) and from Bagdasarian et al. (1973) have provided human Hageman factor in precursor form suitable for biochemical studies. Recently, these methods have been extended and refined (Griffin et al., 1976) to achieve a purification of human Hageman factor of greater than 95% precursor molecules. Briefly, this preparation of human Hageman factor utilizes a heat step followed by sequential column chromatography on DEAE and SP-sephadex. The inclusion of inhibitors of proteolytic enzymes as well as care to avoid bacterial contamination are essential for the preparation of precursor Hageman factor.

Human Hageman factor isolated by this procedure is a single polypeptide chain of molecular weight 80,000 as determined by sodium dodecyl sulfate (SDS) gel electrophoresis (Revak et al., 1974). The amino acid analyses of preparations from two different laboratories are in good agreement (Revak et al., 1974; McMillin et al., 1974). An interesting feature of the amino acid composition is the high content of proline (10%) and the very low content of methionine (0.1–0.3%). Immunologic quantification of levels of Hageman factor in a pool of normal adult plasma demonstrate that it is present at a concentration of 29 μg/ml with an individual range of 15–42 μg/ml.

Activation of Hageman factor may be measured by several different techniques, namely, (1) acceleration of the recalcification clotting time of Hageman factor-deficient plasma, (2) a coupled enzymatic assay with prekallikrein (Revak *et al.*, 1974), or (3) measurement of the hydrolysis of N-α-acetylglycine lysine methylester (Ulevitch *et al.*, 1974). Studies from several laboratories (Cochrane *et al.*, 1973a; Kaplan and Austen, 1971; Revak *et al.*, 1974) have shown that activation of Hageman factor may proceed by two distinct mechanisms. One type of activation is induced by negatively charged polymeric substances, such as kaolin, lipopolysaccharide (LPS), or vascular basement membrane. *In vitro* studies indicate that a specific density of negative charges is required for the activation of Hageman factor by negatively charged polymeric substances. Evidence to support this derives from several different experimental observations. For example, pretreatment of kaolin with hexadimethrene bromide (polybrene), a cationic polymer, did not greatly effect the binding of Hageman factor to kaolin, but did markedly reduce the activation of Hageman factor. It is presumed that pretreatment of kaolin with polybrene reduced the density of negative charges and thus inhibited the activation of Hageman factor. In addition, experiments with bacterial lipopolysaccharide (LPS) preparations with different amounts of phosphate demonstrated a correlation between the phosphate content and the ability to activate Hageman factor (Morrison and Cochrane, 1974), thus providing additional support for the role of negatively charged groups in the activation of Hageman factor. When preparations of Hageman factor activated by negatively charged substances were analyzed by SDS gel electrophoresis, no changes in molecular weight were detected (Ulevitch *et al.*, 1974). Thus, this type of activation is characterized by an interaction of the Hageman factor with the activator, followed by a presumed conformational change in the parent molecule to yield an active enzyme. A recent study (McMillin *et al.*, 1974), which employed circular dichroism measurement of Hageman factor exposed to ellagic acid has provided evidence for an interaction between Hageman factor and the activator. This study suggests that a change in the environment of some basic and tyrosine residues has occurred.

While many of the negatively charged substances capable of activating Hageman factor have little biological importance, substances such as LPS, collagen, and vascular basement membrane may be of great importance. The studies of Wilner *et al.* (1968) indicated that human skin collagen does activate human Hageman factor. However, recently, studies of Griffin *et al.* (1975) and Jaffe (personal communication) using highly purified collagen preparations indicate that another factor associated with collagen is probably required for the activation of Hageman factor. This factor may be a sulfated mucopolysaccharide. A definition of the substances required for collagen activation of Hageman factor is essential for the full understanding of how Hageman factor is activated *in vivo*.

Activation of Hageman factor by proteolytic enzymes is another mechanism by which the precursor molecule is converted to an enzymatically active moeity. The use of SDS gel electrophoresis has allowed the detection of the structural changes associated with enzymatic activation of Hageman factor. Studies with trypsin indicated that the precursor Hageman factor is cleaved to fragments of 52,000, 42,000, and 28,000 molecular weight (Revak *et al.*, 1974). These changes are shown in Figure 2. The same cleavage patterns have also been demonstrated to occur when either kallikrein or plasmin is incubated with precursor Hageman factor. By combining immunologic and structural studies, it has been shown (Revak *et al.*, 1974) that the Hageman factor molecule consists of discrete regions with specific bio-

207

THE CHEMISTRY
AND BIOLOGY OF
THE PROTEINS OF
THE HAGEMAN
FACTOR-ACTIVATED
PATHWAYS

RICHARD J.
ULEVITCH AND
CHARLES G.
COCHRANE

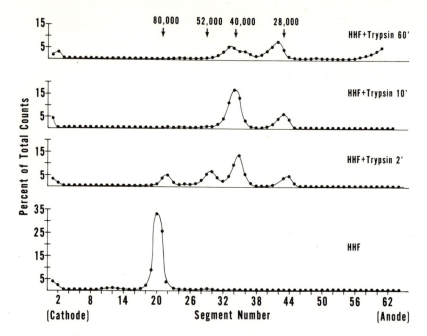

Figure 2. SDS gel electrophoresis of ^{125}I-Hageman factor. Samples were incubated in a 50-μl volume for the specified times with 0.2μg trypsin, and the reaction was stopped by the addition of 10 μg ovomucoid trypsin inhibitor.

chemical functions. These regions, which have been designated *c, d,* and *e,* are shown in Figure 3. The region involved in binding to negatively charged surfaces is contained in fragments *c* and *d,* while the enzymatic site is found in the *e* region.

Hageman factor activated by either enzymatic or nonenzymatic mechanisms is an active protease that is capable of hydrolyzing synthetic esters (Wuepper, 1971; Ulevitch *et al.,* 1974), can activate the three plasma substrates, and is inhibited by DFP (Ulevitch *et al.,* 1974). Although no detailed kinetic analyses have been performed, preliminary evidence from several laboratories suggests that the form of the activated Hageman factor may influence its ability to activate a given substance. For example, the 28,000-molecular-weight fragment may be a better activator of prekallikrein than the active 80,000-molecular-weight fragment. However, definitive proof of this requires the application of the detailed kinetic analysis of substrate activation.

The studies of Forbes *et al.* (1970) and Schreiber *et al.* (1973) have demonstrated that the 28,000-molecular-weight fragment of Hageman factor is inhibited by

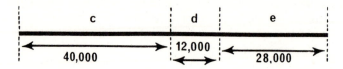

Figure 3. Regions of the Hageman factor molecule identified by structural and immunologic analyses. The enzymatic site is associated with the *e* region, while the *c* and *d* regions contain the sites responsible for binding to negatively charged polymeric substances.

the inhibitor of the first component of complement, C1-INH. Recent work in this laboratory (Revak *et al.*, 1974) has confirmed these observations and further has indicated that when Hageman factor is activated on a negatively charged surface in the presence of normal human plasma, the Hageman factor binds to the surface, but the *e* fragment is rapidly cleaved and released into the supernatant where it interacts with C1-INH and is inactivated. When C1-INH deficient plasma is employed, much of the fragment remains free and active, but a significant amount (20–50%) becomes bound to antithrombin III. Binding to antithrombin III is not observed when activation takes place in normal plasma. At the present time nothing is known about plasma inhibitors of the active 80,000-molecular-weight species. Neither α2-macroglobulin nor α1-antitrypsin has any inhibitory effect on the *e* fragment of Hageman factor.

209

THE CHEMISTRY
AND BIOLOGY OF
THE PROTEINS OF
THE HAGEMAN
FACTOR-ACTIVATED
PATHWAYS

2.2. Prekallikrein

Prekallikrein has been purified from normal human plasma by standard chromotographic techniques. This molecule is a glycoprotein with a molecular weight of 107,000 as measured by SDS gel electrophoresis. Prekallikrein may be activated by either trypsin or active Hageman factor (Wuepper, 1972). The active molecule, kallikrein, has both esterolytic and proteolytic activity. Studies of the kallikrein and prekallikrein on SDS gel electrophoresis demonstrated no detectable fragments of the parent molecule after activation until the activated sample was reduced and alkylated. At present, there have been no additional structural studies of the protein. Immunologic quantitation of the prekallikrein antigen in pooled human plasma has recently been reported by Bagdasarian *et al.* (1974) to be 103 ± 13 μg/ml.

The activity of kallikrein may be measured in several ways, namely, (1) measurement of the hydrolysis of substituted arginine esters (Wuepper and Cochrane, 1972), (2) the production of bradykinin from kininogen, and (3) the hydrolysis of a tripeptide p-NO_2 analide substrate (Svendsen, 1974). This substrate, *n*-benzoyl–Pro–phenylalanine–Arg–$p$$NO_2$-analide represents the synthesis of a specific peptide based upon the carboxy-terminal sequence of bradykinin and provides a specific and sensitive assay for kallikrein. This tripeptide substrate can be used with purified kallikrein as well as substituted for TAME (Ulevitch, personal communication) in the assay system of Colman *et al.* (1969), which is thought to reflect kallikrein concentrations in whole plasma. The principal plasma inhibitors of kallikrein are α2-macroglobulin C1-INH (Bagdasarian *et al.*, 1974), although nothing is known about the relative efficiency of these inhibitors *in vivo*.

The determination of a genetic deficiency of prekallikrein, Fletcher trait (Wuepper, 1972, 1973), has provided new insights into the regulation of the activation of the Hageman factor activated systems. This new concept, reciprocal activation of Hageman factor by plasma proteases, will be discussed in detail in a subsequent section.

2.3. Plasma Thromboplastin Antecedent (Factor XI)

Factor XI was first recognized after the observation of a group of individuals who had a defect in blood thromboplastin formation. This protein has recently been purified from normal human plasma (Wuepper and Cochrane, 1975). SDS gel electrophoresis of the purified protein demonstrated a molecular weight of 160,000. Upon reduction, the native molecule was split into two single polypeptide chains with molecular weights of 80,000. Activation of the precursor molecule with either trypsin or active Hageman factor produced cleavage of the molecule. However, the cleavage was only detected by SDS gel electrophoresis after reduction and alkylation, where fragments of 46,000 and 28,000 were observed. Purified factor XI is capable of hydrolyzing substituted arginine esters. A recent report indicated that the concentration of factor XI in normal plasma is 8–9 μg/ml (Wuepper and Cochrane, 1975).

2.4. Plasminogen Activator

The third substrate of activated Hageman factor, the plasminogen activator, has only recently been subject to detailed investigation. Kaplan and Austen (1972) have reported the separation of the plasminogen activator from both prekallikrein and factor XI. This protein has a molecular weight of approximately 100,000. The purified preparations were not inhibited by the C1-INH but were susceptible to inhibition by α2-macroglobulin and DFP. To date, the 28,000 molecular weight fragment of Hageman factor is the only reported activator of the plasminogen activator. No other studies have been reported on the properties of the plasminogen activator.

Recent reports suggest that the plasminogen activator may also be involved in the reciprocal activation of Hageman factor, and this will be discussed in Section 3.

3. Regulation of the Activation of Hageman Factor—Reciprocal Activation

A new concept concerning the regulation of the activation of Hageman factor first developed from studies of plasma deficient in prekallikrein: Fletcher trait plasma. Previously, the activation of the Hageman factor pathways had been characterized as a unidirectional event, beginning with the activation of Hageman factor and proceeding sequentially with the activation of the plasma substrates. It is now quite clear that these events are not necessarily unidirectional. Many studies have provided evidence for the activation of Hageman factor by one or more of the activated substrates, an event now termed *reciprocal activation*. This activation is induced by proteolytic cleavage of the native Hageman factor molecule and can occur with Hageman factor bound to a negatively charged surface as well as with Hageman factor in solution.

This mechanism of reciprocal activation has been studied in this laboratory by SDS gel electrophoresis of highly purified precursor Hageman factor molecules labeled with [125]I. Addition of kallikrein to precursor Hageman factor molecules in solution or bound to a negatively charged polymeric substance results in the cleavage of the Hageman factor molecule. The cleavage products have been characterized by SDS gel electrophoresis to have molecular weights of 52,000, 40,000, and 28,000. The enzymatic activity is associated with the 28,000-molecular-weight fragment. The observations of Kaplan and Austen (1971) and Burrowes *et al.* (1971) also demonstrate a possible role for plasmin in reciprocal activation of Hageman factor. Exposure of native Hageman factor to plasmin results in the

211

THE CHEMISTRY
AND BIOLOGY OF
THE PROTEINS OF
THE HAGEMAN
FACTOR-ACTIVATED
PATHWAYS

production of the same pattern of proteolysis observed with kallikrein. The possible importance of plasmin in reciprocal activation of Hageman factor is supported by the observation that low concentrations of streptokinase, a plasminogen activator, will correct the coagulation defect of Fletcher trait plasma (Colman *et al.*, 1975).

Reciprocal activation may provide an amplification mechanism to rapidly increase the concentration of activated Hageman factor. This effect may have particular importance in accelerating the activation of Hageman factor by negatively charged substances, a possible mechanism for *in vivo* activation of Hageman factor. Support for this derives from the observation that the coagulation defect of Fletcher trait plasma may be corrected by prolonged exposure of the plasma to kaolin, celite, or glass. However, the addition of as little as 2% of normal plasma or about 2 μg prekallikrein corrects the clotting defect, suggesting that the rate of Hageman factor activation is markedly increased in the presence of kallikrein.

Recently, several different investigators have independently characterized a newly recognized deficiency, which manifests itself in a marked reduction of the activation of Hageman factor (Saito *et al.*, 1975; Colman *et al.*, 1975; Wuepper *et al.*, 1975; Donaldson *et al.*, 1976). This deficiency is associated with a complete absence of high-molecular-weight kininogen and the plasmas are characterized by a complete abrogation surface-activated intrinsic coagulation. The generation of kallikrein, plasmin, and activity of the intrinsic clotting system are completely blocked. Levels of Hageman factor are normal and prekallikrein and plasminogen activator are somewhat reduced, although not to an extent sufficient to explain the defects noted. Replacement with preparations of the high-molecular-weight kininogen correct all the defects. Just how the high-molecular-weight kininogen acts is not understood at present.

4. Biological Activities Associated with the Activated Components of the Hageman Factor Pathways

Besides the direct effects on coagulation via factor XI on vascular permeability via kallikrein cleavage of kininogen, with formation of bradykinin, and fibrinolysis via the plasminogen activator, other biological activities have been demonstrated to result from the activation of the proteins of the Hageman factor pathways. Some of these activities will be discussed in this section.

Activation of the Hageman factor pathways either by exposure of plasma to negatively charged surfaces or by activation of isolated components leads to development of phlogogenic stimuli. Much of this information has been reviewed comprehensively (Ratnoff, 1969), and only portions of the literature before publication of the review, along with more recent data, will be presented.

Application of activated Hageman factor to the vascular beds of guinea pigs led to increased permeability of the vessels and accumulation of leukocytes (Graham *et al.*, 1965). Glass-activated plasma induces pain when applied to an exposed blister base (Armstrong *et al.*, 1953, 1954, and 1957), an effect attributed to polypeptide kinin generated in the plasma. Dilution of plasma of several species in glass vessels causes generation of a factor that increases vascular permeability in the skin upon injection (MacKay *et al.*, 1953; Becker *et al.*, 1959; Elder and Wilhelm, 1958). Generation of the factor, termed *permeability factor of dilution* (PF/dil), requires the presence of Hageman factor (Margolis, 1958, 1959; Ratnoff and Miles, 1964) and

RICHARD J.
ULEVITCH AND
CHARLES G.
COCHRANE

prekallikrein (Wuepper, 1973; Johnston *et al.*, 1974) for its generation. While thought originally to represent a distinct component acting between Hageman factor and prekallikrein, more recent studies in which active PF/dil was removed by exposure to insolubilized antibody to Hageman factor (Johnston *et al.*, 1974) indicated that PF/dil is, indeed, activated Hageman factor. For its generation, high-molecular-weight kininogen is also required (Saito *et al.*, 1975; Wuepper *et al.*, 1975; Colman *et al.*, 1975; Donaldson *et al.*, 1976). As discussed above, both prekallikrein and high-molecular-weight kininogen are essential for adequate activation of Hageman factor.

The accumulation of neutrophilic and monocytic leukocytes by kallikrein and plasminogen activator has been described (Kaplan *et al.*, 1972, 1973) and the chemotactic activity linked to the enzymatic capacity of these proteins. Since a focus of activation is essential for the chemotactic accumulation of leukocytes, it is of interest that kallikrein, like Hageman factor, binds to collagen-rich membranes (Harpel, 1972).

Plasmin activation leads to several changes of potential importance in inflammation. When plasmin is incubated with the third component of complement (C3), a fragment possessing chemotactic properties is released from C3 (Ward, 1967). Plasmin also generates activity of C1s (Lepow *et al.*, 1958; Ratnoff and Naff, 1967), thereby setting in motion the complement sequence. In addition, plasmin cleavage of fibrinogen leads to formation of the degradation products *d* and *e*. These fragments are reported to possess chemotactic and permeability-enhancing activities (Barnhart *et al.*, 1971).

5. Participation of the Hageman Factor Pathways in Experimental and Human Disease

While the Hageman factor pathway has been implicated in the pathogensis of many diseases, few firm data exist that unequivocally link the system to any disease process. Nevertheless, several interesting avenues have been and are currently being explored that, with the benefit of new technical capabilities, may yield significant knowledge.

5.1. Anaphylaxis

In acute anaphylaxis of guinea pigs, levels of kininogen in the circulation were found depleted and free kinin was elevated (Brocklehurst and Lahiri, 1963). Similarly in the dog, bradykinin could be detected in the blood during anaphylactic shock (Beraldo, 1950; Back *et al.*, 1963). Infusion of antigen into perfused lung of sensitized guinea pigs led to the generation of active kallikrein in the perfusate (Jonasson and Becker, 1966). More recently, levels of Hageman factor and other clotting components have been found depleted in rabbits that were sensitized with IgE antibody and shocked with antigen (Halonen and Pinckard, 1975; Pinckard *et al.*, 1975). The mechanisms responsible for activation of the Hageman factor pathway in anaphylaxis are not understood. It is clear that antigen–antibody union is not sufficient to activate Hageman factor (Cochrane *et al.*, 1972), and one must turn to secondary factors resulting from the initial reaction, such as release of activating agents from cells, exposure of membranes that may activate Hageman factor, and others. Further work should delineate such possibilities.

5.2. Gouty Arthritis

213

THE CHEMISTRY
AND BIOLOGY OF
THE PROTEINS OF
THE HAGEMAN
FACTOR-ACTIVATED
PATHWAYS

The participation of the Hageman factor pathways in gouty arthritis has received considerable support. Kinins have been isolated from synovial infusions in this disease (Melmon *et al.*, 1967). Since kinins mediate pain, an increase in vascular permeability and leukocytic accumulation, participation of this peptide may well be suspected in the pathogenesis of gout. This speculation is enhanced by the observation that Hageman factor may be activated by the sodium urate crystals that are found in the synovial fluid during acute attacks.

5.3. Hypotensive Shock Following Injection of Bacterial Lipopolysaccharide

Bradykinin is a potent hypotensive agent. As little as 4 μg/kg, administered intravenously, induces a 30% fall in mean arterial blood pressure in rabbits, and 15 μg/kg has a similar effect in monkeys. The hypotensive response to intravenously injected bradykinin in monkeys is transient and appears in great part to result from a fall in peripheral resistance. Nies *et al.* (1968) measured the levels of kininogen and free bradykinin in rhesus monkeys following injection of lipopolysaccharide (LPS). During the development of hypotension, levels of free bradykinin rose to approximately 10 ng/ml, while levels of kininogen fell correspondingly. Considering the rapid rate that bradykinin is degraded in the circulation ($t_{1/2}$, 20–30 sec), these levels must represent the residual of a large quantity of bradykinin generated. Free bradykinin was measured over a 2-hr period in the blood of the LPS-injected monkeys. A decrease in kininogen levels following injection of LPS or endotoxin was observed by Meyer and Werle (1964), Greeff *et al.* (1966), and Erdos and Miwa (1968). The latter authors discounted the importance of kinin formation in the hypotension of rabbits occurring in the first few minutes after injection of endotoxin in view of the failure of the bradykinin inhibitor carboxypeptidase to block the endotoxin-induced hypotension. It is possible that the early ephemoral hypotension could have been caused by activation of the complement system, as we have observed in our laboratory (Ulevitch, 1976). It would be of interest to examine the effect of administering carboxypeptidase on the hypotension that develops about 1 hr after injection of LPS, at a time when free kinin is measurable (Nies *et al.*, 1968).

In human beings undergoing hypotensive shock in bacteremic states, the levels of free arginine esterase activity rise (Mason and Colman, 1969; Mason *et al.*, 1969). The arginine esterase is postulated to represent free kallikrein. That bacterial LPS can generate activity of the Hageman factor pathways was demonstrated by direct means in this laboratory (Morrison and Cochrane, 1974). In the *nephrotic syndrome* in children, levels of the initial members of the Hageman factor pathways are reportedly diminished (Honig *et al.*, 1971; Lange *et al.*, 1974).

5.4. Disseminated Intravascular Coagulation

The participation of the intrinsic clotting system in disseminated intravascular coagulation (DIC) has been postulated from studies showing a diminution of levels of Hageman factor (Muller-Berghaus and Schneberger, 1971; Lerner *et al.*, 1968). Activation of Hageman factor by injection of ellagic acid in rabbits, together with epsilon-amino caproic acid and norepinephrine, induced DIC (McKay *et al.*, 1969).

In addition, injection of activated Hageman factor in pregnant rats produced intravascular coagulation (McKay *et al.*, 1971). Thus, Hageman factor and the intrinsic clotting system may be intimately involved in the development of DIC. The possibility that activated Hageman factor may activate factor VII (Nemerson, 1975) and the extrinsic clotting system must also be considered.

6. Summary

The proteins of the Hageman factor–activated pathways are all proteolytic enzymes that circulate in the blood in precursor form. Activation occurs by limited proteolysis. A critical role for kallikrein in the reciprocal activation of Hageman factor has been documented. These proteins can initiate diverse biologic effects, such as coagulation, vascular permeability changes, fibrinolysis, and chemotaxis. In addition, although the direct participation of the proteins of the Hageman factor pathways in experimental and human disease has not been demonstrated, suggestive evidence for participation in anaphylactic shock, LPS-induced hypotension, and gouty arthritis has been discussed.

ACKNOWLEDGMENT

This work was supported in part by United States Public Health Service Grants HL 18376, HL 16411, and AI 07007.

References

Armstrong, D., Dry, R. M. L., Keele, C. A., and Markham, J. W., 1953, Observations on chemical excitants of cutaneous pain in man, *J. Physiol. London* **120**:326.

Armstrong, D., Keele, C, A., Jepson, J. B., and Stewart, J. W., 1954, Development of pain-producing substance in human plasma, *Nature London* **174**:791.

Armstrong, D., Jepson, J. B., Keele, C. A., and Stewart, J. W., 1957, Pain-producing substance in human inflammatory exudates and plasma, *J. Physiol. London* **135**:350.

Austen, K. F., 1974, Hageman factor–dependent coagulation, fibrinolysis and kinin generation, *Transplant. Proc.* **6**:39.

Back, N., Munson, A. E., and Guth, P. S., 1963, Anaphylactic shock in dogs, *J. Amer. Med. Assoc.* **183**:260.

Bagdasarian, A., Talamo, R. C., and Colman, R. W., 1973, Isolation of high molecular weight activators of human plasma prekallikrein, *J. Biol. Chem.* **248**:3456.

Bagdasarian, A., Lahiri, B., Talamo, R. C., Wong, P., and Colman, R. W., 1974, Immunochemical studies of plasma kallikrein, *J. Clin. Invest.* **54**:1444.

Barnhart, M. I., Sulisz, L., and Bluhm, G. B., 1971, Role for fibrinogen and its derivatives in acute inflammation, in: *Immunopathology of Inflammation* (B. K. Forscher and J. C. Houek, eds.), p. 59, Excerpta Medica, Amsterdam.

Becker, E. L., Wilhelm, D. L., and Miles, A. A., 1959, Enzymic nature of the serum globulin permeability factors, *Nature London* **183**:1264.

Beraldo, W. T., 1950, Formation of bradykinin in anaphylactic and peptone shock, *Amer. J. Physiol.* **163**:283.

Brocklehurst, W. E., and Lahiri, S. C., 1963, Formation and destruction of bradykinin during anaphylaxis, *J. Physiol. London* **165**:39P.

Burrowes, C. E., Movat, H. Z., and Soltay, M. J., 1971, The kinin system in human plasma. VI. The action of plasmin, *Proc. Soc. Exp. Biol. Med.* **138**:959.

Cochrane, C. G., Wuepper, K., Aikin, B., Revak, S., and Spiegelberg, H., 1972, The interaction of Hageman factor and immune complexes, *J. Clin. Invest.* **51**:2736–2745.

Cochrane, C. G., Revak, S. D., and Wuepper, K. D., 1973a, Activation of Hageman factor in solid and fluid phases. A critical role of kallikrein, *J. Exp. Med.* **138**:1564.

215

THE CHEMISTRY
AND BIOLOGY OF
THE PROTEINS OF
THE HAGEMAN
FACTOR-ACTIVATED
PATHWAYS

Cochrane, C. G., Revak, S. D., Wuepper, K. D., Johnston, A., Morrison, D. C., and Ulevitch, R., 1973b, Activation of Hageman factor and the kinin forming, intrinsic clotting, and fibrinolytic systems, in: *Advances in the Biosciences* (G. Raspe, ed.), p. 237, Pergamon Press, Viowes.

Colman, R. W., Mason, J. W., and Sherry, S., 1969, The kallikreinogen–kallikrein enzyme system of human plasma. Assay of components and observations in disease states, *Ann. Intern. Med.* **71**:763.

Colman, R. W., Bagdasarian, A., Talamo, R. C., Scott, C. F., Seavy, M., Guimaraes, J. A., Pierce, J. V., and Kaplan, M., 1975, Williams trait: human kininogen deficiency with diminished levels of plasminogen proactivator, and pre-kallikrein associated with abnormalities of the Hageman factor dependent pathways, *J. Clin. Invest.* **56**:1650–1662.

Donaldson, V. H., Glueck, H. I., Miller, M. A., Movat, H. Z., and Habal, F., 1976, Kininogen deficiency in Fitzgerald trait: role of high molecular weight kininogen in clotting and fibrinolysis, *J. Cab. Clin. Mol.* **87**(2):327–337.

Elder, J. M., and Willhelm, D. L., 1958, Enzyme-like globulins from serum reproducing the vascular phonemona of inflammation V. Activable permeability factor in human serum, *Br. J. Exp. Pathol.* **39**:335.

Erdos, E. G., and Miwa, I., 1968, Effect of endotoxin shock on the plasma kallikrein–kinin system of the rabbit, *Fed. Proc. Fed. Amer. Soc. Exp. Biol.* **27**:92.

Forbes, C. D., Pinsky, J., and Ratnoff, O. D., 1970, Inhibition of activated Hageman factor and activated plasma thromboplastin antecedent by purified serum C1 inactivator, *J. Lab. Clin. Med.* **76**:809.

Graham, R. C., Jr., Ebert, R. H., Ratnoff, O. D., and Moses, J. H., 1965, Pathogenesis of inflammation. II. In vivo observations of the inflammatory effects of activated Hageman factor and bradykinin, *J. Exp. Med.* **121**:807.

Greeff, K., Scharnagel, K., Luhr, R., and Strobach, H., 1966, Die Abnahme des Kininogengehaltes des Plasmas beim toxischen anaphylaktischen und anaphylaktoiden Shock, *Naunyn-Schmiedeberg's Arch. Exp. Pathol. Pharmakol.* **253**:235–245.

Griffin, J. H., and Cochrane, C. G., 1976, Human factor XII, in: *Methods in Enzymology,* Vol. VL, Part B (L. Lorand, ed.), Academic Press, New York, in press.

Griffin, J. H., Harper, E., and Cochrane, C. G., 1975, Studies on the activation of human blood coagulation factor XII (Hageman factor) by soluble collagen, *Fed. Proc. Fed. Amer. Soc. Exp. Biol.* **34**:3626.

Halonen, M., and Pinckard, R. N., 1975, Intravascular effect of IgE antibody upon basophils, neutrophils, and blood coagulation in the rabbit, *J. Immunol.* **115**:519.

Harpel, P. C., 1972, Studies on the interaction between collagon and a plasma kallikrein-like activity, *J. Clin. Invest.* **51**:1813.

Honig, G. R., and Lindley, A., 1971, Deficiency of Hageman factor (factor XII) in patients with the nephrotic syndrome, *J. Pediatr.* **78**:633.

Johnston, A. R., Cochrane, C. G., and Revak, S. D., 1974, The relationship between PF/dil and activated human Hageman factor, *J. Immunol.* **113**:103.

Jonasson, O., and Becker, E. L., 1966, Release of kallikrein from guinea pig lung during anaphylaxis, *J. Exp. Med.* **123**:509.

Kaplan, A. P., and Austen, K. F., 1971, A prealbumin activator of prekallikrein. II. Derivation of activators of prekallikrein from active Hageman factor by digestion with plasmin, *J. Exp. Med.* **133**:696.

Kaplan, A. P., and Austen, K. F., 1972, The fibrinolytic pathway of human plasma. Isolation and characterization of the plasminogen proactivator, *J. Exp. Med.* **136**:1378.

Kaplan, A. P., Kay, A. B., and Austen, K. F., 1972, A prealbumin activator of prekallikrein. III. Appearance of chemotactic activity for human neutrophils by the conversion of human prekallikrein to kallikrein, *J. Exp. Med.* **135**:81.

Kaplan, A. P., Goetzel, E. J., and Austen, K. F., 1973, The fibrinolytic pathway of human plasma. II. The generation of chemotactic activity by activation of plasminogen proactivator, *J. Clin. Invest.* **52**:2591.

Lange, L. G., Carvalho, A., Badasarian, A., Lahini, B., and Colman, R. W., 1974, Activation of Hageman factor in the nephritic syndrome, *Am. J. Med.* **56**:565–569.

Lepow, I. H., Ratnoff, O. D., and Levy, L. R., 1958, Studies on the activation of a proesterase associated with partially purified first component of human complement, *J. Exp. Med.* **107**:451.

Lerner, R. G., Rappaport, S. I., and Spitzer, J. M., 1968, Endotoxin-induced intravascular clotting: the need for granulocytes, *Thromb. Diath. Haemorrh.* **20**:430.

MacKay, M. E., Miles, A. A., Schacter, C. B., and Wilhelm, D. L., 1953, Susceptibility of the guinea pig to pharmacological factors from its own serum, *Nature London* **172**:714.

RICHARD J.
ULEVITCH AND
CHARLES G.
COCHRANE

Margolis, J., 1958, Activation of a permeability factor in plasma by contact with glass, *Nature London* **181**:635.

Margolis, J., 1959, Hageman factor and capillary permeability, *Aust. J. Exp. Biol. Med. Sci.* **37**:239.

Margolius, A., and Ratnoff, O. D., 1956, Observations on the hereditary nature of Hageman trait, *Blood* **11**:565.

Mason, J. W., and Colman, R. W., 1969a, The role of Hageman factor in disseminated intravascular coagulation of sepsis and neoplasia, *Amer. J. Clin. Path.* **52**:755.

Mason, J. W., Kleeberg, U. R., and Colman, R. W., 1969b, Human plasma kallikrein and Hageman factor in endotoxin shock, *Clin. Research* **17**:371.

McKay, D. G., Muller-Berghaus, G., and Cruse, V., 1969, Activation of Hageman factor by ellasic acid and the generalized Schwartzman reaction, *Am. J. Path.* **54**:393.

McKay, D. G., Latour, J. G., and Lopez, A. M., 1971, Production of the generalized Schwartzman reaction by activated Hageman factor and α-adrenergic stimulation, *Thromb. Diath. Haemorrhag.* **26**:71.

McMillin, C. R., Saito, H., Ratnoff, O. D., and Walton, A. G., 1974, The secondary structure of human Hageman factor (factor XII) and its alternation by activating agents, *J. Clin. Invest.* **54**:1312.

Melmon, K. L., Webster, M. E., Goldfinger, S. E., and Seegmiller, J. E., 1967, The presence of a kinin in inflammatory synovial effusion from arthritides of varying etiologies, *Arthritis Rheum.* **10**:13.

Meyer, A., and Werle, E., 1964, in: *Pathogenese, Diagnostik, Klinik und Therapie der Erkrankungen des Exokrinen Pankreas* (K. Heinkel and H. Schon, eds.), p. 299, Schattauer-Verlag, Stuttgart.

Morrison, D. C., and Cochrane, C. G., 1974, Direct evidence for Hageman factor (factor XII) activation by bacterial lipopolysaccharides (endotoxins), *J. Exp. Med.* **140**:797.

Muller-Berghaus, G., and Schneberger, R., 1971, Hageman factor activation in the generalized Shwartzman reaction induced by endotoxin, *Br. J. Haematol.* **21**:513.

Nies, A. S., Forsyth, R. P., Williams, H. E., and Melmon, K. L., 1968, Contributions of kinins to endotoxin shock in unanesthetized rhesus monkeys, *Cir. Res.* **22**:155.

Pinckard, R. N., Tanigawa, C., and Halonen, M., 1975, IgE-induced blood coagulation alterations in the rabbit: consumption of coagulation factors XII, XI, and IX *in vivo*, *J. Immunol.* **115**:519.

Ratnoff, O. D., 1966, The biology and pathology of the initial stages of blood coagulation, in: *Progress in Hematology* (E. B. Brown and C. V. Moore, eds.), Vol. 5, p. 204, Grune and Stratton, New York.

Ratnoff, O. D., 1969, Some relationships among hemostasis, fibrinolytic phenomena, immunity and the inflammatory process, in: *Advances in Immunology* (F. J. Dixon and H. Kunkel, eds.), Vol. 10, p. 146, Academic Press, New York.

Ratnoff, O. D., and Davie, E. W., 1962, The purification of activated Hageman factor (activated factor XII), *Biochemistry* **1**:967.

Ratnoff, O. D., and Miles, A. A., 1964, The induction of permeability-increasing activity in human plasma by activated Hageman factor, *Br. J. Exp. Pathol.* **45**:328.

Ratnoff, O. D., and Naff, G. G., 1967, The conversion of C'1s to C'2 esterase by plasmin and trypsin, *J. Exp. Med.* **125**:337.

Revak, S. D., and Cochrane, C. G., 1976, The relationship of structure and function in human Hageman factor. The association of enzymatic and binding activities with separate regions of the molecule, *J. Clin. Invest.* **57**:852–860.

Revak, S. D., Cochrane, C. G., Johnston, A. R., and Hugli, T. E., 1974, Structural changes accompanying enzymatic activation of human Hageman factor, *J. Clin. Invest.* **54**:619.

Saito, H., Ratnoff, O. D., and Donaldson, V. H., 1974, Defective activation of clotting, fibrinolytic and permeability-enhancing systems in human Fletcher trait plasma, *Circ. Res.* **34**:641.

Saito, H., Ratnoff, O. D., Waldmann, R., and Abraham, J. P., 1975, Fitzgerald trait. Deficiency in a hitherto unrecognized agent, Fitzgerald factor, participating in surface-mediated reactions of clotting, fibrinolysis, generation of kinins and the property of diluted plasma enhancing vascular permeability (PF/dil), *J. Clin. Invest.* **55**:1082.

Schreiber, A. A., Kaplan, A. P., and Austen, K. F., 1973, Inhibition by C1-INH of Hageman factor fragment activation of coagulation, fibrinolysis and kinin generation, *J. Clin. Invest.* **52**:1402.

Smink, M. M., Daniel, T. M., Ratnoff, O. D., and Stavitsky, A. B., 1967, Immunologic demonstration of a deficiency of Hageman factor-like material in Hageman trait, *J. Lab. Clin. Med.* **69**:819.

Svendsen, L., 1974, The chemistry and biology of the kallikrein–kinin system in health and disease, International Conference Report at Reston, Virginia (October 1974).

Ulevitch, R. J., Letchford, D., and Cochrane, C. G., 1974, A direct enzymatic assay for the esterolytic activity of activated Hageman factor, *Thromb. Diath. Haemorrhag.* **31**:30.

217

THE CHEMISTRY
AND BIOLOGY OF
THE PROTEINS OF
THE HAGEMAN
FACTOR-ACTIVATED
PATHWAYS

Ulevitch, R. J., Cochrane, C. G., Morrison, D. C., and Henson, P. M., 1976, A characterization of hypotensive changes associated with rapid intravascular complement activation, in preparation.

Ward, P. A., 1967, A plasmin-split fragment of C′3 as a new chemotactic factor, *J. Exp. Med.* **126**:189.

Wilner, G. D., Nossel, H. L., and Le Roi, E. C., 1968, Activation of Hageman factor by collagon, *J. Clin. Invest.* **47**:2708.

Wuepper, K. D., 1971, Plasma prekininogenase (prekallikrein) activation: hydrolysis of native and synthetic substrates, *Fed. Proc. Fed. Amer. Soc. Exp. Biol.* **30**:451 (abstract 1427).

Wuepper, K. D., 1972, Biochemistry and biology of components of the plasma kinin-forming system, in: *Inflammation, Mechanisms and Control* (I. H. Lepow and P. A. Ward, eds.), p. 93, Academic Press, New York.

Wuepper, K. D., 1973, Prekallikrein deficiency in man, *J. Exp. Med.* **138**:1345–1355.

Wuepper, K. D., and Cochrane, C. G., 1972, Plasma prekallikrein: isolation, characterization and mechanism of activation, *J. Exp. Med.* **135**:1.

Wuepper, K. D., and Cochrane, C. G., 1975, Purification and characterization of human precursor plasma thromboplastin antecedent, in preparation.

Wuepper, K. D., Miller, D. R., and Lacombe, M. J., 1975, Flaujeac trait: deficiency of kininogen in man, *Fed. Proc. Fed. Amer. Soc. Exp. Biol.* **34**:3623.

11

Isolated Deficiencies of the Complement System in Experimental Animals

HARTMUT GEIGER and NOORBIBI K. DAY

1. Introduction

In addition to the genetic deficiencies of complement (C) components in man, genetically transmitted or experimentally induced deficiencies of individual components of the C system have been described in animals of various species (Table 1). These animals provide a useful model for study of the requirement of complement activation by both the classical and alternative pathway for immune reactions and defense mechanisms *in vivo* and *in vitro*.

2. C1 Deficiency in Chickens

Recently, Gabrielson *et al.* (1974) determined C1 hemolytic activity in hypo-gammaglobulinemic chickens, aged 22–24 days, which had been bursectomized by administration of cyclophosphamide for 3 consecutive days after hatching. Hemoly-tic C1, titrated by three different methods, was found to be significantly reduced when compared to a normal control group (Table 2), thus reflecting, in the experi-mental system, the clinical observation of deficiency in hemolytic C1 and lowered circulating C1q in patients with the infantile X-linked recessive form of agamma-globulinemia (Gewurz *et al.*, 1968; Kohler and Müller-Eberhard, 1969). Recent investigations by Kohler and Müller-Eberhard (1972) with labeled C1q in agamma-globulinemic patients showed that there was no evidence of decreased C1q synthesis in these patients with the disease. The labeled C1q complexed loosely with IgG and was quickly lost from the circulation in the hypogammaglobulinemic patients.

HARTMUT GEIGER • Universitäts-Kinderklinik, Heidelberg, Germany. NOORBIBI K. DAY •
Sloan-Kettering Institute for Cancer Research, New York, New York.

TABLE 1.   Isolated Deficiencies of Complement Components in
Experimental Animals

Deficient component	Species	Comments
C1	Chicken	Reduced hemolytic C1 activity combined with hypogammaglobulinemia after bursectomy
C4	Guinea pig Rat	
"C3"	Guinea pig	Extinct strain Deficiency of components between C3 and C9 not defined
C5	Mouse	
C6	Rabbit Hamster	

Similar studies, which could explain the association of hypogammaglobulinemia and reduced C1 activity in bursectomized chickens, still need to be done (see Table 2).

3.   C4 Deficiency

3.1.   C4 Deficiency in Guinea Pigs

Ellman *et al.* (1970) discovered guinea pigs that had a complete absence of the fourth component of complement while trying to produce, in the guinea pig, antiserum against immunoglobulin allotypes. Since then, complement activation and complement-mediated biological functions have been extensively studied both *in vivo* and *in vitro* in these animals (Frank *et al.*, 1971; Ellman *et al.*, 1971; Root *et al.*, 1972). Guinea pig anti-C4 antiserum prepared by injection of pooled guinea pig serum into C4-deficient guinea pigs gives a single strong line on Ouchterlony analysis with partially purified guinea pig C4. This antiserum has surprisingly little species cross-reactivity, since it does not react with rabbit, mouse, rat, or goat serum and gives only a weak precipitin line against human serum (Frank *et al.*, 1971). Two experiments indicate that C4-deficient guinea pigs are entirely lacking in C4 and that the existence of an immunochemically modified and inactive C4 in these animals is very unlikely. Hartley strain guinea pigs and normal NIH guinea pigs immunized with C4-deficient serum failed to make antibodies to any component in

TABLE 2.   C1 Deficiency in the Chicken
Experimentally Induced by Chemical Bursectomy

Complement titration:	C1 activity reduced Titers of other complement components unknown
Biological functions:	Not studied

the C4-deficient serum, and antibodies to normal C4 in rabbits did not reveal any precipitation against C4-deficient serum on Ouchterlony analysis of the sera of the deficient guinea pigs (Frank *et al.*, 1971). In the sera of C4-deficient guinea pigs, total hemolytic complement and hemolytic C4 are totally undetectable. The hemolytic activity of the serum of the deficient animals is readily restored either by adding normal guinea pig serum or partially purified C4. These findings show that an inhibitor of C4 cannot account for the apparent absence of C4. The titers of C3–9 complex are normal, whereas serum C2 titers are about half the C2 titers of normal animals. Furthermore, approximately 60% of C4-deficient guinea pigs have reduced titers of C1, i.e., 10–20% of normal. The basis for the inconsistent depression of C1 titers remains unclear. By contrast, a reduced synthetic rate of C2 in macrophages from C4-deficient animals was shown to be responsible for the low C2 titers (Colten and Frank, 1972) (Table 3).

Mating studies showed that the C4-deficiency in guinea pigs is transmitted as an autosomal recessive trait. Under normal laboratory conditions, the C4-deficient guinea pigs remain healthy and have normal fertility, and the offspring survive well. The suprisingly good health of the C4-deficient animals may be explained by the persisting ability to overcome the C4 deficiency almost completely through activation of the later C components and the generation of biologically active fragments of C through the intact bypass system. For example, antigen–antibody complexes inactivate C4 deficient sera by 50% of the later C components when compared with comparable challenge of normal guinea pig serum. The degree of fixation of the later components after incubation of the serum with *Escherichia coli* endotoxin is not significantly different for C4-deficient heterozygous and normal guinea pig serum. The *in vitro* generation of polymorphonuclear neutrophilic chemotactic factor was also found to be normal in C4-deficient serum (Frank *et al.*, 1971). As could be expected from the *in vitro* experiments with normal generation of chemotactic activity in C4-deficient serum, the allergic reaction (Arthus phenomenon) in C4 deficient animals (Frank *et al.*, 1971).

The bactericidal and opsonic properties of C4-deficient serum was investigated by Root *et al.* (1972). In studying the bactericidal activity against two strains of *E.*

TABLE 3. C4 Deficiency in the Guinea Pig

Transmission:	Autosomal recessive
Complement titration:	CH50 / C4 } Not measurable
	C1 10–20% of normal in 5 of 8 animals
	C2 50% of normal
	C3–9 titers normal
Biological functions:	Activation of late components by endotoxin normal
	Chemotactic activity normal
	Arthus reaction normal
	Bactericidal and opsonic activity impaired
	Immune clearance impaired
	Impaired antibody production to low concentrations of certain antigens

coli, the latent period was prolonged and the rate was slower in C4-deficient serum as compared to that of the serum of normal or heterozygous guinea pigs. Because of the impaired opsonization, the ingestion rate of ^{14}C-labeled *Staphylococcus aureus,* type 2S pneumococci, *E. coli,* and *Candida albicans* was slower in C4-deficient serum than in normal or heterozygous serum.

These observations show that bacterial opsonization and killing can occur in C4-deficient animals after activation of the later C components through the alternative pathway, but that maximal rate of opsonization and killing may require the activation of the complement sequence through the classical pathway. On the other hand, intravenous challenge with log-phase pneumococci did not disclose a difference in the mortality between C4-deficient and normal guinea pigs. The clearance rate of ^{51}Cr-labeled guinea pig erythrocytes was found to be impaired in C4-deficient animals and could be accelerated by injection of normal guinea pig serum (Ellman *et al.,* 1971). Furthermore, deficient animals showed an impaired antibody production to small doses of ovalbumin or BSA (Frank *et al.,* 1971), which could suggest that complement plays some part in antibody formation. Finally, in turnover studies with ^{125}I-radiolabeled C3, the fractional catabolic rate, the synthetic rate, and the percent of C3 in the plasma pool were the same in C4-deficient and normal animals, suggesting that activation of the classical C pathway is not essential for significant C3 turnover in the resting state (Atkinson *et al.,* 1974). Although the C4-deficient guinea pigs do well under ideal conditions of husbandry in a laboratory environment and seem to have mechanisms that can compensate in large degree for the deficiency of the C component, it seems most likely that life in the wild would reveal, through a high frequency of diseases as yet undefined, the survival advantage of C4.

3.2. C4 Deficiency in Rats

Arroyave *et al.* (1974) reported a genetic deficiency of the fourth component of complement in Wistar rats. From sera of 40 male rats, 12 were found to have values of total hemolytic C activity of 20% or less present in the other rat sera studied. This defect could not be demonstrated in female rats. Single-component analysis revealed the defect to reside in the fourth component of complement. The reduced hemolytic activity in deficient rat serum could be restored by highly purified human C4. No further studies were carried out in this interesting model.

4. "C3" Deficiency in Guinea Pigs

In 1919, a strain of guinea pigs totally lacking hemolytic C activity was discovered at the Vermont Agricultural Station (Moore, 1919). This strain was thought to have a deficiency of the "classical" third component of C, which is now known to include C3, C5, C6, C7, C8, and C9. The hemolytic activity could be restored *in vitro* by heat-inactivated serum and *in vivo* over a 3-day period after injection of normal guinea pig serum into the peritoneal cavity of deficient animals (Hyde, 1923). After injection of viable *Bacillus cholerae suis* into 100 deficient animals, 77 died, whereas 80 of 100 normal guinea pigs survived such a challenge. This observation led to the suggestion that in the C deficient animals, the opsonic capacity of the serum may be impaired (Moore, 1919). In another *in vivo* experiment, skin reactions or a deadly anaphylactoid shock by high doses of Forssman

223

ISOLATED
DEFICIENCIES OF THE
COMPLEMENT
SYSTEM IN
EXPERIMENTAL
ANIMALS

TABLE 4. "C3" Deficiency in the Guinea Pig

Transmission:	Autosomal recessive
Complement titration:	CH50 $\left.\right\}$ Not measurable "C3" piece
Biological functions:	Impaired opsonic activity Forsman shock cannot be produced

antibody did not occur in the C-deficient animals (Hyde, 1932). For unknown reasons, the deficient strain became extinct several decades ago, so that the defect apparently transmitted as an autosomal trait has not been defined in modern terms. Whereas yeast (zymosan)-treated serum did not restore the serum hemolytic activity in the "C3"-deficient strain, the C4-deficient strain of guinea pigs is readily reconstituted with zymosan-treated normal guinea pig serum (Table 4). These findings indicate clearly that these two strains of C-deficient guinea pigs are different (Frank *et al.*, 1971).

5. C5 Deficiency in Mice

In 1964, it was discovered that the serum of certain strains of inbred mice lacked a β-globulin designated hc' (Erickson *et al.*, 1964) or MuB1 (Cinader *et al.*, 1964). The absence of this protein was accompanied by a complete deficiency of hemolytic C activity (Rosenberg and Tachibana, 1962; Erickson *et al.*, 1964; Cinader *et al.*, 1964). Genetic studies revealed that the defect was transmitted in an autosomal recessive trait (Herzenberg *et al.*, 1963; Tachibana *et al.*, 1963). In order to define the missing C component, C1, C2, C4, and C3 were found to be normal in deficient mouse serum (Terry *et al.*, 1964; Linscott *et al.*, 1964). Experiments undertaken by Nilsson and Müller-Eberhard (1967) showed clearly that the deficient globulin was analogous to human C5, because highly purified C5 reconstituted the hemolytic activity of the C-deficient mouse serum. Numerous experiments were undertaken mostly in mice of the line B10 D2/SN (new), which have normal C activity, and the coisogenic line B10 D2/SN (old), which are devoid of C5. The results reported are somewhat conflicting and depend to the same degree on the strain of mice used and on the experimental conditions applied. They may, however, be briefly summarized as follows: Only in the face of rather strong immunologic challenge did the C-deficient mice react in an inferior way to normal mice, whereas under less extreme conditions, usually no difference in inflammatory defense reactions could be observed between the two critical strains. Snyderman *et al.* (1968) found chemotactic activity after incubation with endotoxin or *Serratia marcescens* and *Veillonella alcalescens* only in normal mouse serum and not in C5-deficient serum from the B10 D2/SN (old) strain of mice. Similar results were obtained *in vivo* when *Salmonella typhosa* endotoxin was injected intraperitoneally in C deficient and normal mice (Snyderman *et al.*, 1971). Three, 6, and 24 hr after injection with endotoxin, C deficient animals showed significantly fewer polymorphonuclear leukocytes in peritoneal exudates than normal mice. Furthermore, chemotactic activity in peritoneal exudate supernatants were only detectable in the mice with a normal C system and not in the C-deficient animals (Table 5).

TABLE 5.   C5 Deficiency in the Mouse

Transmission:	Autosomal recessive
Complement titration:	CH50 ⎫
	C5 ⎬ Not measurable
	C1, C4, C2, C3 normal
Biological functions:	Chemotactic activity impaired
	Impaired resistance to the injection of high numbers of tumor cells and bacteria
	Delayed rejection of grafted skin from A/Wy Sn mice
	Mild course of nephrotoxic serum nephritis

Ben-Efraim and Cinader (1964) tested the role of complement in the passive cutaneous anaphylaxis and found an impaired response in C deficient mice when compared to that of normal mice. C5 deficient mice that were challenged with *Corynebacterium kutscheri* showed a weaker resistance to this common mouse pathogen (Caren and Rosenberg, 1966). Interesting results were obtained when sarcoma 1 tumor cells of the mouse strain A/Jax were inoculated intraperitoneally into B10 D2/NB (old) and B10 D2/N3 (new) strains of mice (Phillips *et al.*, 1968): A clear difference in the rejection of tumor cells was demonstrable when more than 5 $\times 10^5$ tumor cells were used. Similar deficiences in resistance were revealed by the experiments of Skin *et al.* (1969), in which the mortality of the C-deficient mice infected with virulent pneumococcus strain increased with the number of bacteria injected intraperitoneally. Skin of CF/1 or C57BL/6J strains of mice transplanted with C-deficient and/or C-sufficient mice were rejected similarly by both groups (Caren and Rosenberg, 1966). When skin of C5-deficient A/WySn strains of mice was used for grafting, rejection was delayed in the C-deficient mice (Weitzel and Rother, 1970).

Unanue *et al.* (1966) studied nephrotoxic serum nephritis in several strains of mice and found no difference in the heterologous or autologous phase of the disease between C-intact and C-deficient mice. These results were not, however, confirmed by Lindberg and Rosenberg (1968), who observed a higher urine protein loss and a 60% mortality in the intact mice during the autologous phase of nephrotoxic nephritis. By contrast, all C-deficient mice survived.

6.   C6 Deficiency

6.1.   C6 Deficiency in Rabbits

In 1961, Rother and Rother discovered a strain of rabbits, the sera of which showed a defect of "classical" C3. The serum of these rabbits, therefore, was not able to lyse sensitized sheep erythrocytes. Further studies revealed that the underlying defect of the C system in these rabbits was due to the complete absence of C6 (Rother *et al.*, 1966). That the genetically determined defect in these animals was due to a complete deficiency of C6 could be concluded from the following observations:

1. No activity of C6 was measurable, even when the most sensitive methods were employed for its detection.
2. Highly purified C6 from rabbit and human sources completely reconstituted the C6-deficient serum.
3. Anticomplementary activity could not be detected in the C6-deficient serum.
4. The injection of purified C6 into C6-deficient rabbits resulted in production of anti-C6 antibodies.

225

ISOLATED
DEFICIENCIES OF THE
COMPLEMENT
SYSTEM IN
EXPERIMENTAL
ANIMALS

In the meantime, two other strains of C6-deficient rabbits have been described, one originating in Mexico (Biro and Garcia, 1965), the other in Cambridge (Lachmann, 1970). The C6 deficiency is inherited in an autosomal recessive pattern. Extensive studies have been undertaken in C6-deficient rabbits to define the biologic role of C6 in inflammation and in the immune defenses. Under conditions of ideal husbandry in the laboratory, C6-deficient rabbits are not unusually susceptible to infections, possibly because of their unimpaired immune adherence and antibody production, normal opsonization, phagocytosis, and immune clearance of bacteria (Rother and Till, 1974). As could be expected, the C6-deficient serum lacks the ability to kill gram-negative bacteria (Rother et al., 1964a). Ward et al. (1965) reported on defective chemotactic activity in C6 deficient serum, whereas Stecher and Sorkin (1969) and Snyderman et al. (1969) found normal chemotactic responses in C6-deficient serum in the presence of endotoxin or immune complexes. Studies of Johnson and Ward (1971), in which normal and C6-deficient rabbits were injected intravenously with 100 mg endotoxin from E. coli 0III:B4, suggested a requirement of C6 for detoxification of bacterial endotoxin. Further, while the passive Arthus reaction was found to be impaired (Rother et al., 1964b), the active Arthus reaction seems to be quite normal in these animals. The delayed hypersensitivity reaction to tuberculin was, however, found to be suppressed (Rother et al., 1967b) and some skin allografts survived longer in C6-deficient than in normal rabbits (Rother et al., 1967a) (Table 6). These findings suggest that the exact role of the later C components

TABLE 6. C6 Deficiency in the Rabbit

Transmission:	Autosomal recessive
Complement titration:	C6 activity absent
	Other complement components normal
Biological functions:	No susceptibility to infection
	Normal
	Immune adherence, opsonization
	Phagocytosis, immune clearance
	Impaired
	Bactericidal activity
	Passive Arthus reaction
	Chemotactic activity (?)
	Tuberculin reaction
	Graft rejection
	Detoxification of endotoxin
	Generation of platelet factor 3 during clotting
	Normal autologous phase of nephrotoxic serum nephritis

in graft rejection need to be defined. After injection of antirabbit kidney antiserum, C6-deficient rabbits developed nephrotoxic nephritis as severe as that of control animals (Rother *et al.*, 1967c) when studied in the autologous phase of the disease. In 1971, Zimmerman *et al.* (1971) described a coagulation defect in C6-deficient rabbit plasma featured by a prolonged blood clotting time and decreased prothrombin consumption, which could be normalized by adding highly purified C6 to the serum. This defect in blood coagulation in C6-deficient rabbits is due to the failure of C6-deficient plasma to generate platelet factor C3 activity during clotting (Brown and Lachmann, 1973).

6.2. C6 Deficiency in Hamsters

Recently Yang *et al.* (1974) observed a deficiency of C6 in some individual strains of Croblen Syrian hamsters, which showed a high incidence of proliferative enteritis. Sera from these hamsters were unable to reconstitute C6-deficient sera (rabbit or human) but reconstituted C1, C2 (human), and C4 (guinea pig) serum. In contrast, normal hamster sera from the same strain reconstitute the above deficient sera. No differences in ability to induce immune adherence or phagocytosis was detectable between deficient and normal hamster sera. The deficient serum was not anticomplementary.

7. Conclusion

A variety of experimental models of complement and complement component deficiencies have been and are available for analysis in an increasing variety of experimental animals. These defects are generally genetically determined faults and, as such, represent experiments of nature from which much useful information about the function of the C system in general and the role of individual C components in the body economy can be gleaned. Although much study has already been carried out using the fascinating experimental models and much useful information has been obtained, these model systems deserve continued attention if the functions and survival roles of the individual complement components are to be fully understood.

ACKNOWLEDGMENT

Noorbibi K. Day is an established investigator of the American Heart Association.

References

Arroyave, C. M., Levy, R. M., and Johnson, J. S., 1974, Genetic deficiency of the fourth component of complement in Wistar rats, *Fed. Proc. Fed. Amer. Soc. Exp. Biol.* **33**:795 (abstract).
Atkinson, J. P., Skin, H., and Frank, M. M., 1974, Metabolic behavior of C3 in normal, C4-deficient (C4D) and cortisone-treated guinea pigs, *J. Immunol.* **113**:1085–1092.
Ben-Efraim, S., and Cinader, B., 1964, The role of complement in the passive cutaneous reaction of mice, *J. Exp. Med.* **120**:925–942.
Biro, C. E., and Garcia, G., 1965, The antigenicity of aggregated and aggregate free human gamma-globulin for rabbits, *Immunology* **8**:411–419.

227

ISOLATED
DEFICIENCIES OF THE
COMPLEMENT
SYSTEM IN
EXPERIMENTAL
ANIMALS

Brown, D. L., and Lachmann, P. J., 1973, The behaviour of complement and platelets in lethal endotoxin shock in rabbits, *Int. Arch. Allergy* **45**:193–205.

Caren, L. D., and Rosenberg, L. T., 1966, The role of complement in resistance to endogenous and exogenous infection with a common mouse pathogen, *Corynebacterium kutscheri, J. Exp. Med.* **124**:689–699.

Cinader, B., Duiski, S., and Wardlaw, A. C., 1964, Distribution inheritance and properties of antigen, MuB1 and its relation to hemolytic complement, *J. Exp. Med.* **120**:897–924.

Colten, H. R., and Frank, M. M., 1972, Biosynthesis of the second (C2) and fourth (C4) components of complement *in vitro* by tissues isolated from guinea pigs with genetically determined C4 deficiency, *Immunology* **22**:991–999.

Ellman, L., Green, J., and Frank, M., 1970, Genetically controlled total deficiency of the fourth component of complement in the guinea pig, *Science* **170**:74, 75.

Ellman, L., Green, J., Judge, F., and Franck, M. M., 1971, *In vivo* studies in C4-deficient guinea pigs, *J. Exp. Med.* **134**:162–175.

Erickson, R. P., Tachibana, D. K., Herzenberg, L. A., and Rosenberg, L. T., 1964, A single gene controlling hemolytic complement and a serum antigen in the mouse, *J. Immunol.* **92**:611–615.

Frank, M. M., Ellman, L., and Green, J., 1971, Studies of immunologic function in C4 deficient guinea pigs, *J. Immunol.* **107**:312 (abstract).

Frank, M. M., May, J., Gaither, T., and Ellmann, L., 1971, *In vitro* studies of complement function in sera of C4-deficient guinea pigs, *J. Exp. Med.* **134**:176–187.

Gabrielsen, A. E., Linna, T. J., Weitekamp, D. P., and Pickering, R. J., 1974, Reduced hemolytic C1 activity in serum of hypogammaglobulinaemic chickens, *Immunology* **27**:463–468.

Gewurz, H., Pickering, R. J., Christian, C. L., Snydermann, R., Mergenhagen, S. E., and Good, R. A., 1968, Decreased C1q protein concentration and agglutinating activity in agammaglobulinemia syndromes, *Clin. Exp. Immunol.* **3**:437–445.

Herzenberg, L. D., Tachibana, D. K., Herzenberg, L. A., and Rosenberg, L. T., 1963, A gene locus concerned with hemolytic complement in *Mus musculus, Genetics* **48**:711.

Hyde, R. R., 1923, Complement deficient guinea pig serum, *J. Immunol.* **8**:267–289.

Hyde, R. R., 1932, The complement deficient guinea pig: a study of inheritable factor in immunity, *Amer. J. Hyg.* **15**:824–836.

Johnson, K. J., and Ward, P. A., 1971, Protective function of C6 in rabbits treated with bacterial endotoxin, *J. Immunol.* **106**:1125–1127.

Kohler, P. F., and Müller-Eberhard, H. J., 1969, Complement-immunoglobulin relation: deficiency of C1q associated with impaired immunoglobulin G synthesis, *Science* **163**:474, 475.

Kohler, P. F., and Müller-Eberhard, H. J., 1972, Metabolism of human C1q. Studies in hypogammaglobulinemia, myeloma and systemic lupus erythematosus, *J. Clin. Invest.* **51**:868–875.

Lachmann, P. J., 1970, C6-deficiency in rabbits, in: *Protides of the Biological Fluids,* (Proceedings of the 17th Colloquium, 1969) (H. Peeters, ed.), pp. 301–309, Pergamon Press, Oxford.

Lindberg, L. H., and Rosenberg, L. T., 1968, Nephrotoxic serum nephritis in mice with a genetic deficiency in complement, *J. Immunol.* **100**:34–38.

Linscott, W. D., and Cochrane, C. G., 1964, Guinea pig 1c-globulin: its relationship to the third component of complement and its alteration following interaction with immune complexes, *J. Immunol.* **93**:972–984.

Moore, H. D., 1919, Complementary and opsonic functions in their relation to immunity: a study of the serum of guinea pigs naturally deficient in complement, *J. Immunol.* **4**:425–441.

Nilsson, U. R., and Müller-Eberhard, H. J., 1967, Deficiency of the fifth component of complement in mice with an inherited complement defect, *J. Exp. Med.* **125**:1–16.

Phillips, M. E., Rother, U., and Rother K., 1968, Serum complement in the rejection of sarcoma I ascites tumor grafts, *J. Immunol.* **100**:493–500.

Root, R. K., Ellman, L., and Frank, M. M., 1972, Bactericidal and opsonic properties of C4-deficient guinea pig serum. *J. Immunol.* **109**:477–486.

Rosenberg, L. T., and Tachibana, D. K., 1962, Activity of mouse complement, *J. Immunol.* **89**:861–867.

Rother, K., and Till, G., 1974, *In vivo*-Störungen des Komplementsystems, in: *Komplement, Biochemie und Pathologie* (K. Rother, ed.), p. 238, Steinkopff, Darmstadt.

Rother, U., and Rother, K., 1961, Über einen angeborenen Komplement-Defekt bei Kaninchen, *Z. Immunitätsforsch.* **121**:224–232.

Rother, K., Rother, U., Petersen, K. F., Gemsa, D., and Mitze, F., 1964a, Immune bactericidal activity of complement: separation and description of intermediate steps, *J. Immunol.* **93**:319–330.

Rother, K., Rother, U., and Schindera, F., 1964b, Passive Arthus-Reaktion bei komplementdefekten Kaninchen, *Z. Immunitätsforsch.* **126**:473–488.

Rother, K., Rother, U., Müller-Eberhard, H. J., and Nilsson, U. R., 1966, Deficiency of the sixth component of complement in rabbits with an inherited complement defect, *J. Exp. Med.* **124**:773–785.

Rother, U., Ballantyne, D. L., Cohen, C., and Rother, K., 1967a, Allograft rejection in C6 defective rabbits, *J. Exp. Med.* **126**:565–579.

Rother, K., McCluskey, R. T., and Rother, U., 1967b, Tuberculin hypersensitivity in C6 deficient rabbits, *Fed. Proc. Fed. Amer. Soc. Exp. Biol.* **26**:787.

Rother, K., Rother, U., Vassalli, P., and McCluskey, R. T., 1967c, Nephrotoxic serum nephritis in C6 deficient rabbits: a study of the second phase of the disease, *J. Immunol.* **98**:965–971.

Skin, H. S., Smith, M. R., and Wood, W. B., 1969, Heat labile opsonins to pneumococcus. II. Involvement of C3 and C5, *J. Exp. Med.* **130**:1229–1240.

Snyderman, R., Gewurz, H., and Mergenhagen, S. E., 1968, Interactions of the complement system with endotoxic lipopolysaccharide; generation of a factor chemotactic for polymorphonuclear leukocytes, *J. Exp. Med.* **128**:259–275.

Snyderman, R., Phillips, J. K., and Mergenhagen, S. E., 1969, Polymorphonuclear leukocyte chemotactic activity in rabbit serum and guinea pig serum treated with immune complexes. Evidence for C5a as the major chemotactic factor, *Infect. Immun.* **1**:521.

Snyderman, R., Phillips, J., Kennedy, J., and Mergenhagen, S. E., 1971, Role of C5 in the accumulation of polymorphonuclear leukocytes (PMNs) in mice treated with endotoxin, *Fed. Proc. Fed. Amer. Soc. Exp. Biol.* **30**:355.

Stecher, V., and Sorkin, E., 1969, Studies on chemotaxis. XII. Generation of chemotactic activity for polymorphonuclear leukocytes in sera with complement deficiencies, *Immunology* **16**:231–239.

Tachibana, D. K., Ulrich, M., and Rosenberg, T. L., 1963, The inheritance of hemolytic complement activity in CF-1 mice, *J. Immunol.* **91**:230–232.

Terry, W. D., Borsos, T., and Rapp, H. J., 1964, Differences in serum complement activity among inbred strains of mice, *J. Immunol.* **92**:576–578.

Unanue, E. R., Mardiney, M. R., and Dixon, F. J., 1966, Nephrotoxic serum nephritis in complement intact and deficient mice, *J. Immunol.* **98**:609–617.

Ward, P. A., Cochrane, C. G., and Müller-Eberhard, H. J., 1965, The role of serum complement in chemotaxis of leukocytes *in vitro, J. Exp. Med.* **122**:327–346.

Weitzel, H., and Rother, K., 1970, Studies on the role of serum complement in allograft rejection and in immunosuppression by antithymocyte serum (ATS), *Eur. Surg. Res.* **2**:310.

Yang, S. Y., Jensen, R., Folke, L., Good, R. A., and Day, N. K., 1974, Complement deficiency in hamsters, *Fed. Proc. Fed. Amer. Soc. Exp. Biol.* **33**:795.

Zimmermann, T. S., Arroyave, C. M., and Müller-Eberhard, H. J., 1971, A blood coagulation abnormality in rabbits deficient in the sixth component of complement (C6) and its correction by purified C6, *J. Exp. Med.* **134**:1591–1600.

12

Inherited Deficiencies of the Complement System

NOORBIBI K. DAY, B. MONCADA, and
ROBERT A. GOOD

1. Introduction

In recent years, studies of genetically determined deficiencies of components of the complement (C) system have begun to yield the same crucial type of information often yielded in the past by other inborn errors of metabolism, e.g., the primary immunodeficiencies as experiments of nature. To date, the deficiencies of the complement system described in man (Tables 1 and 2) are as follows: C1-esterase inhibitor in patients with hereditary angioneurotic edema; C1q in combined immuno-deficiency states; C1r deficiencies associated with infections and a strange vascular disease with lupus-like lesions and chronic glomerulonephritis; C1s with lupus and lupus-like syndrome; C2 with systemic lupus erythematosus, lupus-like syndrome, dermatomyositis, anaphylactoid purpura, increased susceptibility to infections, Hodgkin's disease, and discoid lupus, and recently in a patient with chronic lymphocytic leukemia and dermatitis herpetiformis; C3 with increased frequency of infections, in particular, of the pulmonary apparatus; C4 with lupus erythematosus; C5 deficiency with membranous glomerulonephritis, vasculitis, arthritis, and propensity to bacterial infections; C5 abnormality with Leiner's syndrome, recurrent and persistent gram-negative bacterial skin disease and gastroenteritis; C6 in one individual who is apparently healthy at the moment and in another with repeated episodes of meningococcal meningitis; C7 with Raynaud's phenomenon; C7 in-activator with apparent good health; C8 deficiency with prolonged disseminated gonococcal infection syndrome, and also in three homozygous C8-deficient siblings in a family in which xeroderma pigmentosa is also present. No report to date of C9

NOORBIBI K. DAY and ROBERT A. GOOD • Sloan-Kettering Institute for Cancer Research, New York, New York. B. MONCADA • Universidad Autonoma de San Luis Potosi, San Luis Potosi, S. L. P., Mexico.

NOORBIBI K. DAY,
B. MONCADA, AND
ROBERT A. GOOD

TABLE 1. Genetically Controlled Complement (C) Deficiencies in Man

Author(s)	C component	Disease
Pondman *et al.* (1968)	C1s	Systemic lupus erythematosus (SLE)
Blum *et al.* (1976)	C1s	Lupus-like syndrome
Donaldson *et al.* (1963)	C1s INH	Hereditary angioneurotic edema (HANE)
Pickering *et al.* (1971)	C1s INH	HANE—renal disease
Kohler *et al.* (1974)	C1s INH	HANE—SLE-like disease, two affected male children in a kindred
Donaldson *et al.* (1964)[a]	C1s INH	HANE—discoid lupus in two unrelated individuals
Pickering *et al.* (1970), Day and Good (1975)	C1r	Recurrent infections and chronic glomerulonephritis
Moncada *et al.* (1972), Day *et al.* (1972)	C1r	LE-like syndrome, necrotizing skin lesions, skin infections, arthritis, infections
	C2 (see Table 2)	
Alper *et al.* (1972)	C3	Recurrent infections
Alper *et al.* (1976)	C3	Recurrent infections
Ballow *et al.* (1975)	C3	Recurrent infections
Alper and Davis, (1976)[a]	C3	Recurrent infections
Osofsky *et al.* (1976)	C3	Fevers, skin rash, arthralgias
Torisu *et al.* (1970)	C4	Four unrelated, apparently healthy individuals, no family history
Hauptman *et al.* (1974)	C4	LE-like syndrome
Rosenfeld *et al.* (1976)	C5	SLE and recurrent infections
Miller *et al.* (1968)	C5 dysfunction	Leiner's syndrome, gram-negative skin and bowel infection
Leddy *et al.* (1974)	C6	Mild Raynaud phenomenon; otherwise healthy
Lim *et al.* (1976)	C6	Recurrent meningococcal meningitis
Boyer *et al.* (1975)	C7	Raynaud's phenomenon
Wellek and Opferkuch (1974)	C7 inactivator	Healthy
Gewurz (1976)[a]	C7	Renal disease
Petersen *et al.* (1976)	C8	Prolonged disseminated gonococcal infections
Day *et al.* (1976b)	C8	Xeroderma pigmentosum; no obvious complement related disease
Alper *et al.* (1970)	C3b INH	Recurrent infections

[a]Personal communication.

deficiency has been presented. Although several healthy persons with C2 deficiency have been described, the association of this deficiency with serious disease is now incontrovertible, and the frequency of the deficiency with disease is greater than can be explained by chance alone. Other factors, such as environment and other mechanisms in the host, may be involved in association of disease with the C defect.

2. C1q Deficiency in Man

C1q, a subcomponent of the first component of complement, has been observed to be deficient in some immunodeficiency diseases, in particular, in severe combined immunodeficiency (SCID). Müller-Eberhard and Kunkel (1961) initially

TABLE 2. Inherited C2 Deficiency in Man—Association with Clinical Disease

Author(s)	Propositus age	Clinical disease	Functional C2 (% of normal)
Silverstein (1960)	49	Healthy	4–10
Klemperer et al. (1966)			
Ruddy et al. (1970)	—	Healthy	<1
Klemperer et al. (1967)	—	Healthy	4
Cooper et al. ((1968)	7	Synovitis	<1
Pickering et al. (1971),	12	Membraneous glomerulonephritis	<1
Day et al. (1973)		SLE	
Agnello et al. (1972)	55	SLE-like syndrome	<1
Sussman et al. (1973)	10	Anaphylactoid purpura	<1
Leddy et al. (1975)	59	Fatal dermatomyositis	<1
Douglass et al. (1976)	24	Discoid lupus	<1
Osterland et al. (1975)	18	SLE, hemolytic anemia	<1
Alper et al. (1974)[a]	—	Purpura	—
Leddy et al.[a]	22	Mild membrano proliferative glomerulonephritis	1
Day et al. (1973)[b]	20	Healthy	<1
Stern et al. (1976)	—	Discoid lupus	<1
Wild et al. (1976)	38	Discoid lupus	<1
Day et al. (1976a)	26	Hodgkin's disease	<1
	28 sib.	Hypertension, recurrent septic meningococcal infection	<1
Wolski et al. (1975)	17	SLE-like syndrome	<1
Becker[a]	53	CLL and dermatitis herpetiformis	<1

[a]Personal communication.
[b]Unpublished observation.

reported that some agammaglobulinemic sera were low in C1q. O'Connell et al. (1967) reported absence of C1q from the serum of an infant with SCID (Swiss type or lymphopenic agammaglobulinemia). Gewurz et al. (1969) demonstrated that C1q proteins were reduced in Swiss-type lymphopenic agammaglobulinemia, although mean C1q titers were also decreased in other forms of agammaglobulinemia, but not to the same degree (78 and 46% of normal, respectively). Ballow et al. (1973) showed that C1q was reconstituted in patients with combined immunodeficiency disease (CID) after bone marrow transplantation (BMT). Six patients were studied (Table 3). The diagnosis of CID was made according to the WHO criteria. Serum levels of C1q were quantitated by radial immunodiffusion by the Mancini technique. Matched controls had a mean serum concentration of 20.2 μg N/ml, whereas CID patients had a mean level of 6.3 μg N/ml. Four patients had successful engraftment, partial or full immunologic reconstitution, and an increase in serum C1q to normal following BMT. One patient failed to have a graft "take," had no immunologic reconstitution, and his C1q remained very low. In the sixth patient, the serum levels of C1q fluctuated widely, but despite reconstitution and establishment of full immunologic function, the C1q remained generally deficient. The sixth patient was interesting in that difficulty was encountered in achieving immunologic reconstitution, and seven marrow transplants had to be given from a matched sibling before full immunologic reconstitution was achieved. Despite a normal immune function at present, the serum concentration of C1q remains low even 5 years after the

NOORBIBI K. DAY,
B. MONCADA, AND
ROBERT A. GOOD

TABLE 3.   Reconstitution of C1q Following Bone Marrow Transplantation[a]

Patient	Serum C1q (μg N/ml)[b]		Immunologic reconstitution?	Evidence for engraftment?
	Before	After		
J.F.	5.1	15.9	Yes	Yes
K.S.	6.8	23.0	Yes	Yes (no markers, but rapid reconstitution)
K.R.	9.0	29.5	Yes (partial)	Yes
D.C.	4.6	23.0	Yes	Yes
C.M.	5.6	6.6	No	No
T.T.	6.7	9.4	Yes	?

[a]From Ballow *et al.* (1973) with permission of the journal.
[b]Normal serum C1q (age 6–12 months): 20.2±4.9.

successful marrow transplant. The reason for this is not clear, but it is possible that the specific group of cells necessary for the C1q reconstitution were not successfully engrafted at the same time that the cells responsible for immunologic development were reconstituted. However, enzymatic markers in this patient clearly establish that her lymphoid immunological system has been reconstituted from the cells of the donor. Thus the dissociation of the cells that produce C1q from those responsible for immunologic reconstitution in this patient suggests that C1q deficiency and immunologic deficiency of this patient were based on different cellular developments. Our studies with patients following transplantation suggest that T cells and B cells can be reconstituted while C1q levels remain deficient. In this patient, γ-globulin concentration has returned to normal. It has been demonstrated, however, that C1q is synthesized by lymphoid tissues (Stecher and Thorbecke, 1967; Day *et al.*, 1970). The rise of C1q levels to normal in the patient with several bone marrow reconstitutions could be of donor origin, reconstituted by engraftment of donor cells. The exact definition of the lymphoid cell responsible for C1q production has yet to be determined.

Recently, Kohler and Müller-Eberhard (1972) described an increased rate of C1q catabolism and an increased pool size for C1q in hypogammaglobulinemic patients with multiple myeloma and common variable immunodeficiency. They attributed the low levels of C1q to this metabolic abnormality and showed that a decrease in rate of C1q catabolism was produced by increasing the gammaglobulin concentration. A very similar interpretation was drawn by Gabrielsen *et al.* (1974) from experimental analyses of chickens.

3. C1r Deficiency in Man

Two separate cases of C1r deficiency have been described in man. The first, described by Pickering *et al.* (1970), was in a female patient who also had chronic glomerulonephritis. In a subsequent study of this same case (Day and Good, 1975), it was shown that this patient had a history of multiple episodes of upper respiratory infections, pneumonia, impetigo, unexplained fevers, and gross hematuria. By 10 years of age, her renal disease had progressed to an end-stage and she required a renal transplant. Complement studies performed prior to the transplant indicated that the total hemolytic complement levels were not detectable. C1r was absent, C1s was markedly reduced (30%), and C4 levels were elevated. The increase in C4 was interpreted to indicate that the extreme deficiency of C1r and/or the C1s deficiency was not a consequence of the activation of these subcomponents but due to an inability of these patients to synthesize adequate amounts of C1r and C1s (Pickering *et al.*, 1970). Two years following a successful kidney transplantation, we studied the C activity in this patient (Day and Good, 1975). Table 4 summarizes our findings. The total hemolytic complement was higher than normal and C1 was now readily measurable. The C1s, which was previously reduced, had returned to normal levels as measured immunochemically. Although C1r has not been directly determined, it would appear that it too has been corrected. The implications of these studies are that either one or both of these complement components are synthesized by the transplanted kidney or that the transplanted kidney has a determining effect on the synthesis of complement or complement components at other sites. We have subsequently carried out genetic studies on this family and have demonstrated that the C1r deficiency is inherited (see Chapter 13).

Two members in a second kindred described by Moncada *et al.* (1972) as having an unmeasurable total hemolytic complement, were shown by us to have a C1r deficiency (Day *et al.*, 1972). The brother had numerous infections, especially of the skin, during childhood, and now has clinical manifestations resembling lupus erythematosus, with rather severe consequences of vasculitis. A female sibling in this family also has C1r deficiency, has had numerous upper respiratory infections since infancy, and is troubled with arthritis and rhinobronchitis. Three siblings have died. One brother died at age 12 with lupus erythematosus, which was described by the mother as being similar to the disease studied in the male patient with C1r deficiency. Two other siblings died in infancy, one with gastroenteritis and a stillborn from an unknown cause. Extensive studies of complement were performed on the sera of these patients, and it was demonstrated that C1r is immunochemically undetectable in the serum. When purified C1r was added to serum deficient in C1r, C1 became measurable by hemolytic assays. Further genetic studies using monospecific antiserum against C1r indicated that this deficiency is acquired by an autosomal recessive inheritance, since approximately one-half the values of C1r were present in the parents and other siblings (de Bracco *et al.*, 1974). Detailed genetic studies on this family are also presented in Chapter 13. When complement profiles were performed (Day *et al.*, 1972) on the sera of all family members, it was demonstrated that, whereas total hemolytic complement was elevated in the remaining family members studied, C4 was markedly elevated in the sister's serum.

TABLE 4. Complement Studies of C1r-Deficient Patient

Time	CH50	C1	C1r	C1s
Before transplant	10	100	Absent	16 μg/ml[a]
After transplant	84[b]	1876	Not done	Normal

[a]Normal: 32.8.
[b]Normal: 80.

NOORBIBI K. DAY,
B. MONCADA, AND
ROBERT A. GOOD

The C8 level was consistently elevated in all family members. Studies of the bactericidal and immune adherence functions of the patients deficient in C1r indicated that the bactericidal activity against the rough strain of *Escherichia coli* was markedly impaired in both patients' sera. Immune adherence function was also reduced when the patients' sera were used with sensitized erythrocytes (EA). However, when sensitized cells carrying C1, EAC1 were used, immune adherence activity demonstrated normal values, suggesting the inability of these sera to form EAC1, 4, 2. When the alternate pathways of these patients' sera were studied using bacterial endotoxin and cobra venom, activators of the alternate pathways, the C system of the patients' sera can be engaged in the absence of C1r. The absence of C1r did not completely prevent activation of the C system even by antigen–antibody complexes.

4. Deficiency of C1s Inhibitor

A defect of C1s inhibitor that is genetically transmitted is present in patients with hereditary angioneurotic edema (HANE). C1-esterase inhibitor has important biological functions and inhibits a number of plasma enzymes: C1, kininogenase, plasmin, activated thromboplastin antecedent, PF/dil, and C1r. Several hundred individuals with deficiency of C1 esterase inhibitor have been described since its characterization by Donaldson and Evans (1963). Patients with HANE suffer attacks of nonpainful edema in the subcutaneous tissues in the mucosae of the respiratory or alimentary tract. Extreme discomfort with recurrent abdominal pain and death may ensue because of the risk of laryngeal or tracheal swelling. C1s inhibitor has been isolated (Schultze *et al.,* 1962; Pensky and Schwick, 1969) and is an $\alpha 2$-neuraminoglycoprotein ($\alpha 2$-NGAP). Antibodies have been prepared to this protein (Rosen *et al.,* 1965; Laurell *et al.,* 1969) and are useful in immunochemical determinations. Of all affected kindred, 15% were unusual in that they contained a biologically inactive form of C1 esterase inhibitor, which is immunochemically identical to the normal protein (Rosen *et al.,* 1965). C1-esterase is also assayed functionally by its ability to inhibit hydrolysis of *N*-acetyltyrosine ester (Levy and Lepow, 1959). When plasma from HANE patients was obtained during an attack of angioneurotic edema and injected into HANE patients or guinea pigs, vascular permeability was enhanced. Plasma obtained between attacks did not have this effect (Landerman *et al.,* 1960). Highly purified C1s (Haines and Lepow, 1964) produced angioedema when injected into guinea pig (Ratnoff and Lepow, 1963) or human skin (Klemperer *et al.,* 1969). Permeability in such sera could be generated *in vitro* by incubation at 37°C for 3 hr (Donaldson *et al.,* 1969). The permeability factor has a kinin-like activity, but is not bradykinin, since it differed in amino acid composition (Donaldson *et al.,* 1970). This kinin may be derived from C2 as the kinin-like activity, and generation is inhibited in the presence of antibody to C4 and C2 (Lepow, 1971). A variety of drugs, including aspirin, adrenalin, antihistamine and ACTH, morphine, steroid, UV radiation, vitamins, and autogenous vaccines of intestinal bacteria, has been used to treat patients with HANE without any success (Landerman, 1962). Pickering *et al.* (1969) reported the successful treatment of acute attacks in two patients, one with laryngeal edema and the other with abdominal colic, by infusion of fresh frozen plasma that was assumed to contain the missing inhibitor. Successful treatment by plasma has also been reported by Cohen and attacks has also been reported using the antifibrinolytic agent epsilon aminocaproic acid (EACA) (Lundh *et al.*, 1968; Champion and Lachmann, 1969).

5. Hereditary C1s Deficiency

Isolated C1s deficiency was first described by Pondman *et al.* (1968) in a patient with systemic lupus erythematosus. Another C1s-deficient individual was discovered by Blum *et al.* (1976), and that patient had a lupus-like syndrome. Studies of sera of five siblings and parents in the family of this patient revealed the absence of hemolytic activity in sera of one brother and two sisters due to deficiency of C1, but these siblings did not have lupus.

C4 and C2 levels in the sera of patients with C1s deficiency are higher than normal and C3–9 titers are normal. C1q is absent only in the propositus at the time of diagnosis and it, but not C1s, returned to normal after treatment (Dr. Livia Blum, personal communication). The authors named above have concluded that C1q deficiency in the serum may be due to circulating antigen–antibody complexes, and that hereditary C1s deficiency is present in this family due to the absence of an autosomal dominant allele that governs the synthesis of C1s.

6. Hereditary C2 Deficiency

Several C2-deficient individuals have been now described (see Table 2), and this deficiency probably occurs very frequently. Although the earliest C2-deficient individuals discovered were apparently healthy, it is becoming increasingly evident that many of them have vascular diseases, renal diseases, and manifestations of skin rash. C2 deficiencies have also been associated with Hodgkin's disease, chronic lymphocytic leukemia, infectious fatal dermatomyositis, membranous proliferative glomerulonephritis, and anaphylactoid purpura (see Table 2). More recently, patients with half levels of C2 and concomitant disease are also being reported. The first such patient was described by Fu *et al.* (1975), and recently we, together with Dr. McCrory of Cornell Medical College, have investigated another individual who has both chronic renal disease and approximately half values of C2. Genetic studies in this family indicated that the mother was a heterozygote for C2, and another sibling was also a heterozygote for C2. The discovery of close linkage of the $C2^0$ gene with the major histocompatibility complex, first by Fu *et al.* (1974) and subsequently by Day *et al.* (1975b) and others, has introduced a new modality in the study of C deficiencies (see Chapter 13). Several review articles of C2 deficiencies and their association with disease have been published (Day and Good, 1975; Agnello *et al.*, 1975). Recently, Stern *et al.* (1976) described two females with C2 deficiency and placed particular stress on a description of their skin lesions. Both women presented with an erythematous, raised, scaly rash. In each case, this discoid skin lesion first appeared on the malar area and later became widespread, but in neither case were the hands involved. Both patients were photosensitive; their skin lesions were initiated and subsequently aggravated by sun exposure. Histological examination revealed basal cell deprivation and small areas of liquefaction in the epidermis. Microscopic studies of the skin for immunoglobulins and B_{1c}

were negative in one woman; small amounts of aggregated IgG were present in the other. Both had a past history of recurrent sinopulmonary infections.

7. Hereditary C3 Deficiency

The first reported case of C3 deficiency was that of Alper *et al.* (1972). The patient, a 15-year-old girl, had more than 20 hospital admissions for recurrent infections since infancy. Of these, 14 were for acute lobar pneumonia, 2 were for meningococcal meningitis, and the remainder were for recurrent otitis media, paronychia, and impetigo. Pathogenic bacteria were isolated from her sputum on only a few occasions during her episodes of pneumonia and included *Diplococcus pneumoniae, Streptococcus pyogenes,* and *Klebsiella aerogenes.* All these infections responded to antibiotic therapy. Despite her severe bacterial infections, neutrophilia was not observed. However, there was a normal leukocytosis in response to the injection of typhoid vaccine (Alper *et al.*, 1976). Family history revealed no evidence of increased susceptibility to infections in the patient's six siblings, her parents, her three living grandparents, or other family members. Laboratory tests demonstrated that the concentration of C3 in the patient's serum was less than 0.25 mg/100 ml by immunochemical assay (normal range, 100–200 mg/ 100 ml) and 13 units/ml by hemolytic function (normal range, 15,000–30,000 units/ml). Serum C3 concentrations in the patient's mother and five of her six siblings showed values approximately half the normal. C2, C4, C5, and C6 and C1 esterase inhibitor, C3 inactivator, and properdin Factor B were normal in the patient's serum. These investigators also demonstrated that there was no conversion of properdin Factor B in the serum of the patient upon incubation with zymosan. This confirmed the findings of Götze and Müller-Eberhard (1971) that a fragment of C3b is required for the activation of the alternate pathway (Alper *et al.*, 1972). Further studies on this patient (Alper *et al.*, 1976) of the fractional catabolic rate and synthesis rate of C3 revealed evidence that was consistent with a lack of C3 synthesis as the patient's primary deficit. There was also a mild increase in the rate of conversion of purified C3 added to her serum and incubated at 37°C *in vitro.* Major-blood-group-compatible erythrocytes from a patient with paroxysmal nocturnal hemoglobinuria had the same shortened survival in the C3-deficient patient as in a normal control. The introdermal injection of C1s, which produces a marked increase in vasopermeability in the skin of normal subjects, produced no definite change in the patient, possibly implicating C3 or a protein in the alternative pathway as the normal mediator of this response. C5 inactivation and passive hemolysis of unsensitized guinea pig erythrocytes occurred normally in C3-deficient serum on incubation with cobra venom factor, indicating that C3 is not required for these reactions. The patient's humoral antibody response to both protein and carbohydrate antigens was entirely normal, making it unlikely that C3 is essential for antigen processing or initiation of the immune response.

Alper *et al.* (personal communication) are currently studying a C3-deficient 4-year-old child, a patient of Dr. John Davis of Virginia (personal communication, 1976).

Recently, Ballow *et al.* (1975) reported another C3-deficient individual. This patient, a 4-year-old girl with recurrent infections due to encapsulated bacteria as well as gram-negative organisms, was found to have a complete absence of total hemolytic complement and an absence of C3. Total hemolytic complement was reconstituted by the addition of functionally pure C3. With the exception of a moderately reduced hemolytic C4, all other C components, measured hemolytically and by radial immunodiffusion, were present in normal amounts. By Ouchterlony analysis, the patient's serum contained C3b inactivator and properdin but no antigenic C3. In the paper by Ballow *et al.* (1975), in which a description of the study of this patient is given, there is a typographical error in Table 1. Table 1 should read "hemolytic C3 <10," because no hemolytic C3 was detectable in this patient's serum. Activation of the alternate pathway by purified cobra venom factor and inulin was examined. Neither of these substances led to activation of properdin Factor B → $\overline{B}$. On addition of partially purified Cordis C3, in four of four instances and with different preparations of Cordis C3, activation of Factor B → $\overline{B}$ occurred in the inulin–serum–C3 mixture. By contrast, activation of Factor B → $\overline{B}$ occurred only once in four times with CVF–serum–C3 mixtures. Immune adherence was found to be normal in the patient's serum and could be removed by anti-C4 antiserum or hydrazine treatment. A marked opsonic defect against *E. coli* was present. Serum bactericidal activity against a rough strain of *E. coli* was also defective. The ability to mobilize an inflammatory response was examined by the Rebuck skin window technique. A delay in neutrophil migration occurred until the sixth hour. *In vitro* lymphocyte transformation and serum immunoglobulins were normal. The proportion of peripheral blood T cells forming spontaneous sheep erythrocyte rosettes and the percentage of B cells forming EAC rosettes by the C3 receptor were normal. The significance of the absence of C3 in this patient is emphasized by the increased number of infections with encapsulated bacteria and the decreased functional biological activities of the C system that are important in host defense mechanism(s).

A fourth C3-deficient patient was recently discovered by Osofsky *et al.* (1976). Their patient is a 34-month-old male presenting with fevers, skin rash, and arthralgias, whose blood lacks C3 immunochemically and hemolytically. There are no problems with obvious infections and no infectious agent has been isolated, so that with the exception of the aforementioned symptoms, the child seems quite healthy. Protein levels of C1q, C4, C5, properdin, and C3b-INA and hemolytic activities of complement components C1–C9, except C3, were normal or elevated; total hemolytic complement activity was 13% normal and the defect was corrected by purified C3. As shown by previous studies (Alper *et al.,* 1972), Factor B was not cleaved upon addition of zymosan or cobra venom factor (Ballow *et al.,* 1975). Immune adherence activity was also normal in sera of all three patients studied (Ballow *et al.,* 1975; Alper *et al.,* 1976; Osofsky *et al.,* 1976) and in the killing of *E. coli* by neutrophils in two patients (Ballow *et al.,* 1975; Osofsky *et al.,* 1976). Osofsky's patient's serum was deficient in the generation of C dependent chemotactic factors. The latter property was not reported by Alper *et al.* (1972) or Ballow *et al.* (1975). Genetic studies on C3-deficient patients indicate that the deficiency is inherited as an autosomal codominant trait (Alper *et al.,* 1976; Osofsky *et al.,* 1976).

8. Deficiency of C3b Inactivator

A single patient with C3b inactivator was described by Alper *et al.* (1970). The patient had a history of increased susceptibility to infection with organisms such as hemolytic streptococci, *Hemophilus influenzae,* and *Neisseria meningitides.* His C3 was dramatically reduced to 30 mg/100 ml (normal range, 100–200 mg/100 ml), but of this amount, three-quarters circulated as the inactive conversion product, C3b, and only 7 mg/100 ml was native C3. With the exception of C5, which was slightly low, the other C components were normal. The authors concluded that there was a circulating protease with C3 as its substrate and that the patient might be lacking an inhibitor of this enzyme. A marked increase on functional catabolic rate of about 5 times normal was obtained with the injection of [125]l-labeled C3 into the patient with rapid conversion of the injected labeled C3. Other protease inhibitors, such as α1-antitrypsin, α1-antichymotrypsin, α2-macroglobulin, inter-α-trypsin inhibitor, and C1 inhibitor were present in normal concentrations in the serum.

When 500 ml of normal plasma was infused in the patient, C3b disappeared rapidly and native C3 rose gradually to about 70 mg/100 ml by the fifth day after infusion. The C3 fell and C3b reappeared only after 17 days. A second turnover study with labeled C3 showed a fractional catabolic rate of only about twice normal and no demonstrable conversion of the labeled C3 *in vivo.* These findings by Alper *et al.* (1970) were strong evidence that the patient lacked a protease inhibitor, i.e., C3 inactivator, which allowed continuous activation of components of the alternative pathway. Family studies indicated that this deficiency is inherited.

9. Hereditary C4 Deficiency

Inherited C4 deficiency was first described by Hauptman *et al.* (1974) in an 18-year-old girl showing typical clinical symptoms of systemic lupus erythematosus but atypical biological manifestations. Her serum was totally deficient in C4. This abnormality was found consistently throughout a period of more than 1 year. Immunogenetic analysis showed that this deficiency was linked to HLA (Rittner *et al.,* 1975). No LE cells, antinuclear factors, or immunoglobulin deposits were evident. The patient's serum, however, had cryoglobulins, serum anticomplementary activity, cold lymphocytotoxins, and cutaneous lesions. Two other C4-deficient individuals have been found recently, but to date the studies of these cases have not been published.

10. C5 Dysfunction

Familial C5 dysfunction was first reported in an 18-month-old female (Miller *et al.,* 1968) with a generalized recalcitrant seborrheic dermatitis, persistent diarrhea, recurrent infections due primarily to gram-negative bacteria, and marked dystrophy with failure to thrive. Despite intensive study, no abnormality of humoral or cellular immunity was detected. The patient's serum was defective in the phagocytosis of yeast particles (Miller and Nilsson, 1970), which was related to the C5 abnormality. This serum defect was dramatically improved by plasma transfusion therapy. C5-deficient mouse sera failed to restore the patient's serum, but purified human C5 was found to be effective. Measurement of total hemolytic complement was normal, and the patient's C5 appeared to be normal in amount immunochemically. The mobility and antigenicity of the C5 was demonstrated to be normal by Ouchterlony technique and immunoelectrophoretic analysis. The defect in the serum was present in the patient's mother and several relatives. Although not fully established, C5 defect is probably transmitted as a dominant characteristic.

11. Hereditary C5 Deficiency

Recently, Rosenfeld *et al.* (1976) discovered an individual with hereditary C5 deficiency. The proband, a 20-year-old black female, who has had systemic lupus erythematosus since age 11, lacked serum hemolytic complement activity even during remission. C5 was undetectable in her serum by both immunodiffusion and hemolytic assays. Other C components were normal during remission of lupus but C1, C4, C2, and C3 levels fell during exacerbations. C5 levels of other family members were either normal or approximately half normal, which is consistent with an autosomal codominant inheritance of the gene determining C5 deficiency. The patient has a remarkable propensity for bacterial infections associated with neutrophilia. These infections have occurred even during periods of low-dose or alternate-day corticosteroid therapy, which controls the lupus syndrome, No coagulation defect was present in the serum. The patient's healthy sister has 1–2% of normal levels of C5. Both sera were severely impaired in their ability to generate chemotactic activity.

When these two C5-deficient sera were tested for their capacity to promote phagocytosis of yeast, however, it was found that their opsonic capacity was normal. The reason for the difference between this observation by Rosenfeld *et al.* regarding sera of patients lacking C5 and the observation by Miller and Nilsson (1970) that sera of patients with C5 dysfunction were unable to phagocytose yeast particles is not clear at present. Dr. Miller's explanation for this difference is as follows (personal communication): Over the past 3 years, he and his associates have identified at least 10 additional cases with C5 dysfunction. The sera of these patients regularly fail to opsonize yeast particles. In the course of these studies, a large number of normal sera have also been studied. These workers have shown that, on occasion, normal sera are encountered that contain heat-stable opsonic activity toward yeast particles that is not inhibited by anti-C5, suggesting that C5 need not be the opsonically active factor occurring in human sera.

12. Hereditary C6 Deficiency

Two C6-deficient individuals have now been described. In both cases, it has been established that this deficiency follows a classical Mendelian inheritance. The first reported case was described by Leddy *et al.* (1974) in an 18-year-old black female who was admitted to the University of Rochester Medical Center with a 1-day history of fever, chills, polyarthralgia, and painful fingertip lesions. Past health had been excellent except for one admission to another hospital 13 months earlier for gonococcal arthritis, which responded to penicillin therapy. Other than the gonococcal disease, there was no history of findings suggestive of joint disease, muscle pain or weakness, pleurisy, kidney disease, proteinuria, or skin lesions. The family history was negative for infections. The sixth serum component (C6) of complement was undetectable by both functional and immunochemical assay. Functional titers of all other C components were normal. Addition of functionally pure C6 to the patient's serum restored hemolytic activity to normal, thus showing that the absence of C6 in the patient's serum could not be accounted for by a circulating C6 inhibitor. Both parents of the proband and five of the six siblings available had approximately half the normal levels of functional C6. The other sibling had a normal C6 level.

C-dependent functional properties of C6-deficient serum showed a total absence of bactericidal activity against *Salmonella typhi* 901 and *Hemophilus influenzae* and an inability to mediate lysis of red blood cells from patients with paroxysmal nocturnal hemoglobinuria in either the acidified serum or "sugar water" tests. The C6 deficient serum was, however, able to (1) generate chemotactic activity during incubation with bacterial endotoxin or aggregated IgA, (2) mediate the immune adherence phenomenon, and (3) coat human red cells sensitized by cold agglutinins with C4 and C3. The hemostatic functions were normal, in contrast to observations by Zimmerman *et al.* (1971) and Zimmerman and Müller-Eberhard (1971), who showed a defect in blood clotting in sera of C6-deficient rabbits. The reason for this may be the difference in the two species studied.

The second case of C6 deficiency, described by Lim *et al.* (1976), was in a 6-year-old male with meningococcal meningitis, who responded favorably to ampicillin but suffered two repeated attacks of infections with the same organism (*N. meningitides*, Group Y, Type IV) in the following month. No abnormalities of the otolarynx, skin, or neuroskeleton were found.

Serum bactericidal antibody titers against autologous meningococci were high. Other C-dependent functional properties studied were normal, i.e., chemotaxis, opsonization, and neutrophil function. Specific immunity and the coagulation system were also normal.

13. Hereditary C7 Deficiency

The first case of C7 deficiency was first described by Boyer *et al.* (1975) in a 42-year-old Caucasian woman with Raynaud's phenomenon, sclerodactyly, and telangiectasia. Studies of the family members indicated that this deficiency was inherited by an autosomal mode of inheritance. The half-life of exogenous C7 in the patient (given by transfusion of whole blood) was 91 hr, and there was no evidence of C7 synthesis *in vivo* following transfusion. Both the classical C pathway and an alternative C pathway to the C7 stage were normal. The C7 deficient serum was unable to support the generation of chemotactic factors by antigen–antibody complexes or endotoxin and in the opsonization of unsensitized yeast particles. By addition to the serum of functionally pure C7, both deficiencies were corrected.

C7 deficiency was reported by Wellek and Opferkuch (1974) in a 13-year-old healthy boy. No C7 was detectable by hemolytic or immunochemical methods. A C7-inactivating principle was demonstrated in the C7-deficient serum. This principle inactivated C7 both in the fluid phase and in its cell-bound state.

A third C7-deficient individual with renal disease has just been discovered (Gewurz *et al.*, unpublished observations).

14. Hereditary C8 Deficiency

C8 deficiency has been recently discovered in two families. The first description of a C8-deficient individual was by Peterson *et al.* (1976) in a 23-year-old female with a prolonged disseminated gonococcal infection. C8 was undetectable by hemolytic assays and immunoprecipitation. Addition of purified C8 restored the hemolytic activity. The titers of the remaining C components were normal. Genetic studies indicated that this deficiency was inherited (Merritt *et al.*, 1976). The patient's serum could be activated by both classical and alternative C pathways, was able to support normal opsonization of yeast particles and staphylococci, and had a normal capacity to coat sensitized red blood cells with C3 and C4 and to generate chemotactic activity. The C8 deficient fresh serum did not have any bactericidal activity against *N. gonorrhoae,* but addition of purified C8 restored this activity.

The second individual with C8 deficiency was recently discovered by Day *et al.* (1976b) in a large Tunisian family with xeroderma pigmentosum (see Chapter 13). Three homozygote deficient individuals and five heterozygote individuals are present in two branches of this family. Other studies on sera of these patients are currently under investigation. No disease attributable to the deficiency of this component in these patients has been observed.

15. Conclusion

From these studies, it is clear that isolated deficiencies of the complement system in man are frequently associated with disease, and that these deficiencies regularly reflect functional deficiencies, decreased concentration, or even complete absences of individual components of the complement system. It was predictable from the phylogenetic studies that are reviewed in Chapter 9 that this would be the case. A system like the complement system, which comprises a cascade of interactions, proteins, proenzymes, and enzymes, could not have been maintained against the pressures of genetic drift after several hundred million years unless the system as a whole and each of its major components had survival advantage. When a system such as this has survival advantage, hereditary defects yielding missing or defective components can be expected to be associated with disease. Further, the diseases observed can be expected to reveal the major *raison d'etre* of the system. This set of relationships seems to be in the process of being revealed as we study the association of disease with genetically determined absences or deficiency of the complement components.

The surprising thing about the clinical association of complement component deficiencies with disease is the nature of the diseases that are occurring. The frequency with which the connective tissue, mesenchymal, or so-called collagen–vascular diseases are represented in this context is astonishing. It has been argued that these stimulating clinical and genetic relationships are but an artifice, derived from the fact that the population most intensively studied for complement perturbations is the population with lupus erythematosus, nephritis, and related diseases. Our own experiences, however, with large numbers of healthy, normal people, families of patients with complement component deficiencies, and a very large cancer population and family members of this population indicate that the relationship of collagen–vascular diseases and complement component deficiencies is not fortuitous, based upon sampling error. Deficiencies of the complement system predispose, in a manner as yet not clarified, to collagen–vascular diseases as well as to infections. This suggests, as has long been suspected, that many of the autoimmune and collagen–vascular diseases are indeed infectious or reflect disturbances in immunological handling of consequences of infection, e.g., antigen–antibody complexes.

What has not been anticipated is that some of the primary deficiencies of the complement system would be closely linked to the major histocompatibility complex as was originally discovered by Fu and co-workers. This extraordinary association suggests much speculation, but its meaning will be revealed only by further analysis.

ACKNOWLEDGMENT

Noorbibi K. Day is an Established Investigator of the American Heart Association.

References

Agnello, V., de Bracco, M. M. E., and Kunkel, H. G., 1972, Hereditary C2 deficiency with some manifestations of systemic lupus erythematosus, *J. Immunol.* **108**:837–840.

Agnello, V., Ruddy, S., Winchester, R. J., Christian, C. L., and Kunkel, H. G., 1975, Hereditary C2 deficiency in systemic lupus erythematosus and acquired complement abnormalities in an unusual SLE-related syndrome, in: *Immunodeficiency In Man and Animals* (R. A. Good, J. Finstad, and N. W. Paul, eds.), in: *Birth Defects: Original Article Ser.,* **XI**(1):312–317, Sinauer Associates, Sunderland, Massachusetts.

Alper, C. A., Abramson, N., Johnston, R. B., Jr., Jandl, J. H., and Rosen, F. S., 1970, Increased susceptibility to infection associated with abnormalities of complement-mediated functions and of the third component of complement (C3), *N. Engl. J. Med.* **282**:349–354.

Alper, C. A., Colten, H. R., Rosen, F. S., Rabson, A. R., Macnab, G. M., and Gear, J. S. S., 1972, Homozygous deficiency of the third component of complement (C3) in a patient with repeated infections, *Lancet* **2**:1179–1181.

Alper, . A., Colten, H. R., Gear, J. S. S., Rabson, A. R., and Rosen, F. S., 1976, Homozygous C3 deficiency. The role of C3 in antibody production, C1s-induced vasopermeability, and cobra venom reduced passive hemolysis, *J. Clin. Invest.* **57**: 222–229.

Ballow, M., Day, N. K., Biggar, W. D., Park, B. H., Yount, W. J., and Good, R. A., 1973, Reconstitution of C1q following bone marrow transplantation in patients with severe combined immunodeficiency, *Clin. Immunol. Immunopathol.* **2**:28–35.

Ballow, M., Shira, J. E., Harden, L., Yang, S. Y., and Day, N. K., 1975, Complete absence of the third component of complement in man, *J. Clin. Invest.* **56**:703–710.

Beck, P., Willis, D., Davies, G. T., Lachmann, P. J., and Sussman, M., 1973, A family study of hereditary angioneurotic oedema, *Q. J. Med.* **42**:317–339.

Blum, L., Lee, K., Lee, S. L., Barone, R., and Wallace, S. L., 1976, Hereditary C1s deficiency, *Fed. Proc. Fed. Amer. Soc. Exp. Biol.* **35**(3)(abstract 2480).

Boyer, J. T., Gall, E. P., Norman, M. E., Nilsson, U. R., and Zimmerman, T. S., 1975, Hereditary deficiency of the seventh component of complement, *J. Clin. Invest.* **56**:905–913.

de Bracco, M. M. E., Windhorst, D., Stroud, R. M., and Moncada, B., 1974, The autosomal C1r deficiency in a large Puerto Rican family, *Clin. Exp. Immunol.* **16**:183–188.

Champion, R. H., and Lachmann, P. J., 1969, Hereditary angio-oedema treated with ε-aminocaproic acid. *Br. J. Dermatol.* **81**:763–5.

Cohen, G., and Peterson, A., 1972, Treatment of hereditary angioedema with frozen plasma, *Ann. Allergy* **30**:690–692.

Cooper, N. R., tenBensel, R., and Kohler, P. F., 1968, Studies of an additional kindred with hereditary deficiency of the second component of human complement (C2) and description of a new method for the quantitation of C2, *J. Immunol.* **101**:1176–1182.

Day, N. K., and Good, R. A., 1975, Deficiencies of the complement system in man, in: *Immunodeficiency in Man And Animals* (R. A. Good, J. Finstad, and N. W. Paul, eds.), in: *Birth Defects: Original Article Ser.* **XI** (1): 306–311, Sinauer Associates, Sunderland, Massachusetts.

Day, N. K., Gewurz, H., Pickering, R. J., and Good, R. A., 1970, Ontogenic studies of C1q synthesis in the piglet, *J. Immunol.* **104**:1316–1319.

Day, N. K., Geiger, H., Stroud, R., deBracco, M. M. E., Moncada, B., Windhorst, D., and Good, R. A., 1972, C1r deficiency. An inborn error associated with cutaneous and renal disease. *J. Clin. Invest.* **51**:1102–1108.

Day, N. K., Geiger, H., McLean, R., Michael, A., and Good, R. A., 1973, C2 deficiency: Development of lupus erythematosus, *J. Clin. Invest.* **52**:1601–1607.

Day, N. K., Geiger, H., and Good, R. A., 1975a, Complement, in: *Molecular Pathology* (R. A. Good, S. B. Day, and J. Yunis, eds.), pp. 115–160, Charles C. Thomas, Springfield, Illinois.

Day, N. K., L'Esperance, P., Good, R. A., Michael, A. F., Hansen, J. A., Dupont, B., and Jersild, C., 1975b, Hereditary C2 deficiency: Genetic studies and association with the HL-A system, *J. Exp. Med.* **141**:1464–1469.

Day, N. K., Rubinstein, P., Case, D., Walker, M. E., Tulchin, M., Good, R. A., Dupont, B., Hansen, J. A., and Jersild, C., 1976a, Linkage of gene for C2 deficiency and the major histocompatibility complex (MHR) in man. Family study of a further case, *Vox Sang.* **31**(2):96–102.

Day, N. K., Degos, L., Beth, M., Sasportes, M., Gharbi, R., and Giraldo, G., 1976b, C8 deficiency in a family with xeroderma pigmentosum. Lack of linkage to the HL-A region, in: *HLA and Disease*, Vol. 58, p. 197 (abstract), INSERM, Paris.

Donaldson, V. H., and Evans, R. R., 1963, A biochemical abnormality in hereditary angioneurotic edema: absence of serum inhibitor of C'1 esterase, *Amer. J. Med.* **35**:37–44.

Donaldson, V. H., Ratnoff, O. D., Dias da Silva, W., and Rosen, F. S., 1969, Permeability increasing activity in hereditary angioneurotic edema plasma. II. Mechanism of formation and partial characterization, *J. Clin. Invest.* **48**:642–653.

Donaldson, V. M., Mertee, E., Rosen, F. S., Kretschmer, K. W., and Lepow, J. M., 1970, A polypeptide kinin in hereditary angioneurotic edema plasma; Role of complement in its formation, *J. Lab. Clin. Med.* **76**:986 (abstract).

Douglass, M. C., Lamberg, S. I., Lorincz, A. L., Good, R. A., and Day, N. K., 1976, Lupus erythematosus-like syndrome with a familial deficiency of C2, *Arch. Dermatol.* **112**:671–674.

Fu, S. M., Kunkel, HG., Brusman, H. P., Allen, F. M., Jr., and Fotino, M., 1974, Evidence for linkage between HL-A histocompatibility genes and those involved in the synthesis of the second component of complement, *J. Exp. Med.* **140**:1108–1111.

Fu, S. M., Stern, R., Kunkel, H. G., Dupont, B., Hansen, J. A., Day, N. K., Good, R. A., Jersild, C., and Fotino, M., 1975, LD-7a association with C2 deficiency in five of six families, in: *Histocompatibility Testing 1975*, Proceedings of the 6th International Histocompatibility Workshop, pp. 933–936, Munksgaard A/S, Copenhagen.

Gabrielsen, A. E., Linna, T. J., Weitekamp, D. P., and Pickering, R. J., 1974, Reduced hemolytic C1 activity in serum of hypogammaglobulinemic chickens, *Immunology* **27**:463–468.

Gewurz, H., Pickering, R. J., Naff, G. B., Snyderman, R., Mergenhagen, S. E., and Good, R. A., 1969, Decreased properdin activity in acute glomerulonephritis, *Int. Arch. Allergy* **56**:592.

Götze, O., and Müller-Eberhard, H. J., 1971, The C3 activation system: an alternate pathway of complement activation, *J. Exp. Med.* **134**:90s–108s.

Haines, A. L., and Lepow, I. H., 1964, Studies on human C'1 esterase. II. Function of purified C'1 esterase in the human complement system, *J. Immunol.* **92**:468–478.

Hauptman, G., Grosshans, E., and Heid, E., 1974, Lupus erythemateux aigus et déficits héréditaires en complement. A propos d'un cas par déficit complement en C, *Ann. Dermatol. Syphilgr. Paris* **101**:479–495.

Jaffee, C. J., Atkinson, J. P., Gelfand, J. A., and Frank, M. M., 1975, Hereditary angioedema: the use of fresh frozen plasma for prophylaxis in patients undergoing oral surgery, *J. Allergy Clin. Immunol.* **55**:386–393.

Klemperer, M. R., Woodworth, H. C., Rosen, F. S., and Austen, K. F., 1966, Hereditary deficiency of the second component of complement (C'2) in man, *J. Clin. Invest.* **45**:880–890.

Klemperer, M. R., Austen, K. F., and Rosen, F. S., 1967, Hereditary deficiency of the second component of complement (C'2) in man: further observations of a second kindred, *J. Immunol.* **98**:72–78.

Klemperer, M. R., Rosen, F. S., and Donaldson, V. H., 1969, A polypeptide derived from the second component of human complement (C2) which increases vascular permeability, *J. Clin. Invest.* **48**(Jan.–June):44a–45a (abstract 142).

NOORBIBI K. DAY,
B. MONCADA, AND
ROBERT A. GOOD

Kohler, P. F., and Müller-Eberhard, H. J., 1972, Metabolism of human C1q studies in hypogammaglobu-linemia, myeloma and systemic lupus erythematosus, *J. Clin. Invest.* **51**:868–875.

Kohler, P. F., Percy, J., Campion, W. M., Smyth, C. J., 1974, Hereditary angioedema and "familial" lupus erythematosus in identical twin boys, *Amer. J. Med.* **56**:406–411.

Landerman, N. S., 1962, Hereditary angioneurotic edema. I. Case reports and review of the literature, *J. Allergy* **33**: 316–329.

Landerman, N. S., Webster, M. E., Becker, E. L., and Ratcliffe, H. E., 1960, Hereditary angioneurotic edema. II. Deficiency of inhibitor for serum globulin permeability factor and/or plasma kallikrein, *J. Allergy* **33**:330.

Laurell, A. B., Lindegren, J., Malmros, J., and Martensson, A., 1969, Enzymatic and immunochemical estimation of C1 esterase inhibitor in sera from patients with hereditary angioneurotic edema, *Scand. J. Clin. Lab. Invest.* **24**:221.

Leddy, J. P., Frank, M. M., Gaither, T., Baum, J., and Klemperer, M. R., 1974, Hereditary deficiency of the sixth component of complement in man, *J. Clin. Invest.* **53**:544–553.

Leddy, J. P., Griggs, R. C., Klemperer, M. R., and Frank, M. M., 1975, Hereditary complement (C2) deficiency with dermatomyositis, *Amer. J. Med.* **58**:83–91.

Lepow, I. M., 1971, Permeability producing peptide by product of the interaction of the fourth and second components of complement, in: *Biochemistry of the Acute Allergic Reactions: Second International Symposium* (K. F. Austen and E. L. Becker, eds.), pp. 205–215, Blackwell Scientific Publications, London.

Levy, R., and Lepow, I. H., 1959, Assay and properties of serum inhibitor of C'1 esterase, *Proc. Soc. Exp. Biol. Med.* **101**: 608–611.

Lim, D., Gewurz, A., Lint, T., Ghaze, M., Sepheri, B., and Gewurz, H., 1976, Absence of the sixth component of complement in a patient with repeated episodes of meningococcal meningitis, *J. Ped.* **89**:42–47.

Lundh, B., Laurell, A. B., Wetterqvist, H., White, T., and Granerus, G., 1968, A case of hereditary angioneurotic oedema, successfully treated with ε-aminocaproic acid. Studies on C'1 esterase inhibitor, C'1 activation, plasminogen level and histamine metabolism, *Clin. Exp. Immunol.* **3**:733–745.

Merritt, A. D., Petersen, B. H., Angenieta, A. B., Meyers, D. A., Brooks, G. F., and Hodes, M. E., 1976, Chromosome G: Linkage of the eighth component of complement (C8) to the histocompatibility region (HLA), in: *3rd International Workshop on Human Gene Mapping. Birth Defects XII,* p. 6, Baltimore Conference, The National Foundation, New York, in press.

Miller, M. E., and Nilsson, U. R., 1970, A familial deficiency of the phagocytosing enhancing activity of serum related to a C5 dysfunction of the fifth component of complement (C5), *N. Engl. J. Med.* **282**:354–358.

Miller, M. E., Seals, J., Kaje, R., and Levitsky, L. C., 1968, A familial plasma-associated defect of phagocytosis. A new cause of recurrent bacterial infections, Lancet **2** (July): 60–63.

Moncada, B., Day, N. K., Good, R. A., and Windhorst, D. B., 1972, Lupus erythematosus-like syndrome with a familial defect of complement, *N. Engl. J. Med.* **286**:689–693.

Müller-Eberhard, H. J., and Kunkel, H. G., 1961, Isolation of a thermolabile serum protein which precipitates γ-globulin aggregates and participates in immune hemolysis, *Proc. Soc. Exp. Biol. N. Y.* **106**:291–295.

O'Connell, E. J., Enriquez, P., Linman, J. W., Gleich, G. J., and McDuffie, F. C., 1967, Absence of activity of first component of complement in man: Association with thymic alymphoplasia and defective inflammatory response, *J. Lab. Clin. Med.* **70**:715.

Osofsky, S. G., Thompson, B. H., Lint, T. F., and Gewurz, H., 1976, Hereditary deficiency of the third component of complement in a child with fever, skin rash and arthralgias and response to whole blood transfusion, *J. Ped.,* in press.

Osterland, C. K., Espinoza, L., Parker, L. P., and Schur, P. H., 1975, Inherited C2 deficiency and systemic lupus erythematosus: Studies on a family. *Ann. Intern. Med.* **82**:323–328.

Pensky, J., and Schwick, H. G., 1969, Human serum inhibitor of C'1 esterase: Identity with α_2-neuraminoglycoprotein, *Science* **163**:698–699.

Petersen, B. H., Graham, J. A., and Boroks, G. F., 1976, Human deficiency of the eighth component of complement: The requirement of C8 for serum *Neisseria gonorrhoeae* bactericidal activity, *J. Clin. Invest.* **57**:283–290.

Pickering, R. J., Good, R. A., Kelly, J. R., 1969, Replacement therapy in hereditary angioedema.

Successful treatment of two patients with fresh frozen plasma, *Lancet* **1**:326–330.

Pickering, R. J., Naff, G. B., Stroud, R. M., Good, R. A., and Gewurz, H., 1970, Deficiency of C1r in human serum; effects on the structure and function of macromolecular C1, *J. Exp. Med.* **141**:803–815.

Pickering, R. J., Michael, A. F., Herdman, R. C., Good, R. A., and Gewurz, H., 1971, The complement system in chronic glomerulonephritis: three newly associated aberrations, *J. Pediatr.* **78**:30–43.

Pondman, K. W., Stoop, J. W., Cormane, R. H., and Hannema, A. J., 1968, Abnormal C1 in a patient with systemic lupus erythematosus, *J. Immunol.* **101**:811 (abstract).

Ratnoff, O. D., and Lepow, I. H., 1963, Complement as a mediator of inflammation. Enhancement of vascular permeability by purified human C′1 esterase, *J. Exp. Med.* **118**: 681–697.

Rittner, C. H., Hauptmann, G., Grosse-Wilde, H., Grosshans, E., Tongio, M. M., and Mayr, S., 1975, Linkage between HL-A (major histocompatibility complex) and genes controlling the synthesis of the fourth component of complement, in: *Histocompatibility Testing 1975,* pp. 945–954, Munksgaard, Copenhagen.

Rosen, F. S., Charache, P., Pensky, J., and Donaldson V., 1965, Hereditary angioneurotic edema: two genetic variants, *Science* **148**:957–958.

Rosenfeld, S. I., Kelly, M. E., and Leddy, J. P., 1976, Hereditary deficiency of the fifth component of complement in man, *J. Clin. Invest.* **57**:1626–1634.

Ruddy, S., Klemperer, M. R., Rosen, F. S., Austen, K. F., and Kumate, J., 1970, Hereditary deficiency of the second component of complement (C2) in man; correlation of C2 haemolytic activity with immunochemical measurements of C2 protein, *Immunology* **18**:943–954.

Schultze, H. E., Heide, K., and Haupt, H., 1962, Über ein bisher unbekanntes Saures α_2-Glycoprotein, *Naturwissenschaften* **94**:133.

Silverstein, A. M., 1960, Essential hypocomplementemia: report of a case, *Blood* **16**:1338–1341.

Stecher, U. J., and Thorbecke, C. J., 1967, Sites of synthesis of serum proteins produced by macrophages *in vitro, J. Immunol.* **99**:643.

Stern, R., Fu, S. M., Fotino, M., Agnello, V., and Kunkel, H. G., 1976, Hereditary C2 deficiency: association with skin lesions resembling the discoid lesion of SLE, *Arthritis Rheum.* **19**: 45–50.

Sussman, M., Jones, J. S., Almeida, J. D., 1973, Deficiency of the second component of complement associated with anaphylactoid purpura and presence of mycoplasma in the serum, *Clin. Exp. Immunol.* **14**:531–539.

Torisu, M., Sonozaki, H., Inai, S., and Arata, M., 1970, Deficiency of the fourth component of complement in man, *J. Immunol.* **104**:728–737.

Wellek, B., and Opferkuch, W., 1974, A case of deficiency of the seventh component of complement in man. Biological properties of a C7-deficient serum and description of a C7-inactivating principle, *Clin. Exp. Immunol.* **19**:223–225.

Wild, J. H., Zvaifler, N. J., Müller-Eberhard, H. J., and Wilson, C. B., 1976, Deficiency of the second component of complement (C2) in a patient with discoid lupus erythematosus, *Clin. Exp. Immunol.* **24**:238–248.

Wolski, K. P., Schmid, F. R., and Mittal, K. K., 1975, Genetic linkage between the HL-A system and a deficit of the second component (C2) of complement, *Science* **188**:1020–1022.

Zimmerman, T. S., and Müller-Eberhard, H. J., 1971, Blood coagulation initiation by a complement-mediated pathway, *J. Exp. Med.* **134**:1601–1607.

Zimmerman, T. S., Arroyave, C. M., and Müller-Eberhard, H. J., 1971, A blood coagulation abnormality in rabbits deficient in the sixth component of complement (C6) and its correction by purified C6, *J. Exp. Med.* **134**:1591–1600.

13

Complement and the Major Histocompatibility Systems

CASPER JERSILD, PABLO RUBINSTEIN, and NOORBIBI K. DAY

1. Introduction

Hereditary deficiencies of specific components of the complement (C) system were first discovered in experimental animals (Moore, 1919; Coca, 1920; Hyde, 1923) and later in man (Klemperer *et al.*, 1966). These isolated C deficiencies have been of importance for the understanding of the functional interrelationships between the various C components and in elucidating the biological significance of this complex system. Inherited deficiencies, among other possibilities, may be the outcome of genetically determined defects resulting in any one of the following: (1) total absence of synthesis of one or more of the polypeptides that make up the biologically active component due to the lack of function of either a structural or a regulator gene; (2) the production of a functionally inactive component due to a structural gene defect; or (3) the continuous synthesis or constitutive derepression of a specific inhibitor. Irrespective of which mechanism(s) mentioned is the basis for each specific deficiency, we shall denote genes resulting in deficient C components as C^0 genes; e.g., $C2^0$ is a C2-deficient gene.

The recent progress in the determination and quantitation of specific C components has been instrumental in permitting the study of inherited C deficiencies. These C deficiencies have been shown to be transmitted as autosomal recessive traits. The specific C component is decreased in relatives of C deficient individuals, as measured by immunochemical quantitation and/or functional activities. The C^0

CASPER JERSILD • Tissue Typing Laboratory, Blood Bank and Blood Grouping Department, University Hospital (Rigshospitalet), Copenhagen, Denmark. PABLO RUBINSTEIN • Kimball Research Institute of the New York Blood Center, New York, New York. NOORBIBI K. DAY • Sloan-Kettering Institute for Cancer Research, New York, New York.

CASPER JERSILD,
PABLO RUBINSTEIN,
AND NOORBIBI K.
DAY

heterozygous carriers have approximately half the levels of the component present in uneffected individuals, indicating that the C^0 genes are codominant.

This generalization is based especially on the most common hereditary C deficiency described in man, the C2 deficiency, where a substantial number of families have been studied. However, the clear-cut grouping of family members into C^0 homozygous and normals may not be expected *a priori* to occur in the general population, where additional heterogeneity may obscure the Mendelian nature of the control of serum levels of the respective C component. In the absence of family data, a bimodal distribution of the levels of a particular C component in the general population would support the assumption that these levels are controlled by one gene only, since C levels of the assumed heterozygous C^0 individuals are clearly separated from those of normal individuals.

The suggestion of linkage between genes affecting the level of total hemolytic C in inbred strains of mice and the *H-2* major histocompatibility complex (MHC) of the mouse (Rosenberg and Tachibana, 1969; Hinzova *et al.,* 1972; Demant *et al.,* 1973) added a new perspective to the studies of C deficiencies. It was subsequently found that $C2^0$, $C4^0$, and the genetic polymorphism of Factor B (*Bf* or *B*) are all closely linked to the *HLA* system (Allen, 1974; Fu *et al.,* 1974; Day *et al.,* 1975a; Rittner *et al.,* 1975). Thus, the major histocompatibility system is a genetic marker for some C^0 genes; of greater importance, the normal functions of these C components are probably associated with those of the MHC.

The importance of the *HLA* region in the determination of susceptibility to certain diseases has been intensively investigated and has recently been the subject of several reviews (see, for example, *Transplantation Reviews* **22,** 1975). Although several diseases have shown a striking association with certain *HLA* antigens, the mechanism(s) by which these antigens, or traits genetically linked to them, influences the disease processes is not known. The possibility exists that in at least some of the *HLA*-associated diseases, one of the determining genetic factors might be an abnormality of a particular C component. It is the purpose of this review to focus on the genetic aspects of hereditary C deficiencies and other variants of C components as they relate to the major histocompatibility system in man, rhesus monkey, and mice. Much of this work is very recent, and it is anticipated that new important findings will be added in the very near future.

We are grateful to our colleagues who have readily provided us with pre- and reprints on this topic.

2. Major Histocompatibility Systems

2.1. The *HLA* System of Man

The *HLA* system is by far the most complex genetic system known in man, consisting of several closely linked loci, each with multiple alleles. The *HLA* genes determine antigenic markers, many of which are present on all nucleated cells. These surface antigens are of major importance for the survival of tissue and organ transplants, but the biological significance of this complex system has yet to be elucidated. Two types of antigens belonging to the *HLA* system have been described.

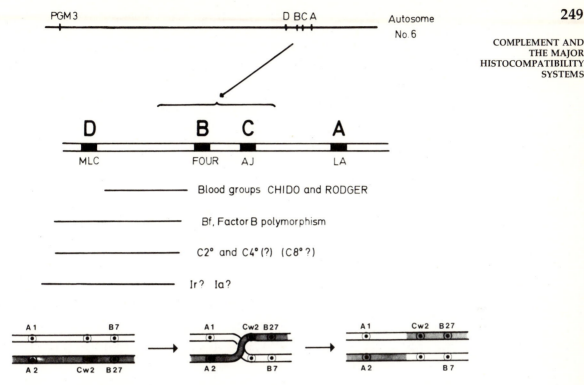

Figure 1. Major histocompatibility system *HLA* in man. Top: Mapping of the various *HLA* loci on Autosome No. 6. The four horizontal lines beneath give tentative mapping of loci for blood groups Chido and Rodgers. Factor B, and $C2^0$ ($C4^0$ and $C8^0$), as well as for postulated Ir and Ia loci. Bottom: Events in the formation of a recombinant *HLA* haplotype, the crossing over being localized between loci A and C.

2.1.1. Serologically Defined (SD) Antigens: *HLA-A, B,* and *C* Antigens

Three loci determining serologically defined (SD) antigens have been identified. These are *HLA-A* (*LA* or first sublocus), *HLA-B* (Four or second sublocus), and *HLA-C* (*AJ* or third sublocus) (Figure 1). The concentration of the corresponding antigens is perhaps highest on peripheral blood lymphocytes. They can therefore be identified by lymphocytotoxicity assays using monospecific antisera against these antigens. The SD antigens are considered to be targets for immune cells and antibodies in the rejection of allografts and may have a normal function in the elimination of viruses.

2.1.2. Lymphocyte-Defined (LD) Antigens: *HLA-D* Determinants

HLA-D determines antigens that may induce a blastogenic response on allogeneic lymphocytes when cocultured *in vitro*. It has only recently been possible to type for LD (*HLA-D*) determinants, using a standardized one-way mixed-lymphocyte-culture (MLC) technique and X-irradiated, *HLA-D* homozygous lymphocytes

CASPER JERSILD,
PABLO RUBINSTEIN,
AND NOORBIBI K.
DAY

of various specificities as stimulating cells. A low MLC response in this technique indicates that one of the *HLA-D* of the responding cells carries the *HLA-D* determinants present on the stimulating (typing) cells (Mempel *et al.*, 1973; Jørgensen *et al.*, 1973; Tweel *et al.*, 1973; Dupont *et al.*, 1973). The *HLA-D* determinants (or closely associated determinants) can also be demonstrated by serological techniques with specific human anti-*HLA-D* sera and highly purified antihuman heavy-chain antiglobulin reagents (van Leeuwen *et al.*, 1973; Winchester *et al.*, 1975; Mann *et al.*, 1975). These antigens are present mainly on B lymphocytes from peripheral blood. The lymphocyte-defined *HLA-D* determinants are responsible for reactivity in mixed leukocyte culture (MLC) *in vitro* and probably for the graft-vs.-host (GVH) reaction *in vivo*.

Figure 1 shows the mapping of the *HLA* loci on the chromosome, and Table 1 gives a list of the various alleles that can now be recognized at each locus. (The newly recommended nomenclature from the Sixth International Histocompatibility Testing Workshop, 1975, is used throughout. Table 1 also gives the previously used nomenclature.)

Table 2 shows the gene frequencies obtained in the normal Danish population. Whereas alleles at the A, B, and C loci have been studied for several years (Staub Nielsen *et al.*, 1975), data on gene frequencies of locus D alleles have been accumulated only more recently (Thomsen *et al.*, 1975, and others). From Tables 1 and 2, it is apparent that *HLA* is a highly polymorphic system, the number of phenotypes being close to 1.5×10^4, while that of possible genotypes is of the order of 10^7.

2.1.3. Linkage Disequilibrium

These closely linked loci are inherited as a unit and each such unit is called a *haplotype*. Table 3 gives the frequencies of some of the more common *HLA* haplotypes, considering solely the HLA-A and HLA-B loci. As shown, certain specific alleles at these two loci are present together more frequently in a haplotype than could be expected from their respective gene frequencies. This phenomenon, called *linkage disequilibrium*, can be expressed as a Δ-value, where $\Delta = h_{ab} - p_a p_b$ and h_{ab} is the frequency with which the haplotype is observed and $p_a p_b$ (the product of the respective gene frequencies) is the expected haplotype frequency. As shown in Table 3, Δ/h is a measure of the linkage disequilibrium. The data given in Table 3 demonstrate that some *HLA* haplotypes occur more frequently than would be expected, and that other combinations are rarer. Linkage disequilibrium, therefore, modifies the extent and practical consequences of the genetic and phenotypic polymorphism as calculated from the gene and antigen frequencies.

In Table 4, similar data on linkage disequilibrium for alleles at the HLA-B and HLA-D loci are presented. Although these data are based on a small number of individuals, some interesting associations can be observed (Thomsen *et al.*, 1975).

2.1.4. Linkage of Genes

Since many genes are located in each chromosome, it is evident that some of them will be sufficiently close together so as to distort the segregation ratios from Mendel's second law (of independent assortment).

TABLE 1. Detectable *HLA* Specificities—New[a] and Previous Nomenclature

Locus A		Locus B		Locus C		Locus D	
New	Previous	New	Previous	New	Previous	New	Previous[b]
HLA-A1	HL-A1	HLA-B5	HL-A5	HLA-Cw1	T1, AJ	HLA-Dw1	LD101, W5a, J. PF
HLA-A2	HL-A2	HLA-B7	HL-A7	HLA-Cw2	T2, 170	HLA-Dw2	LD102, 7a, Pi, SKY
HLA-A3	HL-A3	HLA-B8	HL-A8	HLA-Cw3	T3, UPS	HLA-Dw3	LD103, 8a, SR
HLA-A9	HL-A9	HLA-B12	HL-A12	HLA-Cw4	T4, 315	HLA-Dw4	LD104, W15a, L
HLA-A10	HL-A10	HLA-B13	HL-A13	HLA-Cw5	T5	HLA-Dw5	LD105, Sa.1, IV
HLA-A11	HL-A11	HLA-B14	W14, Maki			HLA-Dw6	LD106, Pr, VIII, pm.
HLA-A28	W28,Ba[a]	HLA-B18	W18, CM			LD107	12a
HLA-A29	W29	HLA-B27	W27, FJH			LD108	W10a
HLA-Aw19	W19, Li	HLA-Bw15	W15, LND				
HLA-Aw23	W23	HLA-Bw16	W16, U18				
HLA-Aw24	W24	HLA-Bw17	W17, MaPi				
HLA-Aw25	W25	HLA-Bw21	W21, ET				
HLA-Aw26	W26	HLA-Bw22	W22, AA				
HLA-Aw30	W30	HLA-Bw35	W5, R[a]				
HLA-Aw31	W31	HLA-Bw37	TY				
HLA-Aw32	W32	HLA-Bw38	W16.1				
HLA-Aw33	W19.6	HLA-Bw39	W16.2				
HLA-Aw34	Malay 2	HLA-Bw40	W10, BB				
HLA-Aw36	Mo[a]	HLA-Bw41	Sabell, MK				
HLA-Aw43	BK	HLA-Bw42	MWA				
		TT,[a] 4A2[a], 12.2,					
		407,[a] JA					

[a] Recommended nomenclature, VI International Histocompatibility Testing Conference, Århus, 1975.
[b] For detailed information, see Joint Report from the Sixth International Histocompatibility Workshop Conference. II. Typing for HLA-D (LD-1 or MLC) Determinants, 1976, in: *Histocompatibility Testing 1975*, Munksgaard, Copenhagen.

CASPER JERSILD,
PABLO RUBINSTEIN,
AND NOORBIBI K.
DAY

TABLE 2. *HLA* Gene Frequencies

Locus A[a]			Locus B[a]			Locus C[a]			Locus D[b]		
Antigen	N	Gene frequency	Antigen	N	Gene frequency	Antigen	N	Gene frequency	Antigen	N	Gene frequency
A1	1967	0.1683	B5	1967	0.0545	Cw1	1291	0.0287	Dw1	95	0.099
A2	1967	0.3228	B7	1967	0.1419	Cw2	1291	0.0496	Dw2	157	0.128
A3	1967	0.1454	B8	1967	0.1274	Cw3	1291	0.1933	Dw3	157	0.112
A9	1967	0.0915	B12	1967	0.1359	Cw4	426	0.0897	Dw4	157	0.091
A10	1967	0.0489	B13	1967	0.0215	Cw5	n.t.		Dw5	34	0.045
A11	1967	0.0520	B14	1967	0.0227	Blank		0.640	Dw6	89	0.094
A28	1967	0.0509	B18	1967	0.0361				D-w10a	157	0.046
A29	426	(0.0228)	B27	1967	0.0440				D-w12a	157	0.049
Aw19	1941	0.0991	Bw15	1967	0.0936				D-Sa.2	34	0.015
Aw23	n.t.		Bw16	1967	0.0273				Blank		0.321
Aw24	n.t.		Bw17	1967	0.0392						
Aw25	1009	(0.0190)	Bw21	1967	0.0177						
Aw26	1009	(0.0297)	Bw22	1967	0.0192						
Aw30	n.t.		Bw35	1967	0.0722						
Aw31	n.t.		Bw37	424	0.0059						
Aw32	1009	(0.0312)	Bw38		(0.0138)						
Aw33	n.t.		Bw39	1009	(0.0135)						
Aw36	n.t.		Bw40	1967	0.0950						
Aw37	n.t.		Bw41	1967	0.0069						
Blank		0.021	Bw42	n.t.							
			4A2*(TT)	1967	0.0059						
			407*	1967	0.0023						
			Blank		0.0310						

[a] From Staub-Nielsen *et al.* (1975).
[b] From Thomsen *et al.* (1975).

The methods for the detection of linkage are based on the frequency of recombinations observed between two genes in a family. In the simplest case, one parent carries both traits under scrutiny and the other is doubly negative. This situation, called a *double backcross,* or *test cross,* provides maximal opportunity to detect linkage: If the genes are indeed closely linked, they will be inherited either almost always together (when in coupling) or separately, i.e., just one or the other (when in repulsion). Other genetic situations are also useful but may be less efficient in providing information. From each family studied, the odds for the comparison between the ratios at different degrees of linkage and those to be observed in the absence of linkage are computed. The logarithms of these odds are added and used to calculate the *lod scores.* Lod scores are usually obtained for different degrees of linkage (i.e., different distances between the genes and, hence, different recombination frequencies).

Details on the methodology employed in these computations have been published (see, for example, Falk *et al., 1975*).

2.1.5. Mapping of the *HLA* Chromosomal Region

HLA has been located on chromosome 6 both by cell hybridization experiments (Jongsma *et al.,* 1973; Van Someren *et al.,* 1974) and by the study of a family with a chromosome 6 marker (pericentric inversion) (Lamm *et al.,* 1975). Segregation analyses of *HLA* antigens in several families have made it possible to observe genetic recombinations and thereby obtain information on the number of loci, their sequence, and their relative distances along the chromosome. Data obtained in teratoma have placed *HLA-D* closest to the centromere (Bodner, 1975).

TABLE 3. Linkage Disequilibrium Between Certain Alleles of Loci A and B of the *HLA* System[a,b]

Haplotype (A, B)		Frequency (h)	Δ/h	α^2 (d.f. = 1)	P
A1,	B8	0.0983	0.7823	699.4	<0.001
A1,	Bw17	0.0145	0.5517	21.1	<0.001
A2,	B12	0.0628	0.3010	21.5	<0.001
A2,	Bw40	0.0500	0.3860	31.5	<0.001
A2,	Bw15	0.0466	0.3498	22.5	<0.001
A3,	B7	0.0539	0.6178	126.5	<0.001
A3,	Bw35	0.0246	0.5732	45.5	<0.001
A10,	Bw16	0.0060	0.7667	32.8	<0.001
A10,	B18	0.0113	0.8496	107.9	<0.001
A11,	Bw35	0.0152	0.7500	78.8	<0.001
A11,	Bw22	0.0030	0.667	8.4	0.0037
Aw19,	B12	0.0246	0.4553	22.1	<0.001
Aw19,	B13	0.0073	0.6986	27.5	<0.001
A28,	B14	0.0045	0.7333	19.8	<0.001
A28,	Bw15	0.0092	0.4783	8.6	0.0033
A28,	Bw16	0.0040	0.6250	9.9	0.00165
A28,	B18	0.0055	0.6546	14.9	<0.001

[a]Calculated from data in Table 2.
[b]From Staub-Nielsen *et al.* (1975).

TABLE 4.   Genetic Linkage Disequilibrium Between Certain Alleles of Loci B and D of the *HLA* Systems[a]

Haplotype	Frequency (*h*)	Δ/*h*	(χ^2) (d.f. = 1)	*P*
B8 Dw3	0.086	0.84	73.8	<0.001
Bw15 Dw4	0.043	0.81	27.6	<0.001
B7 Dw2	0.039	0.67	22.3	<0.001
Bw35 Dw1	0.033	0.83	10.3	0.0013
B12 D-12a	0.017	0.58	2.9	n.s.
Bw40 Dw10a	0.013	0.66	2.7	n.s.
Bw37 Dw3	0.011	0.95	5.4	0.02
Bw37 Dw2	0.010	0.92	3.4	n.s.
B18 Dw2	0.0095	0.47	0.4	n.s.
B13 B-12a	0.0093	0.87	10.8	0.0010

[a]Data obtained from individuals shown in Table 2 from Thomsen *et al.* (1975).

The segregation of other genetic markers has been studied also in such families, and linkage with some of these markers has been observed. Phosphoglucomutase-3 (PGM_3) (Lamm *et al.,* 1971), the blood groups Chido (Middleton *et al.,* 1974) and Rodgers (Bodmer, 1975; James *et al.,* 1976), and the electrophoretic variants of Factor B (Allen, 1974) have all shown linkage to *HLA*. More recently, $C2^0$ (Fu *et al.,* 1974) and $C4^0$ (Rittner *et al.,* 1975) have also been shown to be closely linked to the *HLA* complex.

Investigations of similar associations between the histocompatibility systems in the mouse *(H-2)*, in the monkey *(RhL-A)*, and in the complement system have proved to be particularly informative.

2.2.   The *H-2* System of Mice

Excellent reviews on the *H-2* system of mice have been recently published by Klein (1975) and Shreffler and David (1975).

The *H-2* complex is located on chromosome 17, in the IX linkage group. Five chromosomal regions have been defined within the *H-2* region, each determining at least one "major" marker (Figure 2). These are *H-2 D, Ss-Slp, Ir, X,* and *H-2 K*. The *K* and *D* regions contain the H-2 K and H-2 D loci coding for the serologically detectable K and D antigens. Within the *I* region, three subregions, *Ir-A, Ir-B,* and *Ir-C,* have been defined, each containing various genes that determine immune responsiveness toward specific antigens. The *X* region contains a locus coding for a blood group antigen, originally called *H-2.7* or *G* (Snell and Cherry, 1974). The *S* region contains genes coding for the Ss and Slp serum proteins, and since these proteins seem to be associated with C activity in the mouse, a more detailed discussion of the *S* region is presented in the next section.

2.2.1.   The *S* Region

The major marker in this region is the *Ss-Slp* locus, which controls the production of the Ss and Slp serum proteins. The distribution of this marker in some

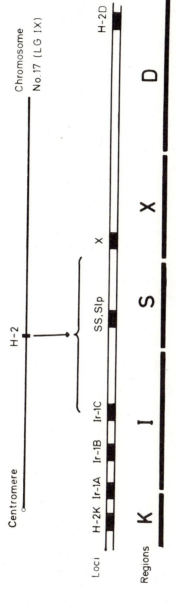

Figure 2. Major histocompatibility system *H-2* in mice. The chromosome regions and marker loci within this H-2 region are shown. The H-2 chromosomal region is located on Chromosome No. 17 of the IX linkage group.

CASPER JERSILD,
PABLO RUBINSTEIN,
AND NOORBIBI K.
DAY

of the more widely used inbred strains is shown in Table 5. The Ss protein (serum serological variant) was first described by Shreffler and Owen (1963). Recently, Capra *et al.* (1975) have isolated this protein and have shown it to have a molecular weight of 150,000 daltons. The isolated Ss protein could be dissociated into two subunits (23,000- and 14,000-dalton subunits). The 14,000 fragment contains no carbohydrate and may be homologous to B-2 microglobulin (Capra *et al.*, 1975). The Slp protein (sex limited protein) also has a molecular weight of approximately 150,000 daltons. Treatment of this protein with 2-mercaptoethanol or dialysis against 1M NaCl, reduces the molecule to two 75,000 dalton units. The electrophoretic mobilities of the Ss and Slp proteins are similar, but Slp is more heat-labile and less stable in 5.5 M KI than Ss (references in Klein, 1975). The actual site of *(in vivo)* synthesis of Slp is unknown, but it is produced in cell cultures of peritoneal macrophages and liver parenchymal cells (Saunders and Edidin, 1974).

The serum levels of the Ss protein are under the control of the *Ss–Slp* locus. The Ss^l and Ss^h determine low (Ss^l) and high (Ss^h) levels of the Ss protein, respectively. Ss^h mice have about 20 times the amount of Ss protein present in Ss^l animals (Shreffler and Owen, 1963). Males tend to have higher levels than females in both Ss^h and Ss^l strains. In addition, males castrated at birth have Ss concentrations similar to those found in normal females of the same strain. Treatment of females (and castrated males) with testosterone increases these levels to those found in normal males. Serum Ss levels also appear to increase in disease and with X-irradiation (Shreffler, 1962; Klein, 1975). Recently, evidences that the Ss protein may be antigenically related to human C4 have been reported (Meo *et al.*, 1975).

The Slp antigens are demonstrable in male sera of certain strains of mice with alloantisera prepared against partially purified Ss protein (Passmore and Shreffler, 1970). Two alleles have been described: Slp^a, coding for the presence of antigen,

TABLE 5. The Ss Slp Types of Some Common Mouse Strains[a,b]

Strain	H2	Ss	Slp
A/J	a	H	a
AKR	k	L	o
B.10 A	a	H	a
Balb/C	d	H	a
B.10 (C57 BL/10)	b	H	o
B.10 D2	d	H	a
B.6 (C57 BL/6)	b	H	o
C3H	k	L	o
CBA	k	L	o
C58	k	L	o
DBA/2	d	H	a
DBA/1	q	H	o
129	b	H	o
RF	k	L	o
SJL	s	H	a

[a]From Passmore and Shreffler (1971).
[b]All mice are maintained at the Jackson Laboratories.

and *Slp⁰*, determining its absence. No instances of genetic recombinants between Ss and Slp have been reported; thus, Ss and Slp are operationally assumed to be the product of a single genetic unit. Ss^h occurs with either Slp^a or Slp^o, whereas Ss^l animals are always Slp^o.

Just as in the case of Ss, the synthesis of Slp antigen is under both genetic and hormonal control; thus, Slp^a (but not Slp^o) females (and castrated males) will develop the Slp antigen upon testosterone treatment.

Further similarities between Ss and Slp have been uncovered by Passmore and Shreffler, who reported on their immunological cross-reactivity (Passmore and Shreffler, 1971) and concluded that all Slp molecules seem to carry Ss sites, while not all Ss molecules carry Slp sites.

The effects of testosterone on the Ss and Slp proteins led Ivanyi *et al.* (1973) to study the levels of testosterone and testosterone-binding protein in mouse serum. These authors concluded that testosterone metabolism is under complex control and that a gene of major importance in its regulation appeared to be linked to *H-2*. This postulated gene was designated *hormone-metabolism-1*, or *Hom-1*.

2.3. The Rhesus Major Histocompatibility Complex *(RhLA)*

Evidence to date has demonstrated important homologies between *RhLA* and human *HLA*. Two series of lymphocyte and platelet antigens have been demonstrated, using cytotoxicity and C fixation methods (Balner, 1973). A third series, controlling MLC reactivity, has been observed (Balner *et al.*, 1973). There is evidence that this locus controls an important parameter of histocompatibility (Balner *et al.*, 1973; Dorf *et al.*, 1975). As in the mouse, close linkage to *Ir* genes has recently been demonstrated.

3. Evidence of Genetic Association between the H and C Systems

3.1. Introduction

The association of *H-2* linked Ss protein and hemolytic C was first suggested by Hinzova *et al.* (1972) and supported by evidence presented by Demant *et al.* 1973. Using an entirely different approach, Allen (1974) demonstrated that the genetic polymorphism of Factor B in man is controlled by a gene linked to the major histocompatibility region. At the same time, Fu *et al.* (1974) presented evidence that the gene responsible for C2 deficiency in man is also linked to *HLA*. These observations stimulated interest in studies of the relationship between *HLA* and C, and numerous papers on C2 deficiency and *HLA* and also of other C deficiencies have been published by several investigators (Section 3.3.2). The results obtained in these studies locate $C2^0$, $C4^0$, and Bf in close proximity to *HLA* in man. Recently, Meo *et al.* (1975) presented evidence that a protein precipitating with antihuman $C4^0$ in mouse serum is associated with the Ss protein and, thus, linked to *H-2*. Confirmatory data were presented by Lachmann *et al.* (1975) and Curman *et al.* (1975). Shevach *et al.* (1975) have observed linkage between $C4^0$ and MHC in guinea pigs.

CASPER JERSILD,
PABLO RUBINSTEIN,
AND NOORBIBI K.
DAY

3.2. Genetic Considerations

The frequency with which the C^0 homozygous state is found depends mainly on the respective gene frequency. Without extensive population studies, an approximation can be gained from the frequency of consanguinity among the parents of the homozygotes. If no consanguinity is apparent, the C^0 gene frequency should be much higher than when it is always present. It can be, therefore, assumed that the frequency of the $C2^0$ gene is relatively high.

Two approaches can be used for estimating C^0 gene frequencies: (1) the frequency with which the homozygous deficiency state can be detected in the random population; and (2) the frequency of heterozygosity, when quantitative studies allow the identification of individuals with decreased levels of the component under study. If these decreases are known to be due to heterozygosity for a C^0 gene, the frequency of such a gene may easily be calculated. Thus, it is essential, especially when using the second approach, to study the family of the individual with the decreased C component level and ascertain whether the condition is inherited.

In the event that no deficiencies are found, it is still possible to calculate a maximal value for the frequency of the corresponding gene at a given level of significance. Then, given the number of investigated individuals, among whom no deficiency state was observed, and given the level of significance required of the estimate, it is possible to calculate the maximal values for the gene frequency. These calculations are made by applying the binomial distribution, which can be expressed as

$$p_n = \binom{N}{n} p^n (1 - p)^{N-n} \qquad \text{Eq. (1)}$$

where p_n is the probability of finding n cases among N individuals investigated.

If $n = 0$ (the number of observed deficiency cases), we can reduce the formula to

$$p_o = (1 - p)^N \qquad \text{Eq. (2)}$$

where p_o is the significance level and p is the maximal gene frequency for this level of significance.

Table 6 gives the maximal gene frequency for a C^0 gene after observing 0 cases among N individuals and choosing the significance level of $P = 0.05, 0.01, 0.005$,

TABLE 6. Maximal Gene Frequency at Different Levels of Significance (P) if No Homozygous Cases Have Been Observed among N Individuals

N	Significance level (P)			
	0.05	0.01	0.005	0.001
100	0.1718	0.2122	0.2272	0.2584
250	0.1091	0.1351	0.1448	0.1651
500	0.0773	0.0958	0.1027	0.1171
1,000	0.0547	0.0678	0.0727	0.0830
2,500	0.0346	0.0429	0.0460	0.0525
10,000	0.0173	0.0215	0.0230	0.0263

and 0.001, respectively. If some homozygous cases had been observed, the formula and tables given by Bailey (1975) could have been used.

3.3.   *HLA*-Linked Traits

3.3.1.   Electrophoretic Polymorphism of Factor B (*B, C3PA,* GBG, *Bf*)

Boenisch and Alper (1970) isolated a glycoprotein from plasma with $\beta2$ mobility, which they named *glycine-rich β_2-glycoprotein,* or GBG, because of its high glycine content. In 1971, Alper *et al.* observed the electrophoretic variation of GBG and found that this polymorphism was genetically determined. They described two common alleles, Gb^F and Gb^S, and two rare alleles, Gb_1^F and Gb_1^S (Alper *et al.,* 1972). Alper *et al.* (1973) were able to demonstrate that GBG was immunochemically identical to Factor B of the properdin system, originally described by Pillemer *et al.* (1954). Proof of their functional identity was given by Goodkofsky and Lepow (1971).

Nomenclature. At the Second International Congress of Immunology, the WHO Committee on nomenclature of complement proposed the term *B factor of Bf* for the protein and *Bf* for the locus. The alleles are called Bf^S, Bf^F, etc. At the Fifth International Complement Workshop and Workshop 39 of the Second International Congress of Immunology, Brighton, England, Factor B was further shortened to "B." To avoid confusion, since the symbol *B* already denotes the Four locus of *HLA* and one of the human blood group antigens, we shall continue to call it *Bf.*

Genetics. In 1974, Allen reported linkage between *Bf* and *HLA*. In a study of 12 two-generation families segregating for *Bf,* none of the 44 informative children showed recombinations between these two loci, suggesting a very close linkage. Allen also noted that linkage disequilibrium between Bf^F and *HLA-B12* could be possible, having observed these two alleles occurring together more frequently than expected among the 32 unrelated parents in the families studied.

On the other hand, Rittner *et al.* (1975) reported five *HLA-Bf* recombinants in 82 informative meiotic divisions. These data were reinterpreted at the Sixth International Histocompatibility Testing Workshop, 1975, by the same group (Albert *et al.,* 1975) and the recombination frequency was then estimated to be 1.66%. The observed recombination frequency suggests that the *Bf* locus is located between the *D* and the *B* locus. Albert *et al.* (1975) also suggested linkage disequilibrium with certain *HLA-B* specificities.

In agreement with these conclusions, Teisberg *et al.* 1975 studied 23 families with no apparent *Bf-HLA* recombinations occurring in the 40 informative offspring. In addition, they investigated two three-generation pedigrees with recombination between *HLA-A* and *HLA-B*. Three recombinants in these two families were informative and indicated that *Bf* went with the *HLA-B* alleles. Similarly, a recent study of a family with five children, one of which showed recombination between the HLA-B and HLA-D loci, demonstrated that the *Bf* locus was contained in the *HLA-A-C-B* segment of the chromosome (Lamm *et al.,* personal communication). However, a different sequence has been demonstrated in a family with a crossover between *HLA-A* and *HLA-B: Bf* went with *HLA-A* (Rubinstein *et al.,* in preparation).

The gene frequencies for *Bf* have been obtained very recently in a study of 199 unrelated individuals. They are Bf^F: 0.239; Bf^S: 0.731; Bf^F1: 0.005; and Bf^S1: 0.025. All these individuals have been typed for *HLA*, and linkage disequilibrium of Bf^F with *HLA-B12* has been again observed (Allen *et al.*, unpublished observation).

3.3.2. Hereditary C2 Deficiency

Low levels of C2 were first described by Silverstein in 1960 in a healthy 35-year-old Caucasian male. C2 levels in this individual were followed for 7 years and recorded throughout as one-tenth of normal values. His two siblings and his two children have normal C2 levels. Hässig *et al.* (1964) tested 41,083 young males at 20 years of age and were able to detect abnormally low levels of C activity, but a few cases were also low in C1 and C4. When 80 family members of 13 probands were studied, low C activity could be demonstrated in only two individuals. These authors were unable to establish a genetic pattern.

In 1966, Klemperer *et al.* described the hereditary deficiency of C2. Using the method of Austen and Beer (1964), they were able to detect three cases of C2 deficiency (C2 levels functionally less than 3 and immunochemically less than 6 μg/ml) within a three-generation family, and also to define 14 members within the family as partially deficient of C2. They concluded the following: "The defect appears to be transmitted as an autosomal recessive characteristic, although individuals who are heterozygous for the defect are easily detectable by virtue of the fact that their sera have approximately half the normal serum complement activity and C2 titers." Since this observation, several other kindreds of C2 deficient individuals have been described. Although the first individual with C2 deficiency was healthy, the other C2-deficient individuals described since have clinical diseases, most of them present as diseases of the mesenchymal tissues (see Chapter 12).

C2 deficiency is the most frequently observed deficiency of C components in man (see Chapter 12). The relatively high frequency of the $C2^0$ genes has facilitated studies on the genetic association with *HLA*, which were described for the first time by Fu *et al.* (1974). In their C2-deficient family, the $C2^0$ genes segregated in close linkage with a particular haplotype, the C2-deficient patient being *HLA-A10, B18* homozygous. These observations were confirmed by Day *et al.* (1975a). Only one of the $C2^0$ genes was associated with an *HLA-A10, B18* haplotype; the other was carried by a rare *HLA-A2, B4A2** haplotype (Figure 3). Of additional interest in this study was that a recombinant between the $C2^0$ and the *HLA-A2, B4A2** was also observed (Day *et al.*, 1975a). Several other $C2^0$-deficient pedigrees (Figures 4 and 5) and their association with *HLA* have been since reported and are presented in Table 7.

In most cases studied thus far, *C2*-carrying *HLA* haplotypes include the *HLA-Dw2* determinant (Fu *et al.*, 1975a,b; Friend *et al.*, 1976; Day *et al.*, unpublished observation) (see Table 7). Thirteen of the 18 *HLA-B* genes were *Bw18*. Eleven of these 18 were also HLA-A10. It should be emphasized that the apparently very strong linkage disequilibrium between *A10, B18*, and *Dw2* is detectable only in the presence of the $C2^0$ gene.

Two possible explanations occur to us for these phenomena. Either all or most of the $C2^0$-carrying haplotypes are derived from a single mutant gene, copies of which are shared by affected families (i.e., founder effect), or, alternatively, the $C2^0$, *Dw2, B18, A10* configuration is associated with other characteristics, possibly of the C system, that are able to compensate the consequences of the C2 deficiency.

$C2^0$ mutants on other *HLA* haplotypes would thus be deleterious even in the heterozygote, and those genes would tend not to be maintained in the population. This last possibility seems less likely, since the heterozygotes are symptom-free, although most of the heterozygote $C2^0$ deficiencies observed so far do carry the *A10,B18,Dw2* haplotype. Since the recombination frequency is low, but not very

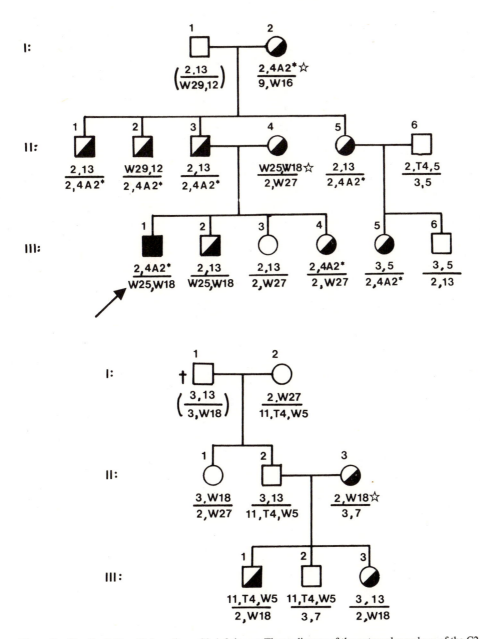

Figure 3. Family *R.K.* with hereditary C2 deficiency. The pedigrees of the paternal members of the C2-deficient SLE patient are shown. The shaded areas represent the hemolytic C2 values. These levels were 2 SDs below the normal mean (normal mean of 40 healthy adults: 1,350 CH50 U/ml ± 500). The *HLA* typing is represented below each individual.

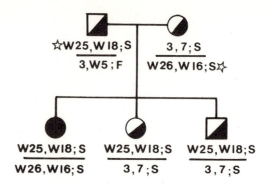

Figure 4. Family G.J. with hereditary C2 deficiency. The pedigrees of the paternal and maternal members of a C2-deficient individual with discoid lupus are shown.

low (two recombinants have been detected among 76 informative individuals), if the first possibility is correct, the mutation must have occurred relatively recently.

In Chapter 12, the clinical conditions observed in the homozygous individuals have been presented. Most of them seem to be diseases of the mesenchymal tissues, but there is no specific clinicopathological consequence of genetic C2 deficiency. This contrasts with the acquired type of C2 deficiency, which is usually associated with the existence of circulating antigen–antibody complexes.

The differential diagnosis between inherited and acquired C2 deficiency is still dependent on genetic data in the family. However, inherited and acquired C2 deficiencies differ in other respects: the genetic type lacks only C2, whereas the acquired cases usually reveal decreased levels of other early-acting components. Another and perhaps a fundamental difference is the association with the *HLA* system. While $C2^0$ maintains a very significant linkage disequilibrium with the *B18-Dw2* haplotype, no such association is detectable in acquired C2 deficiencies such as that found in systemic lupus erythematosus (SLE) (see Kissmeyer-Nielsen *et al.*, 1975).

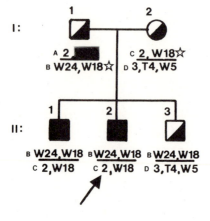

Figure 5. Family F.A. with hereditary C2 deficiency. The pedigree of the maternal and paternal C2-deficient patient with Hodgkin's disease is shown.

TABLE 7. *HLA* Haplotypes Associated with a *C2°* Gene

Authors	HLA-A	HLA-B	HLA-D	Remarks		Clinical disease
Fu *et al.* (1975a)	A10	B18	Dw2	(M)	Family S	Discoid lupus
	A10	B18	Dw2	(P)		
	A10	B18	Dw2	(M)	Family C	Discoid lupus
	A9	B5	Dw2	(P)		
Fu *et al.* (1975b)	A10	B18	Not Dw2	(P)	Family G	No diseases
Day *et al.* (1975a)	A2	Bw44	Dw2	(M)	Family Gr	SLE
	Aw25	B18	Dw2	(M)	Family K	SLE
	A2	B18	n.t.	(P)		
	Aw24	B18	Dw2	(M)	——	
(unpublished observation)	A2	B18	Dw2	(M)	Family A	Hodgkins disease
	Aw25	B18	Dw2	(P)		
	Aw26	Bw38	Dw2	(M)	Family J	SLE-like syndrome
Friend *et al.* (1976)	A10	B18	Dw2	(M)	Family 1	Polyarteritis
	A10	B18	Dw2	(P)		
	A10	B18	Dw2	(M)	Family 2	Membranoproliferative GN
Wolski *et al.* (1975)	Aw30	B13	n.t.	(M)	Family SHK	SLE-like syndrome
	A3	B5	n.t.	(P)		

CASPER JERSILD,
PABLO RUBINSTEIN,
AND NOORBIBI K.
DAY

3.3.3. C4 Deficiency

Complete deficiency of the fourth component of complement (C4) was discovered in an 18-year-old German girl with a disease clinically typical of SLE. Although she presented most of the anomalies usually found in SLE, the most characteristic biological signs were lacking, i.e., absence of LE cells and lack of immunoglobulin or C3 deposits in the skin biopsy. Family studies indicated that the C4 deficiency was inherited as an autosomal recessive trait (Hauptmann *et al.*, 1974), and further studies suggested close linkage between $C4^0$ and *HLA* (Rittner *et al*, 1975). The $C4^0$ gene was inherited together with the *HLA* haplotype *HLA-A2, Bw40, Cw3; BfS*, the propositus probably being homozygous for this haplotype. No other genetic markers were studied.

In another, and larger, family with a C4-deficient patient, Ochs was also able to demonstrate close linkage between the C4 and *HLA* (Ochs, personal communication). In this family, the $C4^0$ was carried on *HLA-A2, B12; Bfs* (maternal) and *HLA-A2, B15; BfS* (paternal).

3.3.4. C8 Deficiency

Deficiency of the eighth component of complement (C8) was first described by Petersen *et al.* (1976) in an American black family. The proband, a 24-year-old woman, had three disseminated gonococcal *(Neisseria gonorrhoeae)* infections. The detection of approximately half-normal levels of C8 in the proband's parents and children was consistent with the interpretation that C8 deficiency is an autosomal codominant trait (Petersen *et al.*, 1976). *HL-A* studies indicate that in this family, C8 deficiency is closely linked to the MHC (Merritt *et al.*, 1976).

We have recently discovered another C8-deficient family (23 members) (Figure 6) with xeroderma pigmentosum (Day *et al.*, 1976). The C8 deficiency was inherited as an autosomal codominant trait. In contrast to the genetic studies described by Merritt *et al.* (1976), no linkage of C8 gene and *HL-A* was evident in these families. It is attractive to speculate at this point that due to the fact that C8 is made up of three polypeptides (Müller-Eberhard, 1975), the C8-deficient family described by Merritt *et al.* lacks one polypeptide chain, which is closely linked to *HL-A,* whereas our family lacks a polypeptide chain of C8, which is not closely linked to the MHC. The study of a third C8 deficient family, when possible, would be of great importance in the understanding of these differences.

3.4. Non-*HLA*-Linked Traits

3.4.1. Hereditary C1r Deficiency

Deficiency of C1r has been reported in two families (C.C. and M.F.) (Day and Good, 1975). Genetic studies in both families indicate that this deficiency is inherited as an autosomal recessive trait (de Bracco *et al.*, 1974; Day *et al.*, 1975b). The genetic data (*HLA* typing and MLC studies) indicate that the $C1r^0$ gene is not closely linked to the major histocompatibility complex (Day *et al.*, 1975b) (Figures 7 and 8).

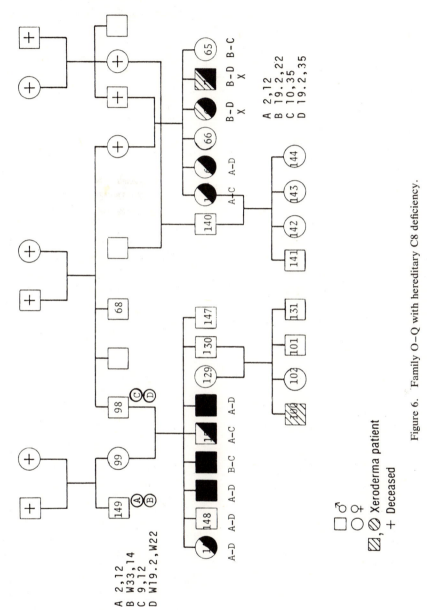

Figure 6. Family O–Q with hereditary C8 deficiency.

CASPER JERSILD,
PABLO RUBINSTEIN,
AND NOORBIBI K.
DAY

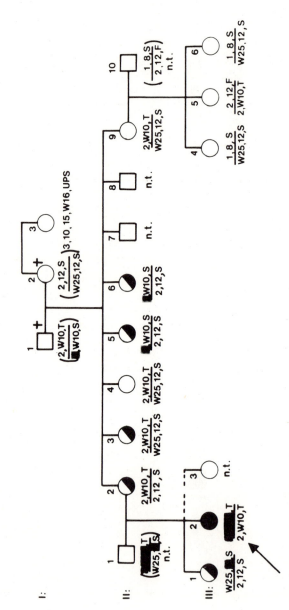

Figure 7. Family C. C. with hereditary C1r deficiency. The pedigree of the maternal members of the C1r-deficient patient are shown. The shaded areas represent the immunochemical C1r determinations.

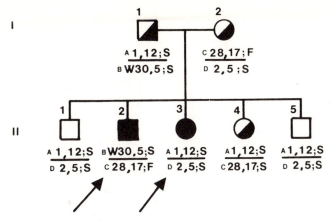

Figure 8. Family M.F. with hereditary C1r deficiency. The pedigree of the paternal and maternal members of C1r-deficient individuals are shown.

It is of interest that the Clr-deficient person (C.C., III:2, Figure 7) was homozygous for the *HLA* and *Bf* type *HLA2, W10, S1*. Three aunts (II:3, II:4, and II:9) had the haplotypes *HLA2,W10/W25,12* and carried the *Bf* alleles *S* and *S1*. The MLC studies were consistent with the *HLA* and *Bf* typing, showing that cells from the proposita (III:2) stimulated weakly cells from individuals II:2, II:3, and II:4 (Table 8). On the other hand, II:2 does stimulate II:5 *(HLA2,W10)*, and thus supports the finding of two distinct *HLA2,W10* haplotypes by *Bf* typing, one being associated with *S1* (III:2) and the other being associated with *S* (II:5 and II:6). These data are not consistent with close linkage of $C1r^0$ with *HLA*.

In the C1r-deficient family M.F., *HLA* typing indicated, again, lack of close

TABLE 8. MLC Responses among Members of Family C.C., and Serum C1r Levels

Responders	Stimulators						C1r (μg/ml)
	$(III:2)_X$	$(II:2)_X$	$(II:3)_X$	$(II:4)_X$	$(II:5)_X$	$(III:1)_X$	
III:2	119[a]	3579	5909	2967	3319	6296	< 12[b]
II:2	1199	250	7398	6615	6629	7105	70[c]
II:3	1874	8777	533	217	8032	8433	70[c]
II:4	683	2580	442	179	4608	2244	107
II:5	4140	6946	9901	7839	683	8323	67[c]
III:1	6035	5862	6103	3618	8075	234	75[c]
						I:3	114
						II:6	65[c]
						II:9	95
						III:4	97
						III:5	112
						III:6	95

[a] Median of raw CPM.
[b] Homozygous C1r-deficient.
[c] Heterozygous C1r-deficient.

CASPER JERSILD,
PABLO RUBINSTEIN,
AND NOORBIBI K.
DAY

linkage between $C1r^0$ and *HLA* (Figure 8). In addition, MLC studies showed strong mutual reactivity between the two homozygous C1r-deficient siblings (II:2 and II:3), and *HLA* identical siblings (II:2, II:3, and II:5) showed MLC nonreactivity. All other combinations were strongly positive in MLC (Table 9). LD typing in this family showed good agreement with the *HLA-SD* typing.

3.4.2. Deficiency of C1s Inhibitor

This deficiency is associated with hereditary angioneurotic edema (HANE). The deficiency has been shown to be transmitted as an autosomal dominant trait. Several kindreds have now been described since the original finding by Donaldson and Rosen (1964). It is remarkable that two forms of the disorder are known, one being characterized by a complete absence of the production of the C1-INH, the other by the synthesis of an abnormal nonfunctional protein (for a more detailed review of this topic, see Shokeir, 1973).

The study of two kindreds, including 11 HANE patients, 15 individuals with abnormal laboratory findings but without symptoms, and 33 normal individuals with *HLA* markers were recently presented by Oheta *et al.* (1975). No association between *HLA* and clinical signs or laboratory findings concerning C1s-INH and *HLA* could be demonstrated.

3.4.3. Genetic Polymorphism of C3

This topic has recently been reviewed by Alper and Rosen (1971) and Alper (1973), whose papers should be consulted for detailed information.

In 1967, Wieme and Demeulenaere found two electrophoretic bands corresponding to C3 and in 1968, Azen and Smithies (1968) and, independently, Alper and Propp (1968) described the genetic polymorphism of this C component.

Two common variants can be detected by different electrophoretic techniques, $C3^F$ and $C3^S$. Sixteen other electrophoretic variants have been observed, all with low frequency. The classification of rare C3 alleles has been described by Alper *et al.* (1973).

TABLE 9. MLC Responses among Members of Family M.F., and Serum C1r Levels

Responders	Stimulators							C1r (μg/ml)
	$(II:2)_X$	$(II:3)_X$	$(I:1)_X$	$(I:2)_X$	$(II:1)_X$	$(II:4)_X$	$(II:5)_X$	
II:2	3078[a]	9025	9880	11465	14648	10898	19107	<12[b]
II:3	2707	13	1957	1574	63	1396	120	<12[b]
I:1	5063	4729	1874	8774	7662	5123	7124	69[c]
I:2	5497	2356	8464	880	5445	4848	5717	69[c]
II:1	9296	194	7805	7443	1047	8566	3209	117
II:4	5572	4503	6439	7995	7508	463	9273	73[c]
II:5	12758	650	12636	10287	1559	12618	2097	102

[a] Median of raw CPM.
[b] Homozygous C1r-deficient.
[c] Heterozygous C1r-deficient.

The extensive use of the alleles of C3 as genetic markers has firmly established that their mode of inheritance is autosomal and codominant. C3 polymorphism has also been studied in several different populations and in various racial groups.

The chemical structure of C3 has recently been the subject of extensive study (Bokisch *et al.*, 1975). The C3 molecule consists of two polypeptide chains, alpha and beta, which are linked by disulphide bonds and by noncovalent forces. The molecular weights are 120,000 and 75,000 daltons, respectively. Detailed information on the structure–function interrelationship is also available (Bokisch *et al.*, 1975). However, the molecular basis for the genetic variation has yet to be elucidated.

The chromosomal assignment of the C3 gene has been suggested by indirect evidence: (1) Weitkamp *et al.* (1975) has presented evidence suggesting linkage with the Lewis blood groups; the recombination fraction is in the order of 6–22%. (2) Linkage also exists between the ACP-1 locus (acid phosphatase-1 or erythrocytes) and the Lewis locus (Nguyen and Moullec, 1971) and between the MNSs blood group locus and ACP-1 (Ferguson-Smith *et al.*, 1973). The MNS locus (German and Chaganti, 1973) and ACP-1 are both located on chromosome 2. As expected from these data, the C3 polymorphism has been shown to segregate independently of several other genetic markers, including *HLA* (Lamm *et al.*, 1975), *Bf,* and the C6 polymorphism (Hobart *et al.*, 1975).

The biological significance of the C3 polymorphism is unknown. Recent investigations seem to indicate functional differences between the two variants *in vivo* as they are reflected in disease susceptibility associated with one of them (Farhud and Walter, 1973). Analysis of C3 activity *in vitro* has so far not provided any evidence of functional differences between the two variant forms. Total C activities in individuals with various C3 phenotypes are identical (Alper and Propp, 1968; Colten and Alper, 1972), and also no difference in the levels of C3 determined immunochemically could be measured in such individuals (Alper and Propp, 1968; Agarwal *et al.*, 1972; Brönnerstam and Cedergren, 1973). The conversion rate of $C3^F$ and $C3^S$ as measured *in vitro* also seems to be identical (Teisberg, 1971; Brönnerstam, 1973). Recent studies by Arvilommi (1974), however, seem to indicate that the binding of C3 to the C3 receptor of monocytes is influenced by the C3 type. Using monocytes isolated from a $C3^S$ individual, Arvilommi found that more monocytes were able to bind erythrocytes coated with fresh human serum of $C3^F$ type than if coated with serum of $C3^S$ type.

In studies of C3 polymorphism in different diseases, an increased frequency of $C3^F$ was observed in sera of patients with rheumatoid arthritis (Farhud and Walter, 1973; Brönnerstam, 1973), hepatitis (Farhud and Walter, 1973; Sørensen and Dissing, 1976), arteriosclerosis (Dissing *et al.*, 1972; Sørensen and Dissing, 1976), and possibly in patients with leprosy (Agarwal *et al.*, 1974). In sera of healthy donors with only occasional episodes of common cold or influenza, the $C3^F$ variant was more frequent than among healthy donors with recurrent episodes of common cold and influenza (Sørensen and Dissing, 1976). Finally, the $C3^S$ gene was significantly increased among mothers of ABO-incompatible children who have lytic anti-A or anti-B antibodies (Brönnerstam and Cedergren, 1973). These observations suggest that the C3 polymorphism might contribute to the modulation of some immunological processes. An important role of C3 in the induction of some types of immunity has recently been demonstrated by Pepys, 1974, and very recent studies of Arnaiz-Villena and Festenstein (1975) demonstrate that it is possible to block the capacity of human lymphocytes to form EAC rosettes (complement-dependent) by specific anti-4^a or 4^b antisera (anti-*W4* and anti-*W6*). (These rosettes most likely attach to the $C3^d$ receptor of lymphocytes, as shown by Ross *et al.*, 1973.)

3.5. Nonhuman Species

3.5.1. Mice

H-2 Linked C Components. The Ss protein and what is known of its relation to C has been described in Section 2.2.1. It should be added that other investigators have found reduced levels of C1, C2, and C4 in Ss-low as compared to Ss-high mice (Goldman and Goldman, 1975) Preliminary data from our laboratories show a similar variation in the serum level of mouse Factor B. For these reasons, coincidence in serum level of a particular C component with that of the Ss protein should not be considered proof of the identity of that component with the *Ss* trait. Moreover, functional assays of C2 and C4 in Ss^h and Ss^l strains fail to disclose any significant differences (Day and Rubinstein, in preparation).

Non-H2 Linked Components. The first genetically controlled variation of complement levels in mice was reported by Rosenberg and Tachibana (1969) and shown to be controlled by a single gene, *Hc* (hemolytic complement). This gene was shown to be independent of *H-2* and its product to be identical to the antigen MuB1 (Cinader *et al.*, 1964), which determines a discrete complement component (Nilsson and Müller-Eberhard, 1967). Cinader *et al.* (1964) further showed that this component (which can be detected by iso- and heteroantisera) exhibits important variations in serum levels according to sex. MuB1 has been shown to be C5 (Nilsson and Müller-Eberhard, 1967): the hormonal control of MuB1 levels has been demonstrated (Urbach and Cinader, 1966), thus providing a possible functional link to the MHC through the HOM-l locus (Ivanyi *et al.*, 1973).

3.5.2. The Rhesus Monkeys

Evidence obtained so far demonstrates important homologies between the *RhL-A* and *HLA*. With respect to genetic polymorphism of Factor B or *Bf* in rhesus monkeys, it has been shown to be controlled by a single autosomal locus (Ziegler *et al.*, 1975a). These authors were able to detect six codominant alleles, Bf^F, Bf^{F1}, Bf^{F2}, Bf^S, Bf^{S1}, and Bf^{S2} and to show that the *Bf* locus is linked to the *RhL-A* (Ziegler *et al.*, 1975b).

4. Conclusions

The discovery of genetic linkage between the MHC and some of the components of C has opened a new and intriguing facet of the role of the MHC systems in the control and regulation of immune responses.

That this linkage is of some physiologic significance may be suggested by the existence of linkage disequilibrium, clear-cut between $C2^0$ and the *A10,B18,Dw2* haplotype and possible between alleles at the *Bf* locus and certain *HLA-B* alleles. Similarly, the *Ss* alleles are distinctly associated with *H-2* genes, at least within unbred strains.

The genetic association between the C components that activate C3 and the MHC suggests a physiologic relationship that may have distinct evolutionary significance: studies on the relation between the activation of C3, the MHC, and the control of immune responses and of the linkage of MHC and C genes during phylogeny are now clearly indicated.

ACKNOWLEDGMENTS

Noorbibi K. Day is an Established Investigator of the American Heart Association.

This study was supported in part by Public Health Service Research Grant NIH CA 18488-01A1 and American Heart Association Grant AHA 75-912.

References

Agarwal, D. P., Benkmann, H.-G. and Goedde, H. W., 1972, Genetic polymorphism of the third component of complement (C3) and levels of β_lC/β_lA—globulin in sera of German and Spanish populations, *Hum. Hered.* **22**:356.

Agarwal, D. P., Benkmann, H. -G., Goedde, H. W., Rohde, R., Delbrück, H., and Rougemont, A., 1974, Levels of serum β_lC/β_lA—globulin (C3) and its polymorphism in leprosy patients and healthy controls from Ethiopia and Mali, *Humangenetik* **21**:355–359.

Albert, E. D., Rittner, C., Grosse-Wilde, H., Netzel, B., and Scholz, S., 1975, Recombination frequency and linkage disequilibrium between HL-A and Bf, in: *Histocompatibility Testing 1975,* pp. 941–944, Munksgaard, Copenhagen.

Allen, F. H., Jr., 1974, Linkage of HL-A and GBG, *Vox Sang.* **27**:382–384.

Alper, C. A., 1973, Genetics and the C3 molecule, *Vox Sang.* **25**:1–8.

Alper, C. A., and Propp, R. P., 1968, Genetic polymorphism of the third component of human complement (C3), *J. Clin. Invest.* **47**:2181–2191.

Alper, C. A., and Rosen, F. S., 1971, Genetic aspects of the complement system, *Adv. Immunol.* **14**:251–290.

Alper, C. A., Boenisch, T., and Watson, L., 1971, Glycine-rich beta-glycoprotein (GBG). Evidence for relation to the complement system and for genetic polymorphism in man, *J. Immunol.* **107**:323 (abstract).

Alper, C. A., Boenisch, T., and Watson, L., 1972, Genetic polymorphism in human glycine-rich beta glycoprotein, *J. Exp. Med.* **135**:68–80.

Alper, C. A., Goodkofsky, II, and Lepow, I. H., 1973, The relationship of glycine-rich beta-glycoprotein to Factor B in the properdin system and to the cobra factor-binding protein of human serum, *J. Exp. Med.* **137**:424–437.

Arnaiz-Villena, H., and Festenstein, H., 1975, 4a(W4) and 4b(W6) human histocompatibility antigens are specifically associated with complement receptors, *Nature London* **258**:732–734.

Arvilommi, H., 1974, Capacity of complement C3 phenotypes to bind onto mononuclear cells in man, *Nature London* **251**:740–741.

Austen, K. F., and Beer, F., 1964, Measurement of the second component of human complement (C2^{hu}) by its interaction with EAC'Ia^{9P}4^{9P} cells, *J. Immunol.* **92**:946–957

Azen, E. A., and Smithies, O., 1968, Genetic polymorphism of C'3 (IC-globulin) in human serum, *Science* **162**:905.

Bailey, B. J. R., 1975, On estimating the frequency of a recessive gene in a random mating population, *Ann. Hum. Genet. London* **38**:351–354.

Balner, H., 1973, Current knowledge of the histocompatibility complex of rhesus monkeys, *Transplant. Rev.* **15**:50–61.

Balner, H., Dorf, M. E., de Groot, M. L., and Benacerraf, B., 1973, The histocompatibility complex of rhesus monkey. III. Evidence for a major MLR locus and histocompatibility-linked Ir genes, *Transplant. Proc.* **5**:1555–1560.

Bodmer, W. F., 1975, Report on chromosome 6, 3rd Conference on Human Gene Mapping, Baltimore.

CASPER JERSILD,
PABLO RUBINSTEIN,
AND NOORBIBI K.
DAY

Boenisch, T. and Alper, C. A., 1970, Isolation and properties of a glycine-rich beta-glycoprotein of human serum, *Biochim. Biophys. Acta* **221**:529–535.

Bokisch, V. A., Dierich, M. P., and Müller-Eberhard, H. J., 1975, Third component of complement (C3): structural properties in relation to functions, *Proc. Nat. Acad. Sci. U.S.A.* **72**:1989–93.

de Bracco, M. M. E., Windhorst, D., Stroud, R. M., and Moncada, B., 1974, The autosomal recessive mode of inheritance of C1r deficiency in a large Puerto Rican family, *Clin. Exp. Immunol.* **16**:183–188.

Brönnerstam, R., 1973, Studies of the C3 polymorphism. Relationship between C3 phenotypes and rheumatoid arthritis, *Hum. Hered.* **23**:206–213.

Brönnerstam, R., and Cedergren, B., 1973, Studies of the C3 polymorphism. Relationship between C3 phenotypes and antibody titers, *Hum. Hered.* **23**:214–219.

Capra, J. D., Vitetta, E. S., and Klein, J., 1975, Studies on the murine Ss protein. I. Purification, molecular weight and subunit structure, *J. Exp. Med.* **142**:664–672.

Cinader, B., Dubiski, S., and Wardlow, A. C., 1964, Distribution, inheritance and properties of an antigen, MuBl, and its relation to hemolytic complement, *J. Exp. Med.* **120**:897–924.

Coca, A. F., 1920, A study of the serum of complement-deficient guinea-pigs, *Proc. Soc. Exp. Biol. N.Y.* **18**:71.

Colten, H. R., and Alper, C. A., 1972, Hemolytic efficiencies of genetic variants of human C3. *J. Immunol.* **108**:1184–7.

Curman, P., Östberg, L., Sandberg, L., Malmheden-Ericksson, I., Stalenheim, C., Rask, L., and Peterson, P. A., 1975, H-2 linked Ss proteins is C4 component of complement, *Nature London* **258**:243–245.

Day, N. K., and Good, R. A., 1975, Deficiencies of the complement system in man, in: *Immunodeficiency in Man and Animals* (R. A. Good, J. Finstad, and N. W. Paul, eds.), p. 306, Sinauer Associates, Sunderland, Massachusetts.

Day, N. K., L'Esperance, P., Good, R. A., Michael, A. F., Hansen, J. A., Dupont, B., and Jersild, C., 1975a, Hereditary C2 deficiency: genetic studies and association with the HL-A system, *J. Exp. Med.* **141**:1464–1469.

Day, N. K., Rubinstein, P., de Bracco, M., Moncada, B., Hansen, J. A., Dupont, B., Thomsen, M., Svejgaard, A., and Jersild, C., 1975b, Hereditary C1r deficiency: lack of linkage to the HL-A region in two families, in: *Histocompatibility Testing 1975*, pp. 960–962, Munksgaard, Copenhagen.

Day, N. K., Degos, L., Beth, M., Sasportes, M., Gharbi, R., and Giraldo, G., 1976, C8 deficiency in a family with xeroderma pigmentosum. Lack of linkage to the HL-A region, in: *HLA and Disease*, Vol. 58, p. 197 (abstract), INSERM, Paris, France.

Demant, P., Capkova, J., Hinzova, E., and Joracova, B., 1973, The role of the histocompatibility-2-linked Ss-Slp region in the control of mouse complement, *Proc. Nat. Acad. Sci. U.S.A.* **70**:863–4.

Dissing, J., Lund, J., and Sorensen, H., 1972, C3 polymorphism in a group of old arteriosclerotic patients, *Hum. Hered.* **22**:466–472.

Donaldson, V. H., and Rosen, F. S., 1964, Action of complement in hereditary angioneurotic edema: the role of C'l-esterase, *J. Clin. Invest.* **43**:2204–2213.

Dorf, M. E., Balner, H., and Benacerraf, B., 1975, Mapping of the immune response genes in the major histocompatibility complex of the rhesus monkey, *J. Exp. Med.* **142**:673–693.

Dupont, B., Jersild, C., Hansen, G. S., Nielsen, L. S., Thomsen, M., and Svejgaard, A., 1973, Typing for MLC-determinants by means of LD-homozygote and LD-heterozygote test cells, *Transplant. Proc.* **5**:1543–1549.

Falk, C. T., Walker, M. E., Martin, M. D., and Allen, F. H., Jr., 1975, Autosomal linkage in humans, *Ser. Hematol.* **8**:154–237.

Farhud, D. D., and Walter, H., 1973, Polymorphism of C3 in German, Bulgarian, Iranian and Angola populations, *Humangenetik* **17**:161–4.

Ferguson-Smith, M. A., Newman, B. F., Ellis, P. M., Thomson, D. M. G., and Riley, I. D., 1973, Assignment by deletion of human red cell acid phosphatase gene locus to the short arm of chromosome 2, *Nature London* **243**:271–273.

Friend, P. S., Hamberger, B. S., Yong-Kikim, A., Michael, A. F., Yuris, E. J., 1976, C2 deficiency in man: genetic relationship to a mixed lymphocyte reaction determinant(7a*), *Immunogenetics* **2**(6):569–576.

Fu, S. M., Kunkel, H. G., Brusman, H. P., Allen, F. M., Jr., and Fotino, M., 1974, Evidence for linkage between HL-A histocompatibility genes and those involved in the synthesis of the second component of complement, *J. Exp. Med.* **140**:1108–1111.

Fu, S. M., Stern, R., Kunkel, H. G., Dupont, B., Hansen, J. A., Day, N. K., Good, R. A., Jersild, C., and Fotino, M., 1975a, Mixed lymphocyte culture determinants and C2 deficiency: LD-7a associated with C2 deficiency in four families, *J. Exp. Med.* **142**:495–506.

Fu, S. M., Stern, R., Kunkel, H. G., Dupont, B., Hansen, J. A., Day, N. K., Good, R. A., Jersild, C., and Fotino, M., 1975b, LD-7a association with C2 deficiency in five of six families, in: *Histocompatibility Testing 1975,* pp. 933–936, Munksgaard, Copenhagen.

German, J., and Chaganti, R. S. K., 1973, Mapping of human autosomes: assignment of the MV locus to a specific segment in the long arm of chromosome no. 2., *Science* **182**:1261–1262.

Goldman, M. B., and Goldman, J. N., 1975, Relationship of levels of early components of complement to the H-2 complex of mice, *Fed. Proc. Fed. Amer. Soc. Exp. Biol.* **34** (3) (abstract 4309).

Goodkofsky, I., and Lepow, I. H., 1971, Functional relationship of factor B in the properdin system to C3 proactivator of human serum, *J. Immunol.* **107**:1200–4.

Hässig, A. V., Borel, J. F., Ammaun, P., Thöui, M., and Bütler, R., 1964, Essentielle Hypokomplementämie, *Pathol. Microbiol.* **27**:542–547.

Hauptman, G., Grosshans, E., and Heid, E., 1974, Lupus erythemateux aigus et déficits héréditaires en complement. A propos d'un cas par déficit complement en C4, *Ann. Dermatol. Syphiligr. Paris* **101**:479–495.

Hinzova, E., Demant, P., and Ivanyi, P., 1972, Genetic control of haemolytic complement in mice: association with H-2, *Folia Biol. Prague* **20**:237–243.

Hobart, M. J., Lachmann, P. J., and Alper, C. A., 1975, Polymorphism of human C6, in: *Protides of the Biological Fluids* (H. Peters, ed.), pp. 575–580, Pergamon Press, New York.

Hyde, R. R., 1923, Complement-deficient guinea-pig serum, *J. Immunol.* **8**:267.

Ivanyi, P., Gregorova, S., Mickova, M., Haupt, R., and Storka, L., 1973, Genetic association between a histocompatibility gene (H-2) and androgen metabolism in mice, *Transplant. Proc.* **5**:189–92.

James, J., Stiles, P., Boyce, F., and Wright, J., 1976, The HL-A type of Rg(a−) individuals, *Vox Sang* **30**:214–216.

Jongsma, A., van Someren, H., Westerveld, A., Hagemeijer, A., and Pearson, P., 1973, Localization of genes on human chromosomes by studies of human-chinese hamster somatic cell hybrids. Assignment of PGM_3 to chromosome C6 and regional mapping of the PGD, PGM_1 and Pep-C genes on chromosome A1, *Humangenetik* **20**:195–202.

Jørgensen, F. H., Lamm, L. U., and Kissmeyer-Nielsen, F., 1973, Mixed lymphocyte cultures with inbred individuals: an approach to MLC typing, *Tissue Antigens* **3**:323–39.

Kissmeyer-Nielsen, F., Kjerbye, K. E., Andersen, E., and Halberg, P., 1975, HL-A antigens in systemic lupus erythematosus, *Transplant. Rev.* **22**:164–167.

Klein, J., 1975, Biology of the mouse histocompatibility-2 complex, in: *Principles of Immunogenetics Applied to a Single System,* p. 498, Springer-Verlag, Berlin, Heidelberg, New York.

Klemperer, M. R., Woodworth, H. C., Rosen, F. S., and Austen, K. F., 1966, Hereditary deficiency of the second component of complement (C'2) in man, *J. Clin. Invest.* **45**:880–890.

Lachman, P. J., Grennan, D., Martin, A., and Demant, P., 1975, Identification of Ss protein as murine C4, *Nature London* **258**:242–243.

Lamm, L. U., Svejgaard, A., and Kissmeyer-Nielsen, F., 1971, PGM3:HL-A is another linkage in man, *Nature London New Biol.* **231**:109–10.

Lamm, L. U., Thorsen, I. -L., Petersen, G. B., Jorgensen, J., Henningsen, K., Bech, B., and Kissmeyer-Nielsen, F., 1975, Data on the HL-A linkage group, *Ann. Hum. Gene. London* **38**:383–390.

Mann, D. L., Abelson, L., Harris, S., and Amos, D. B., 1975, Detection of antigens specific for B-lymphoid cultured cell lines with human alloantisera, *J. Exp. Med.* **142**:84–89.

Mempel, W., Grosse-Wilde, H., Baumann, P., Netzel, B., Steinbauer-Rosenthal, I., Scholz, S., Bertrams, J., and Albert, E. D., 1973, Population genetics of the MLC response: typing for MLC determinants using homozygous and heterozygous reference cells, *Transplant. Proc.* **5**:1529–1534.

Meo, T., Krasteff, T., Schreffler, D. C., 1975, Immunochemical characterization of murine H-2 controlled Ss protein through the identification of its human homologue as the fourth component of complement, *Proc. Nat. Acad. Sci. U.S.A.* **72**:4536–4540.

Merritt, A. D., Petersen, B. H., Angenieta, A. B., Meyers, D. A., Brooks, G. F., and Hodes, M. E., 1976, Chromosome 6: linkage of the eighth component of complement (C8) to the histocompatibility region (HLA), in: 3rd International Workshop on Human Gene Mapping, *Birth Defects* XII, 6, Baltimore Conference (1975), The National Foundation, New York.

Middleton, J., Crookston, M., Falk, J. A., Robson, E. B., Cook, P. J. L., Batchelor, J. R., Bodmer, J.,

CASPER JERSILD,
PABLO RUBINSTEIN,
AND NOORBIBI K.
DAY

Ferrara, G. B., Festenstein, H., Harris, R., Kissmeyer-Nielsen, F., Lawlwe, S. D., Sachs, J. A., and Wolf, E., 1974, Linkage of Chido and HL-A, *Tissue Antigens* **4**:366–373.

Moore, H. D., 1919, Complement and opsonic functions in their relation to immunity (A study of guinea-pigs naturally deficient in complement), *J. Immunol.* **89**:425.

Müller-Eberhard, H. J., 1975, Complement, *Annu. Rev. Biochem.* **44**:697–724.

Nguyen, V. -C., and Moullec, J., 1971, Linkage probable entre les groupes de phosphatase acide des globules rouges et le system Lewis, *Ann. Genet.* **14**:121–125.

Nilsson, U. R., and Müller-Eberhard, H. J. 1967, Deficiency of the fifth component of complement in mice with an inherited complement defect, *J. Exp. Med.* **125**:1–16.

Ochs, H. D., Rosenfeld, S. I., Thomas, E. D., Giblett, E. R., Alper, C. A., Dupont, B., Hansen, J. A., Grosse-Wilde, H., and Wedgwood, R. J., 1976, Linkage between the gene(s) controlling the synthesis of C4 and the major histocompatibility complex, in: *HLA and Disease,* Vol. 58, p. 208 (abstract), INSERM, Paris, France.

Oheta, K., Tiilikainen, A., Kaakinen, A., and Rasanen, J., 1975 (abstract), XIV Congress of the International Society of Blood Transfusion, Helsinki.

Passmore, H. C., and Shreffler, D. C., 1970, A sex limited serum protein variant in the mouse. Inheritance and association with the H-2 region, *Biochem. Genet.* **4**:351–65.

Passmore, H. C., and Shreffler, D. C., 1971, A sex-limited serum protein variant in the mouse: hormonal control of phenotypic expression, *Biochem. Genet.* **5**:201–9.

Pepys, M. B., 1974, Role of complement in induction of antibody production *in vivo.* Effect of cobra factor and other C3 reactive agents on thymus-dependent and thymus-independent antibody responses, *J. Exp. Med.* **140**:126–45.

Petersen, B. H., Graham, J. A., and Brooks, G. F., 1976, Human deficiency of the eighth component of complement: the requirement of C8 for serum *Neisseria gonorrhoeae* bactericidal activity, *J. Clin. Invest.* **57**(2):283–290.

Pillemer, L., Blum, L., Lepow, I. H., Ross, O. A., Todd, E. W., and Wardlaw, A. C., 1954, The properdin system and immunity. I. Demonstration and isolation of a new serum protein, properdin, and its role in immune phenomena, *Science (Washington, D.C.)* **120**:279–85.

Rittner, C. H., Hauptmann, G., Grosse-Wilde, H., Grosshans, E., Tongio, M. M., Mayr, S., 1975, Linkage between HL-A (major histocompatibility complex) and genes controlling the synthesis of the fourth component of complement, in: *Histocompatibility Testing 1975,* pp. 945–954, Munksgaard, Copenhagen.

Rosenberg, L. T., and Tachibana, D. K., 1969, On mouse complement: genetic variants, *J. Immunol.* **103**:1143–1148.

Ross, G. D., Palley, M. J., Rabellino, E. M., and Grey, H. M., 1973, Two different complement receptors on human lymphocytes. One inactivator cleaved C3b, *J. Exp. Med.* **138**:798–811.

Saunders. D., and Edidin, M., 1974, Sites of localization and synthesis of Ss protein in mice, *J. Immunol.* **112**:2210–8.

Shevach, E., Green, I., and Frank, M. M., 1975, Linkage of C4 deficiency to the major histocompatibility locus in the guinea pig (abstract), Sixth International Complement Workshop, Sarasota, Florida.

Shokeir, M. H., 1973, The genetics of hereditary angioedema: a hypothesis, *Clin. Genet.* **4**:494–499.

Shreffler, D. C., 1962, Serum protein types in X-irradiated mice treated with homologous hematopoietic tissues, *Transplant. Bull.* **30**:146–151.

Shreffler, D. C., and David, C. S., 1975, The H-2 major histocompatibility complex and the 1 immune response region: genetic variation, function and organization, *Adv. Immunol.* **20**:125–195.

Shreffler, D. C., and Owen, R. D., 1963, A serologically detected variant in mouse serum: inheritance and association with the histocompatibility-2 locus, *Genetics* **48**:9.

Silverstein, A. M., 1960, Hypercomplementemia: report of a case, *Blood* **16**:1338.

Snell, G. D., and Cherry, M., 1974, Haemagglutination and cytotoxic studies of H-2. IV. Evidence that there are 3-like antigenic sites determined by both the K and D crossover regions, *Folia Biol. Prague* **20** (2):81–100.

Sorensen, H., and Dissing, J., 1976, C3 polymorphism in relation to age, *Hum. Hered.* **25**:284.

Staub Nielsen, L., Jersild, C., Ryder, L. P., and Svejgaard, A., 1975, HL-A antigen, gene and haplotype frequencies in Denmark, *Tissue Antigens* **6**:70–76.

Teisberg, P., 1971a, The distribution of C3 types in Norway, *Hum. Hered.* **21**:154.

Teisberg, P., 1971b, The C3 types of Norwegian Lapps, *Hum. Hered.* **21**:162.

Teisberg, P., Olaisen, B., Gedde-Dahl, T., Jr., and Throsby, E., 1975, On the localization of the Gb locus within the MHS region of chromosome no. 6, *Tissue Antigens* **5**:257–261.

Thomsen, M., Jacobsen, B., Platz, P., Ryder, L. P., Staub Nielsen, L., and Svejgaard, A., 1975, LD typing, polymorphism of MLC determinants, in: *Histocompatibility Testing,* pp. 509–518, Munksgaard, Copenhagen.

Tweel, J. G., van den, Blusse, A., van, O. A., Keuning, J. J., Goulmy, E., Termijtelen, A., Bach, M. L., and Rood, J. J., van, 1973, Typing for MLC(LD) I. Lymphocytes from cousin marriage offspring as typing cells, *Transplant. Proc.* **5**:1535–1538.

Urbach, G., and Cinader, B., 1966, Hormonal control of MuB1 concentration, *Proc. Soc. Exp. Biol. Med.* **123**:779–782.

Van Leeuwen, A., Schuit, H. R. E., and Rood, J. J., van, 1973, Typing for MLC II. The selection of non-stimulator cells by MLC inhibition tests using SD identical stimulator cells (MISIS) and fluorescent antibody studies, *Transplant. Proc.* **5**:1539–1553.

Van Someren, H., Westerveld, A., Hagemeijer, A., Mees, J. R., Khan, P. M., and Zaalberg, O. B., 1974, Human antigen and enzyme markers in man–chinese hamster somatic cell hybrids: evidence for synteny between the HL-A, PGM_3, ME_1 and IPO-B loci, *Proc. Nat. Acad. Sci. U.S.A.* **71**:962–965.

Weitkamp, L. R., Lowien, E. W., Olaisen, B., Feuger, K., Gedde-Dohl, T., Jr., Sorensen, S. A., Conneally, P. M., Bias, W. B., and Ott, J., 1975, in: *Human Gene Mapping 2,* Rotterdam Conference (1974), p. 276, (D. Bergsma, ed.), S. Karger, Basel, Switzerland.

Wieme, R. J., and Demeulenaere, 1967, Genetically determined electrophoretic variant of the human complement component C3, *Nature (London)* **214**:1042–1043.

Winchester, R. J., Fu, S. M., Wernet, P., Kunkel, H. G., Dupont, B., and Jersild, C., 1975, Recognition by pregnancy serums of non-HL-A alloantigens selectively expressed on B-lymphocytes, *J. Exp. Med.* **141**:924–929.

Wolski, K. P., Schmid, F. R., and Mittal, K. K., 1975, Genetic linkage between the HL-A system and a deficit of the second component (C2) of complement, *Science* **188**:1020–22.

Ziegler, J. B., Watson, L., and Alper, C. A., 1975a, Genetic polymorphism of properdin factor B in the Rhesus: evidence for single subunit structure in primates, *J. Immunol.* **114**:1649–1653.

Ziegler, J. B., Alper, C. A., and Balner, H., 1975b, Properdin factor B and histocompatibility loci linked in the Rhesus monkey, *Nature (London)* **254**:609–610.

14

Complement in Cancer

ROBERT L. KASSEL, WILLIAM D. HARDY, JR., and
NOORBIBI K. DAY

1. Introduction

The concept of immunological surveillance as a major host defense against foreign cells has been used to explain both graft rejection and the recognition and elimination of cancer cells (Thomas, 1959; Burnett, 1970). Simply stated, this theory proposes that lymphocytes possess the ability to recognize and destroy cells of a foreign graft or cancer cells that are recognized as nonself by the host. The rapid development of this area of investigation into cancer immunology was so heavily weighted in the direction of cell-mediated immune reactions as to neglect the role of humoral immune parameters in the host response. Recent experiments have demonstrated that complement can play a limiting role in both graft rejection (Koene *et al.*, 1973) and tumor cell destruction (Old *et al.*, 1967; Kassel *et al.*, 1973). These results emphasize the need to reevaluate our present concepts of tumor immunology. This was done in a recent review by Nishioka (1976), who reiterates the need to take an overview of the entire immune system and the interplay of its component parts in the tumor–host relationship. Nishioka divides the immunological surveillance system into four segments: (1) the classical pathway of the complement system; (2) the C3 shunt or alternate pathway of complement; (3) the cell-mediated immunity (mainly lymphocytes) system; and (4) the immunoglobulin-mediated system. The stress placed on the role of the lymphocyte-mediated system in tumor immunology thus covers only one-fourth of the host defense mechanism, whereas the complement system works synergistically with those segments of the immune system involving immunoglobulins, lymphocytes, macrophages, granulocytes, erythrocytes, and platelets. Nishioka suggests a major role for C3 that may be activated by either classical or alternate pathways. The resultant formation of C3a

ROBERT L. KASSEL, WILLIAM HARDY, JR., and NOORBIBI K. DAY • Sloan-Kettering Institute for Cancer Research, New York, New York.

ROBERT L. KASSEL,
WILLIAM D. HARDY,
JR., AND NOORBIBI K.
DAY

and C3b (and possibly C5a and C5b) produces components that are capable of interacting to cause (1) immune adherence (Nishioka, 1967), (2) immune phagocytosis of antigen particles by macrophages and granulocytes (Nelson, 1953; Henson, 1971), (3) antibody production in T–B cell cooperation (Pepys, 1974), (4) antigen-induced lymphocyte transformation (Pepys and Butterworth, 1974), (5) complement-mediated immune cytolysis, and (6) lymphocyte-mediated cytotoxicity (Perlman and Hölm, 1969). Although Nishioka's hypothesis appears to overemphasize the central role of C3, his evidence supports the contention that the effectiveness of the immune system depends on a dynamic interplay of all its components.

It is now known that most neoplastic cells bear tumor-specific antigens. The demonstration of antigen–antibody complexes in the kidneys of tumor-bearing animals (Oldstone *et al.,* 1972; Pascal *et al.,* 1973; Markham *et al.,* 1972; Sutherland and Mardiney, 1973) suggests that circulating antigen–antibody complexes must also be present in these hosts. In experimental animals bearing tumors, changes in C levels have been reported by Harveit (1969) and Drake *et al.* (1973a,b). Increasing evidence in our laboratories indicates that hypocomplementemia occurs in patients with untreated operable cancer. The reason(s) for this is currently under investigation.

The purpose of this review is to present recent experimental data that strongly suggest an important role for complement as a participant in the phenomena of cancer growth and tumor-cell destruction. It will not consider the general field of cancer immunology, which has been reviewed most adequately by Old and Boyse (1973), Nishioka (1967, 1975), Alexander (1974), and Wilson *et al.* (1974).

2. Complement in Tumor-Bearing Animals

The demonstration that the incubation of lymphoma cells with specific antisera leads to a higher degree of cell destruction only if complement is present led Winn (1960) to state that "complement can become a limiting factor in immune reactions allowed to proceed *in vivo.* . . ." The role of complement as a limiting reagent was further demonstrated by Old *et al.* (1967), Negroni and Hunter (1973), Drake *et al.* (1973), Koene *et al.* (1973), and Harveit and Cater (1971). In each of the model systems studied, the addition of a complement source resulted in tumor-cell kill or graft rejection. Work by Old *et al.* (1967) demonstrated that tumors grow progressively even if the tumor cells are sensitized with alloantibody. However, injection of guinea pig serum to provide additional complement can bring about rapid and complete rejection of these otherwise fatal fibrosarcomas.

Reports by various investigators of changes in complement levels in the sera of tumor-bearing animals are presented below. The observations are conflicting and difficult to evaluate, since they originated in different laboratories and involved different assay systems, animal strains, and tumors.

Yoshida and Ito (1968) studied the effects of the growth of Shope papilloma, VX2 and VX7, on complement activity in domestic rabbits and reported a two- to threefold increase in total hemolytic complement levels 2 weeks after transplantation. The rise of C levels continued as tumor growth proceeded in the host, finally reaching a maximum of five- to eightfold the normal C level. In the Shope papilloma, no correlation was observed between the C level and induction, growth, or regression. These results were in agreement with the finding of a premortal rise in C levels in rats bearing Walker 256 carcinosarcoma (Weimer *et al.*, 1964).

The particular properties of mouse C, which was thought to have little activity *in vitro* (Amos, 1960), were probably responsible for the lack of intensive investigations into C changes during tumor induction and tumor growth in this species. Harveit (1969), using Ehrlich ascites and Bergen A4 ascites carcinoma in mice, studied C1 titers during tumor growth. Changes in C levels could not be determined with certainty in the first 7 days after tumor transplantation, but as tumor growth continued, there was a significant drop in C1 level with both tumor types, which either may be a reflection of a host immune response or may have resulted from a decreased C1 production. Harveit and Cater (1971), using the Ehrlich ascites tumor, implicated C as a mediator of the acute inflammatory response observed following the injection of these tumor cells.

Sizenko *et al.* (1972) reported that when DMBA was injected into rats, there was a rise in C levels during the period of carcinogenesis. As the tumor grew, the C levels fell to values below normal and ultimately to levels below the sensitivity of the assay system.

In three strains of mice (C57BL/6, BALB/c, and C3H/He), Drake *et al.* (1973a) measured both immune adherence and hemolytic activity as a function of time after intraperitoneal (i.p.) or subcutaneous (s.c.) injection of six transplantable tumors. The hemolytic data indicated that host complement activity was depressed in all mice following tumor transplantation. Immune adherence studies indicated that, in some instances, the reduction of hemolytic activity could not be attributed to depletion of the early C components. The authors suggested that these results, in contrast to those with the rabbit and the rat, may reflect a phenomenon related to transplantable tumors in the mouse.

Other studies (Drake *et al.*, 1973b; Drake and Mardiney, 1974) on C57BL/6 mice bearing either EL4 lymphoma or B16 melanoma showed that total complement levels were progressively depleted with the increase in tumor burden. Animals bearing EL4 lymphoma i.p. showed a rapid decrease in complement levels to zero 10 days after tumor induction (day 10) in mice with a mean survival time (MST) of 14 days. After s.c. transfer of EL4 or B16 melanoma, the decrease in complement levels was more gradual, being detectable at levels of 20–25% hemolysis on day 20 in animals with an MST of 23 days. These investigators were able to demonstrate that there was an actual decrease in C levels that was not due to the generation of C inhibitors. The i.p. injection of guinea pig complement (0.5 ml) into C57BL/6, AKR, or DBA/2 mice was found to raise C titers to a high level, with a maximum about 9 hr after the injection and little residual activity 15 hr after injection. The injection of anti-EL4 antiserum into mice bearing the EL4, 7-day-old tumors, caused a significant decrease in C levels, while the injection of anti-EL4 antiserum with C prolonged the survival of these animals. The authors point out the need to consider host C levels before attempting serotherapy.

Segerling *et al.* (1975; also cited in Chapter 1, Section 4.6) reported that two guinea pig hepatomas were more sensitive to killing by antibody and complement after treatment, *in vitro*, with chemotherapeutic drugs. The effect was dependent on drug dose, was reversible, and did not appear to be due to increased antigen expression or fixation of the early-acting components of guinea pig complement.

The authors suggest that the beneficial effects of various drugs in the treatment of cancer may be due, in part, to their ability to increase the susceptibility of tumor cells to killing by antibody and complement.

Currently, investigations are being carried out in our laboratories with the objective of developing complement component assays in sera of the mouse and the cat. Changes of C levels during tumor growth in both transplanted and spontaneous tumors will make it possible to understand the complement perturbations that occur as a cause or as a result of the neoplastic process.

3. Complement in AKR Leukemia

The importance of the complement system as an integral part of the body's defense mechanism stems from the study of both congenital and acquired deficiencies in man and in experimental animals (Lachmann, 1972, Day and Good, 1975; Day *et al.*, 1975a; Chapters 11 and 13). One strain of mice genetically deficient in the fifth component of complement, the AKR leukemia strain, has been used recently in experiments that have contributed to an understanding of the role of complement in the destruction of leukemia cells *in vivo* (Kassel *et al.*, 1973).

It was a widely held view that the AKR mouse is immunologically tolerant of the antigens associated with its indigenous leukemia virus (Old and Boyse, 1965). Although this conclusion was based on what appeared to be substantial evidence, we now know that the failure to detect antibody in the serum of infected mice does not exclude a specific immune response. Specific antibody can be demonstrated in the glomeruli of these infected mice, trapped there as antigen–antibody complexes (Mellors *et al.*, 1969; Oldstone *et al.*, 1972; Markham *et al.*, 1972; Pascal *et al.*, 1973). Southerland and Mardiney, 1973 have found similar kidney deposits in lymphomatous patients.

Studies by Graff *et al.* (1970), Kassel (1970), and Kassel *et al.* (1972) reported that there was a marked reduction of leukemia in AKR mice 24 hr after treatment with tissue-culture interferon. Extension of these studies (Kassel *et al.*, 1973) resulted in the observation that normal serum from a variety of species, including the mouse, mimics the effect of interferon. The evidence obtained points strongly to the fifth component of the complement system as the antileukemic factor in normal mouse serum.

Infusion of serum was necessary to effect leukemia cell destruction, which was not observed when serum was given as a single injection. AKR mice with advanced leukemia were infused with serum from Swiss mice or from mice of seven inbred strains possessing the complete spectrum of complement components (Swiss, C57BL/6, B10D2 new, and SJL/J) and those lacking C5 (AKR, A, B10D2 old, and DBA/2). The results of these infusions, measured as the percentage reduction in the size of inguinal, mesenteric, and cervical lymph nodes and spleen 24 hr after infusion, are shown in Figure 1. It is evident that serum from mouse strains with the full spectrum of components can cause reduction in the size of the lymph nodes and spleen, whereas the serum of C5-deficient mice was usually ineffective. The antileukemic activity was abolished by heating Swiss serum to 56°C for 30 min or by incubation with cobra venom factor (CVF) before infusion. The results following infusion of serum from horse, man, guinea pig, and C4-deficient guinea pig are shown in Figure 2. Nine complement components from guinea pig or human serum

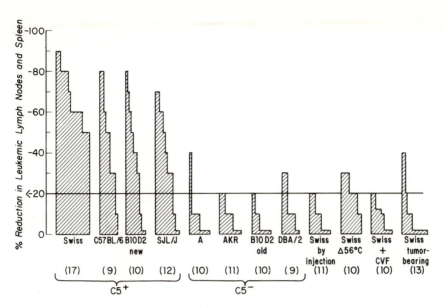

Figure 1. AKR leukemic mice infused with normal serum from C5⁺ and C5⁻ mouse strains. Mice evaluated at 24 hr postinfusion. Reduction greater than 20% considered significant. The numbers in parentheses are the numbers of leukemic mice tested. Results: C5⁺ mouse serum causes reduction in leukemic lymph nodes and spleens; C5⁻ mouse serum is inactive. The antileukemic factor in Swiss mouse serum is (1) not demonstrable by injection (in contrast to infusion), (2) heat-labile, (3) inactivated by CVF *in vitro,* and (4) reduced in tumor-bearing mice. Reprinted with permission from *The Journal of Experimental Medicine,* **138**(4):925–938 (Oct. 1, 1973).

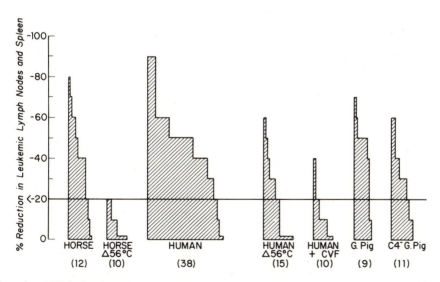

Figure 2. AKR leukemic mice infused with normal serum from heterologous species. The numbers in parentheses are the numbers of leukemic mice tested. Results: Horse, human, and guinea pig sera cause reduction in leukemic lymph nodes and spleen. The antileukemic factor is (1) heat-labile (horse and human sera) and (2) inactivated by CVF *in vitro* (human serum). Reprinted with permission from *The Journal of Experimental Medicine,* **138**(4):925–938 (Oct. 1, 1973).

ROBERT L. KASSEL,
WILLIAM D. HARDY,
JR., AND NOORBIBI K.
DAY

were tested individually for antileukemic activity by infusion in AKR leukemic mice receiving C5$^+$ serum showed varying degrees of lethargy, ruffled coat, and spleen. The eight other complement components were generally ineffective (Figure 3). Highly purified C5 preparations (courtesy of Dr. H. J. Müller-Eberhard) were active and C5 showed a dose-dependent antitumor activity over a range of 200 U/ mouse to 2000 U/mouse. Infusion of purified C5 was necessary to demonstrate the effect, and heating to 56°C for 30 min abolished the antileukemic activity.

The infusion of normal saline, C5-deficient mouse serum, or heat-inactivated homologous or heterologous serum was tolerated with little toxicity. In contrast, mice receiving C5$^+$ serum showed varying degrees of lethargy, ruffled coat, and decreased food intake during the 12–24 hr postinfusion period. Within 24–36 hr, all toxicity associated with serum infusion disappeared. By the fifth day postinfusion, a resurgence of the disease was observed in most leukemic mice.

Recently we have observed that plasma obtained from heparinized C5$^+$ mice has about 4 times the activity of serum obtained from mice of the same age, sex, and strain. Heparinized C5$^-$ plasma has no antileukemic effect, suggesting that heparin is not acting on the tumor cells, but may enhance activity by preventing loss of C components. Plasma prepared with ACD has no activity, and heparinized plasma loses its antileukemic activity if once frozen and thawed. We are attempting to correlate the changes in activity with changes in the complement profiles in plasma. The antileukemic effects of C5 are further reinforced by the observation that the C58 leukemic mouse (C5$^+$) is not affected by similar infusions.

Thus, the infusion of normal serum from homologous or heterologous sources leads to the rapid destruction of leukemia cells. That this observation is made in mice with spontaneously developing disease rather than a transplanted leukemia

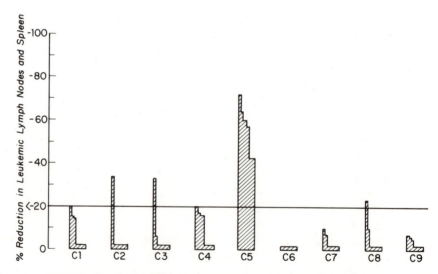

Figure 3. AKR leukemic mice infused with complement components from guinea pig serum and from human serum. Each of the complement components was tested in 4 AKR leukemic mice. The findings for individual components from the two species were identical and were therefore plotted together. Results: C5 is the antileukemic complement component in normal guinea pig and human serum. Reprinted with permission from *The Journal of Experimental Medicine* **138**(4):925–938 (Oct. 1, 1973).

adds considerable significance to its possible clinical application. Prolonged infusion is critical in demonstrating the effect. Comparable amounts of serum given by rapid injection rather than by infusion were inactive, which is a likely reason why the phenomenon has not been observed previously.

At present, the evidence points to a component of the complement system as the antileukemic factor. The evidence is as follows: (1) CVF abolishes the antileukemic effect of normal serum. CVF depletes complement by activating C3, initiating the step-by-step consumption of C3–C9 (Müller-Eberhard and Fjellstrom, 1971). (2) Leukemia cell destruction was induced by serum from four mouse strains, possessing all components of the complement system, but not by serum from four strains of mice with a genetically determined deficiency of C5. (3) Fractions rich in C5 from both human and guinea pig sera showed antileukemic activity, whereas other C fractions (C1-4 and 6–9) had no effect. (4) C58 mice (C5$^+$) with leukemia do not show any leukemia cell destruction following infusions of heparinized Swiss mouse plasma, which is very active in destroying AKR leukemia cells.

The mode of action of C5 appears to be a direct effect on the leukemia cells by providing the missing complement link, which allows cytotoxic antibody produced by the host to cause cell lysis. This may not be surprising, since AKR mice are genetically C5 deficient (Cinader *et al.*, 1964; Erickson *et al.*, 1964; Nilsson and Müller-Eberhard, 1967). Apparently, the mouse is limited in its capacity to generate sufficient C when called upon to reject large numbers of tumor cells. A number of previous studies have suggested that complement may act as a limiting factor in both tumor and skin graft rejection (Kalfayan and Kidd, 1953—Brown-Pearce tumors; Old *et al.*, 1967—mouse ascites sarcoma; Koene *et al.*, 1973—skin graft rejection; Negroni and Hunter, 1973—polyoma-induced neoplasms; Drake *et al.*, 1973—EL4). Thus, complement deficiency (whether relative or absolute) can be viewed as a mechanism whereby tumor cells escape the consequences of their antigenicity. In this regard, reduced levels of complement have been found in the sera of tumor-bearing mice (Harveit, 1969; Drake *et al.*, 1973a,b; Drake and Mardiney, 1974). The possibilities that C5 may react at some other site (causing the release of other biological mediators of leukemia cell destruction) or that C5 acts in a manner independent of a preexisting immune response have not been totally eliminated. We are, at present, attempting to identify C5 receptor sites on the surface of leukemic cells.

4. Feline and Canine Lymphosarcomas (Leukemias)

4.1. Feline Lymphosarcoma

Lymphosarcoma (LSA) is the term commonly used to describe lymphoid tumors in the cat originating from the lymphocytes. The cat is particularly susceptible to LSA, having the highest incidence of naturally occurring lymphoreticular malignancies of any animal (Dorn *et al.*, 1967). LSA accounts for one-third of all feline neoplasms and for 90% of all feline hematopoietic malignancies (Engle and Brodey, 1969).

The domestic cat is an excellent model for the study of viral carcinogenesis in man, since, like man, the cat is an outbred species living in its natural environment (Hardy, 1971). Moreover, feline LSA is known to be caused by an oncornavirus, the

ROBERT L. KASSEL,
WILLIAM D. HARDY,
JR., AND NOORBIBI K.
DAY

feline leukemia virus (FeLV) (Jarrett et al., 1964). FeLV can cause both neoplastic and nonneoplastic diseases in pet cats. The virus has been shown to cause LSA, nonregenerative anemia, thymic atrophy, and a panleukopenia-like syndrome (Hardy et al., 1973a,b). It is also associated with various myeloproliferative disorders and some fetal abortion and resorption syndromes (Hardy and McClelland, 1974; Herz et al., 1970). LSA is a rapidly fatal disease and is not usually treated, because most cats with LSA are infected with FeLV, which will remain even after therapeutic reduction of the disease (Hardy, 1974). Thus, cats in clinical remission could act as carriers and spread the virus to other cats.

FeLV is transmitted from one cat to another by contagion or infection (horizontally) (Hardy et al., 1973b). It is present in the blood, urine, and saliva of infected cats and thus may be transmitted to other cats by licking, biting, and through the use of communal litter pans or possibly by bloodsucking insects. Healthy, uninfected cats living with an FeLV infected cat(s) are susceptible to FeLV infection and have a 35% chance of being infected with FeLV. Once infected, healthy cats have a greatly increased chance of developing LSA (888 times) and the other diseases caused by the virus. The period of disease development is variable, and some cats may not die of disease for 3 years or longer (Hardy et al., 1973b). Those infected cats that are able to develop antibodies to the feline oncornavirus-associated cell-membrane antigen are healthy carriers of FeLV and are a constant source of infection for susceptible cats.

Investigations into the antileukemic effects of normal mouse serum (Kassel et al., 1973) have been extended to cats with naturally occurring LSA. In order to determine whether interferon was responsible for antileukemic activity in the cat, both interferon-containing normal cat serum and normal cat serum (NCS) without interferon were tested for oncolytic activity. Cat serum containing 30,000–70,000 U interferon was prepared by injecting Newcastle disease virus intravenously into cats and harvesting the serum 6 hr later. NCS was obtained by cardiac puncture of healthy stray cats. Cats with LSA brought to our clinics for treatment were given either NCS containing interferon or NCS containing no interferon. It was found that NCS containing no interferon was as effective as interferon containing NCS in causing disease regression. Thus, it appears that interferon is not responsible for the oncolytic activity of NCS. In order to investigate the phenomenon of serum-mediated cancer-cell destruction, further experiments using other blood constituents, in addition to NCS, were begun.

Cats with naturally occurring LSA were treated with the following blood constituents (BC): (1) normal cat serum (NCS), (2) heat-inactivated NCS, (3) CVF-inactivated NCS, (4) whole feline blood, (5) fresh and stored (frozen) plasma, and (6) leukemic cat serum (Table 1). It was found that the phenomenon of serum-mediated leukemic cell destruction was not limited to the mouse. Of the 9 cats with LSA treated with NCS (100 cc NCS/cat diluted in 100 cc phosphate-buffered saline, PBS), 5 had complete regressions (see Figure 4), 3 had partial regressions, and only 1 cat had no disease regression at all. Leukemic cat serum, however, was unable to produce any disease regression in 3 cats and, in fact, made the disease worse in 2 of the cats. Seven cats were treated with whole feline blood (50–100 cc/cat given IV), which was found to be as effective as NCS in controlling the disease, but normal, frozen, stored cat plasma (20–50 cc/cat) was not as effective as either serum or whole blood in the two evaluable cases treated. To date, 4 cats have been given low

TABLE 1. Treatment of Feline Lymphosarcoma with Feline Blood Constituents

Blood constituent treatment	Number of cats treated	Response			FeLV status
		Complete regression	Partial regression	No response	
Normal cat serum	9	5	3	1	All positive
Heat-inactivated[a]	6	4	2	0	All positive
CVF-treated[b]	4	0	3	1	All positive
Normal cat plasma					
Frozen[c]	2	0	1	1	All positive
Fresh[d]					
Low dose	4	0	0	4	All positive
High dose	6	2	1	3	All positive
Whole blood	7	5	1	1	6 positive
					1 FeLV negative[e]
Leukemic cat serum	3	0	0	3[f]	All positive

[a] Heat inactivation: 56°C for 1 hr.
[b] Cobra venom factor (CVF)–treated: 0.1 ml CVF/100 ml normal cat serum incubated at 37°C for 1 hr.
[c] Frozen plasma: frozen at 70°C before administration.
[d] Plasma given fresh—not frozen.
[e] This FeLV negative cat with lymphosarcoma has been in complete regression for the past 6 months.
[f] Two of the cats showed worsening of disease.

doses of fresh feline plasma (10–15 cc/cat) and none has responded. This may have been due to the small dose of plasma, since 2 of 6 cats given high doses of fresh feline plasma (50 cc/cat) responded well, while 1 cat had a partial disease regression, and 3 cats did not respond. We have found differences between the antileukemic activity of cat and mouse sera. For instance, of 6 cats treated with feline serum, which had been heated at 56°C for 60 min to destroy the heat-labile complement components, 4 cats had complete disease regressions and 2 had partial regressions. Also, 4 cats were treated with CVF inactivated NCS, and although there was no response in 1 cat, 3 cats had partial disease regressions. In contrast, heated or CVF-inactivated mouse serum was completely ineffective when given to leukemic AKR mice. The reason for the differences in the response to this treatment in the two species is currently under investigation.

All except 1 cat died within 3 months of blood-constituent therapy (BCT), including those with complete disease regressions. The cause of death in these cases was difficult to determine. In the cats that had no response to BCT, death was usually due to progressive disease. In the cats with complete disease regression, death may have been due to an intravascular coagulation syndrome caused by the large quantities of serum or, possibly, in some cases, to progressive anemia caused by FeLV. The actual cause of death is still uncertain, and studies are in progress to discover why these responding cats died after BCT and how this can be avoided in the future.

4.2. Canine Lymphosarcoma

Lymphosarcoma is the most common lymphoreticular malignancy and is the fourth most common cancer in dogs, accounting for 5–7% of all canine tumors. The

ROBERT L. KASSEL,
WILLIAM D. HARDY,
JR., AND NOORBIBI K.
DAY

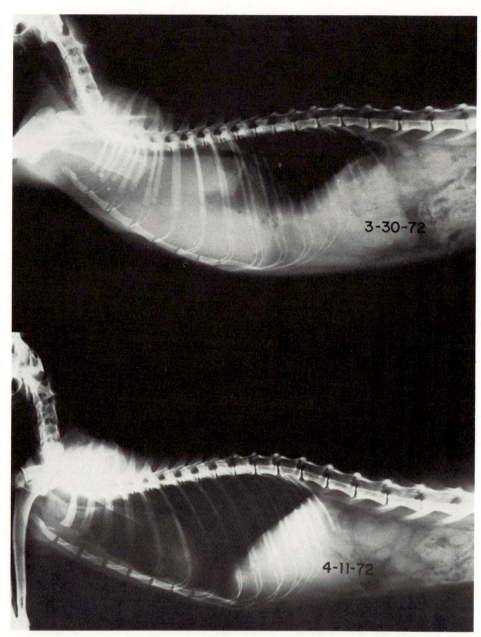

Figure 4.   Radiographs of a cat with advanced lymphosarcoma treated with interferon-containing cat serum, taken: (3-30-72) before treatment, showing extensive obliteration of the thoracic cavity by a lymphoma: (4-11-72) 12 days later, after 5 days of treatment; the chest mass has almost totally disappeared, Reprinted with permission from *The Harvey Lectures Series* **67**:273–315 (1973).

annual incidence is 24 cases for every 100,000 dogs in the population at risk. Both sexes are equally susceptible to LSA, but there is an increased disease incidence in dogs over 5 years of age (Hardy, 1974). There is no known single cause of canine LSA, and many factors are probably involved. Unlike feline LSA, no evidence of a viral involvement has been obtained, and there have been no reports of clustering of cases. However, experiments have shown that canine LSA can be induced in newborn puppies by FeLV.

Limited data on the biological behavior of canine LSA are available. The median survival time for 33 untreated dogs with LSA, as calculated from the time of histological diagnosis to the time of death, was 22 days (Bloom and Meyer, 1945; Brick et al., 1968; Moldovanu et al., 1966; Backgren, 1965; Hardy and Old, 1970; Hardy et al., unpublished results). Thus, once diagnosed, canine LSA appears to be a rapidly fatal disease. There have been several studies into the effectiveness of different forms of chemotherapy for canine LSA (Hardy et al., unpublished data; Squire et al., 1973; Theilen and Worley, 1974). The limited trials using different chemotherapeutic agents and protocols have not yielded conclusive results, since staging of disease and randomization of patients for comparative studies were not adequately controlled. However, some dogs have been kept in remission for extended periods with chemotherapy, although most have eventually come out of remission and died of the disease. The longest average remission time obtained to date is 184 days (Squire et al., 1973). The effectiveness of another therapeutic agent, the enzyme L-asparaginase, has been studied in 29 dogs with LSA (Hardy and Old, 1970). Of these dogs, 55% went into remission with a median remission time of 59 days and a median survival time of 158 days. Whole-body radiation therapy is clinically impracticable and does not appear to be any more effective than chemotherapy (Johnson et al., 1969). Thus, the best that can currently be achieved by therapy is some prolongation of life.

Dogs with naturally occurring LSA were treated with normal frozen dog serum, whole fresh blood, and fresh plasma at both high and low doses (Table 2). The one dog that was given frozen serum showed no response, but survived only 3 days and received only two treatments; it was therefore not considered an evaluable case. However, of the 4 dogs given fresh whole canine blood, 1 showed an 80% regression of disease, 1 had a 60% regression, and the other 2 had a 30–50% disease regression. None of the 4 dogs given fresh canine plasma at low dosages (1–3 cc/lb) had disease regressions, but of the 4 dogs given fresh plasma at higher dosages (3.9–9 cc/lb), 2 had complete (100%) disease regressions, 1 had a 75% regression, and 1 showed a 40% response. These investigations into the response of canine LSA to

TABLE 2. Treatment of Canine Lymphosarcoma with Canine Blood Constituents

Blood constituent treatment	Number of dogs treated	Response		
		Complete regression	Partial regression	No response
Fresh plasma				
Low dose	4	0	0	4
High dose	4	2	2	0
Whole blood	4	0	4	0

ROBERT L. KASSEL,
WILLIAM D. HARDY,
JR., AND NOORBIBI K.
DAY

normal blood constituents are continuing in order to determine whether there are differences in the response of canine and feline LSA to the various blood constituents.

5. Complement Levels in Human Cancer

Increased C levels in the sera of patients with Hodgkin's disease and other malignant lymphomas have been reported (Schier *et al.*, 1956; Rottino and Levy, 1959; Hamladji *et al.*, 1972). An increase of C3 (Masi and Vivarelli, 1971a,b; Masi *et al.*, 1973) was observed in sera of children with acute lymphatic leukemia (ALL) and Hodgkin's disease during the active phase. Lower but not normal levels were observed during remission. Southam and Siegel (1966) observed slight increases in the level of C2 in sera of some cancer patients, which they considered to be insignificant. Zarco *et al.* (1964) and McKenzie *et al.* (1967) used the immune adherence and immune hemolysis tests to evaluate changes in C levels in sera of cancer patients. Higher titers than normal were observed during active disease. In further analyses of the nine C components, it was found that the elevated C levels were due to an increase of C8 and C9. High levels of total C observed by Wohl and Ghossein (1971) remained unchanged following radiotherapy.

In contrast to the consistently high C values described in the preceding reports, Nelson (1963) and Yoshikawa *et al.* (1969) found a wide variation of high to low C levels in sera of patients with ALL, especially during exacerbation of a trend toward normal levels during the stage of remission. Low total C levels in leukemic sera obtained from children (Kubiková-Kouřilová, and Běluša, 1970) and low C3 levels were found in Hodgkin's disease, CLL, and in 71 patients with malignant diseases of the lymphoid cell series with a tendency to return to normal values during remission (Meier and Grob, 1972). Lokhatjuk *et al.* (1974) reported reduced levels of properdin and C in 105 patients with gastric cancer. Recently, Caldwell *et al.* (1972—2 patients), Hauptman *et al.* (1974—1 patient) reported an unusual C profile in patients with lymphosarcoma. C1, C4, C2, and functional C1-INH were diminished. The investigators (Caldwell *et al.*, 1972) felt that the C1-INH deficiency was acquired, most likely as a result of its interaction with C1.

Irie *et al.* (1975) used mixed hemadsorption techniques to demonstrate antibody and complement fixed *in vivo* to the surface of human cancer cells. Positive reactions ranging from 10 to 34% of cells were found on the surface of tumors from 12 cancer patients, while normal tissues from cancer patients or patients with other diseases rarely exhibited distinct mixed hemadsorption reactivity.

Our laboratories have conducted a survey of 5000 cancer patients for total hemolytic complement C1q and C3 levels. Approximately one-third of the patients were found to have either low C, low C1q, or low C3. The correlation of the low C levels with stage of disease, therapy, and/or infections are currently under investigation. One patient with untreated CLL has been studied in greater detail (Day *et al.*, 1975b). Unmeasurable hemolytic C was observed in the serum of a patient with untreated CLL and recurrent nonhereditary angioedema. Immunochemical analysis of C components demonstrated a marked reduction of C1q and C1s inhibitor, undetectable C1s, and elevated B. Hemolytic C1, C4, and C2 were only 5% of normal levels. The levels of C components C3–C9 were normal. Functional C1s inhibitor was unmeasurable. A C1q precipitin and a cryoglobulin were present in the serum; the latter was shown not to be responsible through *in vivo* precipitation for the observed C depletion. A cold-reactive IgM antilymphocyte antibody, determined by both C dependent cytotoxicity and indirect immunofluorescence, exhibited specificities for both autologous lymphocytes and lymphocytes from normal donors. Cytotoxic activity for autologous leukemic cells was removed by absorption with normal isologous tonsil lymphocytes. Specific enrichment of this antibody, relative to the serum level, was demonstrated in the serum by gel diffusion using specific rabbit antilymphocyte antiserum. These data suggest the presence of pathogenetically significant complexes of lymphocyte antigen and specific antibody in certain patients with CLL. We have extended this observation to a study of the sera of patients with various forms of malignancies and have observed C1q binding substances in the sera of a number of cancer patients. Two methods have been used: (1) the modified agar diffusion by Agnello *et al.* (1970) and (2) the C1q deviation test of Sobel *et al.* (1975). The significance and identification of these reactants are currently under investigation.

6. Complement and Therapy

Much of our knowledge of cancer in man will be derived from extensive studies of cancer in animals. The antileukemic effects of serum, whole blood, or heparinized plasma in the mouse, cat, and dog suggest that a similar mechanism for leukemia cell destruction may occur in man, which could explain the rare but undeniable improvement reported after blood transfusion in some patients with leukemia. Extensive clinical trials of exsanguino-transfusion in leukemia patients by Bessis (1949) were "based on the hypothesis that there is an antileukemic substance in normal blood." This hypothesis predated the major developments of modern immunology and may have anticipated the role of tumor-specific antibodies and/or complement in tumor-cell destruction or the antitumor activity of activated "T" cells. Bessis reported that in 38 patients with leukemia treated by repeated exsanguino-transfusion, total or partial remissions were not at all rare. In the 20 children and 18 adults treated, the following results were reported: (1) the general condition was immediately improved in all cases; (2) in 30 cases, there was a clinical remission consisting of the disappearance of adenopathy, hepatosplenomegaly, temperature, pain, and bleeding; (3) in 15 cases, the clinical remission was accompanied by normalization of the blood, and in 6 of these, there was complete clinical, blood, and marrow remission. The remission generally lasted 3 weeks to 3½ months; however, only 2 of these 38 were alive and in remission after 11 months.

Several technical points were raised in the Bessis report that may have some bearing on recent experimental observations in our laboratories. Although the initial Bessis' treatment involved the use of fresh citrated blood, the technique was modified by the use of heparin. It is interesting that fresh, heparinized plasma was used by Bessis in patients with leukemia over 25 years before it was found to be active in the mouse, cat, and dog. Although the use of heparin seems to be a minor technical change, it may prove to be of critical importance in any clinical attempt at complement replacement therapy.

The first case of leukemia reported by Bessis is quoted directly (with permission, from *Blood* 4:324–337, 1949), since it bears comparison with some recent observations.

ROBERT L. KASSEL,
WILLIAM D. HARDY,
JR., AND NOORBIBI K.
DAY

The first case treated was a dying leukemic child of 6 years of age. He was suffering from acute leukemia which presented a complete clinical picture of the disease: high temperature, gingival lesions, bleeding, hepatosplenomegaly, generalized adenopathy, a clear-cut hemotologic picture of low RBC, absent platelets, 86,000 WBC, 98% lymphoblasts and a marrow of 99% lymphoblasts. The replacement transfusions were started when the patient was moribund. Seven liters were transfused. In a few days the clinical condition of the patient was completely changed and the symptoms disappeared rapidly. The blood and marrow returned to normal in 3 weeks. However, this patient later relapsed, and the results of replacement transfusions were less marked. An osteosarcoma of the femur appeared and the patient died.

In 1975, Kochen *et al.* reported an unusual response in a patient with acute lymphatic leukemia (ALL) in relapse, who experienced a precipitous decrease in leukocyte count after each infusion of plasma from a healthy, multiparous female donor with no history of disease or previous transfusion. The patient was a 9-year-old boy with typical ALL (1972) in whom remission was induced and maintained with conventional chemotherapy. Relapse occurred in June, 1974, and for the next 2 months the patient showed little response to drugs. The family requested that he receive no further chemotherapy, and 5 weeks later he was hospitalized in acute relapse with WBC greater than 120,000/mm^3. Because of continuing epistaxis, he was infused with platelet concentrates (platelet-rich plasma, 500 ml) from ten unrelated donors, and in the next 5 days, his WBC decreased to 8500/mm^3 with marked clinical improvement. Serum from one of the donors was found to be cytotoxic to the patient's lymphoblasts but not to his parents' lymphocytes. The patient was given a total of 12 infusions of this plasma during the next 50 days and on three other occasions, his WBC of greater than 100,000 fell precipitously, although the blood was never free of blast cells. For several days, his WBC remained at a low level following daily infusions of 50 ml of plasma from the same donor. The child died of massive bleeding after platelet infusions became ineffective.

The specific role of cytotoxic antibody and complement in this antileukemic response has not been clearly defined, but both are being investigated in this donor's plasma at the present time. If Bessis and Kochen were observing the same phenomenon, then a major role for the cellular elements included in the exsanguinotransfusion technique (e.g., allogeneic lymphocytes that might stimulate an immune response) has been eliminated. During the intervening period of time, immunological techniques have been extensively developed, and an understanding of the interplay of many of the parameters of the immune response is beginning to emerge. The unexpected response to transfusion in a few leukemic patients may be a reflection of the immune response that is going on in the host, and closer examination of the donor contribution might reveal the immunologic deficit that prevents the host from destroying the neoplastic growth. It is time that we use the most advanced techniques available in the armamentarium of the immunologist to evaluate these dramatic responses to "normal" blood or plasma therapy. It is time to examine again, in the light of modern immunology, the Bessis hypothesis that "there is an antileukemic substance in normal blood."

7. Conclusion

The results we have summarized strongly suggest the need for a re-evaluation of dogma minimizing the role of humoral effectors in the restriction of tumor growth and/or tumor-cell destruction. The mechanisms proposed to explain how cancer cells escape immunological inhibition range from simple outpacing of immune responses to the shedding of tumor antigens. The plasma-mediated leukemia cell destruction observed in AKR leukemic mice and lymphomatous cats and dogs has led us to consider that complement, rather than specific antibody, may be a crucial limiting factor in the immune destruction of tumor cells. This suggestion is reinforced by the large number of deficits in total complement and/or individual complement in our survey of 5000 cancer patients. The central role of complement in the delicate interplay of all sectors of the immune system should lead us to place greater emphasis on the interdependence of the components in the total picture of host immunity. The potential use of plasma as another modality in the immunotherapy of cancer makes continued investigation of the role of complement imperative.

References

Agnello, V., Winchester, R. J., and Kunkel, H. G., 1970, Precipitin reactions of the C1q component of complement with aggregated gammaglobulin and immune complexes in gel diffusion, *Immunology* **19**:909–919.

Alexander, P., 1974, Escape from immune destruction by the host through shedding of surface antigens: is this a characteristic shared by malignant and embryonic cells?, *Cancer Res.* **34**:2077–2082.

Amos, B. D., 1960, Possible relationships between the cytotoxic effects of isoantibody and host cell function, *Ann. N.Y. Acad. Sci.* **87**:273–292.

Backgren, A. W., 1965, Lymphatic leukosis in dogs, *Acta Vet. Scand.* **6**(Suppl.): 1–80.

Bessis, M., 1949, The use of replacement transfusion in diseases other than hemolytic disease of the newborn, *Blood* **4**:324–337.

Bloom, F., and Meyer, G. M., 1945, Malignant lymphoma (so-called leukemia) in dogs, *Amer. J. Pathol.* **21**:683–715.

Brick, J. O., Roenigk, W. J., and Wilson, G. P., 1968, Chemotherapy of malignant lymphoma in dogs and cats, *J. Amer. Vet. Med. Assoc.* **153**:47–52.

Burnet, F. M., 1970, The concept of immunological surveillance, *Prog. Exp. Tumor Res.* **13**:1–27.

Caldwell, J. R., Ruddy, S., Schur, P. H., and Austen, K. F., 1972, Acquired CT inhibitor deficiency in lymphosarcoma, *Clin. Immunol. Immunopathol.* **1**:39–52.

Cinader, B., Dubinski, S., and Wardlaw, A. C., 1964, Distribution, inheritance and properties of an antigen, MuB1, and its relation to hemolytic complement, *J. Exp. Med.* **120**:897–924.

Day, N. K., and Good, R. A., 1975, Deficiencies of the complement system in man, in: *Immunodeficiency in Man and Animals* (D. Bergsma, R. A. Good, J. Finstad, and N. W. Paul, eds.), p. 306, Sinauer Associates, Sunderland, Massachusetts.

Day, N. K., Geiger, H., and Good, R. A., 1975a, Complement, in: *Molecular Pathology* (R. A. Good, S. B. Day, and J. J. Yunis, eds.), p. 115, Charles C Thomas, Springfield, Illinois.

Day, N. K., Winfield, J. B., Winchester, R. J., Gee, T. S., and Kunkel, H. G., 1975b, Evidence for immune complexes involving antilymphocyte antibodies associated with hypocomplementemia in chronic lymphocytic leukemia (CLL), *Clin. Res.* **23**:289a.

Dorn, C. R. Taylor, D. O. N., and Hubbard, H. H., 1967, Epizootiologic characteristics of canine and feline leukemia and lymphosarcoma, *Amer. J. Vet. Res.* **28**:993–1001.

Drake, W. P., and Mardiney, M. R., Jr., 1974, Parameters of serum complement in relation to tumor therapy, *Biomedicine* **21**:206–209.

Drake, W. P., LeGendre, S. M., and Mardiney, M. R., Jr., 1973, Depression of complement activity in three strains of mice after tumor transfer, *Int. J. Cancer* **11**:719–724.

Drake, W. P., Ungaro, P. C., and Mardiney, M. R., Jr., 1973a, Passive administration of antiserum and complement in producing anti-EL4 cytotoxic activity in the serum of C57BL/6 mice, *J. Nat. Cancer Inst.* **50**:909–914.

Drake, W. P., Ungaro, P. C., and Mardiney, M. R., Jr., 1973b, The measurement and manipulation of hemolytic complement levels in tumor bearing C57BL/6 mice, *Biomedicine* **18**:284–289.

Engle, G. C., and Brodey, R. S., 1969, A retrospective study of 395 feline neoplasms, *Anim. Hosp.* **5**:21–23.

Erickson, R. P., Tachibana, D. K., Herzenberg, L. A., and Rosenberg, L. T., 1964, A single gene controlling hemolytic complement and a serum antigen in the mouse, *J. Immunol.* **92**:611–615.

Graff, S., Kassel, R., and Kastner, O., 1970, Interferon, *Trans. N.Y. Acad. Sci.* **32**:545–556.

Hamladji, R. M., Belhani, M., Irunberry, J., and Colonna, P., 1972, Serum complement level in Hodgkin's disease, *Nouv. Rev. Fr. Hematol.* **12**:673–682.

Hardy, W. D., Jr., 1971, Feline lymphosarcoma: a model of viral carcinogenesis and significance related to human neoplasia, *Anim. Models Biomed. Res.* **IV**:11–26.

Hardy, W. D., Jr., Management of lymphosarcoma, in: *Current Veterinary Therapy V* (R. W. Kirk, ed.), pp. 381–387, W. B. Saunders Co., Philadelphia.

Hardy, W. D., Jr., and McClelland, A. J., 1974, Feline oncornaviruses, in: *Handbook of Laboratory Animal Science II* (E. C. Melby, Jr., and N. H. Altman, eds.), pp. 12–21, CRC Press, Cleveland.

Hardy, W. D., Jr., and Old, L. J., 1970, L-Asparaginase in the treatment of neoplastic diseases of the dog, cat and cow, *Recent Results Cancer Res.* **33**:131–139.

Hardy, W. D., Jr., Hirshaut, Y., and Hess, P., 1973a, Detection of the feline leukemia virus and other mammalian oncornaviruses by immunofluorescence, in: *Unifying Concepts of Leukemia* (R. M. Dutcher and L. Chieco-Bianchi, eds.), pp. 778–799, S. Karger, Basel.

Hardy, W. D., Jr., Old, L. J., Hess, P. W., Essex, M., and Cotter, S. M., 1973b, Horizontal transmission of feline leukemia virus, *Nature London* **244**:266–269.

Harveit, F., 1969, The complement content of the serum of normal as opposed to tumour-bearing mice, *Br. J. Cancer* **18**:714–720.

Harveit, F., and Cater, D. B., 1971, Interaction of transplants of the Ehrlich carcinoma. Lack of local reaction to subcutaneous transplants in the presence of late intraperitoneal tumour, *Acta Pathol. Microbiol. Scand. Sect. A* **79**:423–431.

Hauptman, G., Grosshans, E., and Heide, E., 1974, Systemic lupus erythematosus and hereditary complement deficiencies. A case with total C4 deficiency, *Ann. Dermatol. Syphiligr.* **101**:479–496.

Henson, P. M., 1971, The immulogic release of constituents from neutrophile leukocytes. I. The role of antibody and complement on non-phagocytable surfaces or phagocytable particles, *J. Immunol.* **107**:1535–1546.

Herz, A., Theilen, G. H., Schalm, O. W., and Munn, R. J., 1970, C-type virus in bone marrow cells of cats with myeloproliferative disorders, *J. Nat. Cancer Inst.* **44**:339–348.

Irie, K., Irie, R. F., and Morton, D. L., 1975, Detection of antibody and complement complexed *in vivo* on membranes of human cancer cells by mixed hemadsorption techniques, *Cancer Res.* **35**:1244–1248.

Jarrett, W. F. H., Crawford, L. M., Martin, W. B., and David, F., 1964, A virus-like particle associated with leukemia (lymphosarcoma), *Nature (London)* **202**:567–569.

Johnson, R. E., Cameron, T. P., and Kincaid, R., 1969, Total body irradiation of canine lymphoma, *Radiat. Res.* **36**:629–632.

Kalfayan, B., and Kidd, J. G., 1953, Structural changes produced in Brown-Pearce carcinoma cells by means of a specific antibody and complement, *J. Exp. Med.* **97**:145–163.

Kassel, R. L., 1970, Carcinolytic effects of interferon, *Clin. Obstet. Gynecol.* **13**:910–927.

Kassel, R. L., Pascal, R. R., and Vas, A., 1972, Interferon-mediated oncolysis in spontaneous murine leukemia, *J. Nat. Cancer Inst.* **48**:1155–1159.

Kassel, R. L., Old, L. J., Carswell, E. A., Fiore, N. C., and Hardy, W. D., Jr., 1973, Serum-mediated leukemia cell destruction in AKR mice, *J. Exp. Med.* **138**:925–938.

Kochen, J., Radel, E., and Nathenson, G., 1975, Transfusion-induced partial remission in acute leukemia, *Pediatr. Res.* **9**:792.

Koene, R. A. P., Gerlag, P. G. G., Hagemann, F. H. M., van Haelst, U. J. G., and Wijdeveld, P. G. A. B., 1973, Hyperacute rejection of skin allografts in the mouse by the administration of alloantibody and rabbit complement, *J. Immunol.* **111**:520–526.

Kubiková-Kouřilová, A., and Běluša, M., 1970, Isohaemagglutinin anti-A and anti-B, and serum complement levels in children with leukemia, *Acta Paediatr. Acad. Sci. Hung.* **11**:319–322.

Lachmann, P. J., 1972, Genetic deficiencies of the complement system, in: *Ontogeny of Acquired Immunity* (R. Porter and J. Knight, eds.) pp. 193–208, Associated Scientific Publishers, Amsterdam.

Lokhatjuk, A. S., Smoljyaninov, E. S., Kazantsev, N. P., and Nemirovskaya, L. Ya., 1974, The properdin and complement activity in patients with gastric cancer, *Questions Oncol.* **XX**:22–25.

Markham, R. V., Sutherland, J. C., Cimino, E. F., Drake, W. P., and Mardiney, M. R., 1972, Immune complexes localized in the renal glomeruli of AKR mice: the presence of MuLV gs-1 and C-type RNA tumor virus gs-3 determinants, *Rev. Eur. Étud. Clin. Biol.* **XVII**:690–694.

Masi, M., and Vivarelli, F., 1971a, I livelli sierici C'3 (β-1-c/β-1-a globulina) in corso di leucosi linfoblastica dell' infanizia, *Clin. Paediatr.* **53**:175–182.

Masi, M., and Vivarelli, F., 1971b, I livelli sierica di C'3 (β-1-c/β-1-a globulina) in corso di linfogranuloma maligno dell' infanzia, *Clin. Paediatr.* **53**:201–207.

Masi, M., Vivarelli, F., and Vecchi, V., 1973, Serum C3 levels in normal and diseased children, *Minerva Pediatr.* **23**:731–735.

McKenzie, D., Colsky, J., and Hetrick, D. L., 1967, Complement reactivity of cancer patients: measurements by immune hemolysis and immune adherence, *Cancer Res.* **27**:2386–2394.

Meier, E. C., and Grob, P. J., 1972, Determination of β1 c/a (complement factor 3) in malignant lymphoma, myeloma and Waldenström's disease, *Dtsch. Med. Wochenschr.* **97**:967–971.

Mellors, R. C., Aoki, T., and Huebner, R. J., 1969, Further implication of murine leukemia-like virus in the disorders of NZB mice, *J. Exp. Med.* **129**:1045–1062.

Moldovanu, G., Friedman, M., and Miller, D. G., 1966, Treatment of canine malignant lymphoma with surgery and chemotherapy, *J. Amer. Vet. Med. Assoc.* **148**:153–156.

Müller-Eberhard, H. J. and Fjellstrom, K. E., 1971, Isolation of the anticomplementary protein from cobra venom and its mode of action on C3, *J. Immunol.* **107**:1666–1672.

Negroni, G., and Hunter, E., 1973, Rejection of polyoma virus-induced neoplasms in mice inoculated with complement and antiserum, *J. Nat. Cancer Inst.* **51**:265–268.

Nelson, R. A., Jr., 1953, The immune adherence phenomenon, *Science* **118**:733–737.

Nelson, R. A., Jr., 1963, Complement and body defense, *Transfusion* **3**:250–259.

Nilsson, U. R., and Müller-Eberhard, H. J., 1967, Deficiency of the fifth component of complement in mice with an inherited complement defect, *J. Exp. Med.* **125**:1–16.

Nishioka, K., 1967, Complement and tumor immunology, *Adv. Cancer Res.* **14**:231–291.

Nishioka, K., 1975, Complement system and tumor immunity, in: *Host Defense Against Cancer and Its Potentiation* (D. Mizuno, G. Chihara, F. Fukuoka, T. Yamamoto, and Y. Yamamura, eds.), pp. 83–97, University of Tokyo Press, Tokyo.

Old, L. J., and Boyse, E. A., 1965, Antigens of tumors and leukemias induced by viruses, *Fed. Proc. Amer. Soc. Exp. Biol.* **24**:1009–1017.

Old, L. J., and Boyse, E. A., 1973, Current enigmas in cancer research, *Harvey Lect.* **67**:273–315.

Old, L. J., Stockert, E., Boyse, E. A., and Geering, G., 1967, A study of passive immunization against a transplanted G+ leukemia with specific antiserum, *Proc. Soc. Exp. Biol. Med.* **124**:63–68.

Oldstone, M. B. A., Aoki, T., and Dixon, F. J., 1972, The antibody response of mice to murine leukemia virus in spontaneous infection: absence of classical immunologic tolerance, *Proc. Nat. Acad. Sci. U.S.A.* **69**:134–138.

Pascal, R. R., Koss, M. N., and Kassel, R. L., 1973, Glomerulonephritis associated with immune complex deposits and viral particles in spontaneous murine leukemia, *Lab. Invest.* **29**:159–165.

Pepys, M. B., 1974, Role of complement in induction of antibody production *in vivo*, *J. Exp. Med.* **140**:126–145.

Pepys, M. B., and Butterworth, A. E., 1974, Inhibition by C3 fragments of C3-dependent rosette formation and antigen induced lymphocyte transformation, *Clin. Exp. Immunol.* **18**:273–282.

Perlmann, P., and Hölm, G., 1969, Cytotoxic effects of lymphoid cells *in vitro*, *Adv. Immunol.* **11**:117–193.

Pincus, S., Bianco, C., and Nussenzweig, J., 1972, Increased proportion of complement-receptor lymphocytes in the peripheral blood of patients with chronic lymphocytic leukemia, *Blood* **40**:303–310.

Rottino, A., and Levy, A. L., 1959, Behavior of total serum complement in Hodgkin's disease and other malignant lymphomas, *Blood* **14**:246–254.

Schier, W. W., Roth, A., Ostroff, G., and Schrift, M. H., 1956, Hodgkin's disease and immunity, *Amer. J. Med.* **20**:94–99.

Segerling, M., Ohanian, S. H., and Borsos, T., 1975, Chemotherapeutic drugs increase killing of tumor cells by antibody and complement, *Science* **188**:55–57.

Sizenko, S. P., Latiy, N. P., and Ivanov, I. F., 1972, The complementary blood serum activity in rats in intravenous injection of 9,10-dimethyl-1,2-benzanthracene, *Questions Oncol.* **18**:76–80.

Sobel, A. T., Bokisch, V. A., and Müller-Eberhard, H. J., 1975, C1q deviation test for the detection of immune complexes, aggregates of IgG, and bacterial products in human serum, *J. Exp. Med.* **142**:139–150.

Southam, C., and Siegel, A., 1966, Serum levels of second component of complement in cancer patients, *J. Immunol.* **97**:331–337.

Sutherland, J. C., and Mardiney, M. R., Jr., 1973, Immune complex disease in the kidneys of

ROBERT L. KASSEL,
WILLIAM D. HARDY,
JR., AND NOORBIBI K.
DAY

lymphoma-leukemia patients: the presence of an oncornavirus antigen, *J. Nat. Cancer Inst.* **50**:633–644.

Squire, R. A., Busch, M., Melby, E. C., Neeley, L. M., and Yarbrough, B. 1973, Clinical and pathologic study of canine lymphoma. Clinical staging, cell classification and therapy, *J. Nat. Cancer Inst.* **51**:565–574.

Theilen, G. H., and Worley, M. B., 1974, Diagnosis and treatment of cancer in small animals, *Amer. Anim. Hosp. Assoc. Proc.* **141**:342–358.

Thomas, L., 1959, Reactions to homologous antigens in relation to hypersensitivity, in: *Cellular and Humoral Aspects of the Hypersensitive States* (H. S. Lawrence, ed.), pp. 529–532, Hoeber-Harper, New York.

Weimer, H. E., Miller, J. N., Meyers, R. L., Baxter, D., Roberts, D. M., Godfrey, J. F., and Carpenter, C. M., 1964, The effects of tumor growth, nutritional stress, and inflammation on serum complement levels in the rat, *Cancer Res.* **24**:847–854.

Wilson, R. E., Alexander, P., Rosenberg, S. A., and Simmons, R. L., 1974, Horizons in tumor immunology, *Arch. Surg.* **109**:17–29.

Winn, H. J., 1960, Immune mechanisms in hemotransplantation, I. The role of serum antibody and complement in the neutralization of lymphoma cells, *J. Immunol.* **84**:530–538.

Wohl, H., and Ghossein, N. A., 1971, Complement levels before and after radiotherapy in cancer patients, *Oncology* **25**:344–346.

Yoshida, T. O., and Ito, Y., 1968, Studies on serum complement levels in rabbits bearing tumors of Shope papilloma-carcinoma complex, *Immunology* **14**:879–887.

Yoshikawa, S., Yamada, K., and Yoshida, T. O., 1969, Serum complement levels in patients with leukemia, *Int. J. Cancer* **4**:845–851.

Zarco, R. M., Flores, E., and Rodriquez, F., 1964, Serum complement levels in human cancer, *J. Philipp. Med. Assoc.* **40**:839–846.

15

Perturbations of Complement in Disease

IRMA GIGLI

1. Introduction

Alterations in the complement (C) system in human pathology have been recognized for many years, but only within recent years have measurements of serum C components become clinically available. In view of the apparent different biological properties of each component of the C system (Ruddy *et al.,* 1972a; Müller-Eberhard, 1975), a proper understanding of the role of C in disease requires an analysis not only of the whole hemolytic C, but also of its components. Immuno-chemical measurements using monospecific antibodies against C proteins are available, but fail to distinguish between native proteins and those that have been rendered inactive either because they have participated in the C reaction sequence or because they have been incorrectly synthesized *de novo.* Stoichiometric hemolytic titrations provide sensitive assessment of the functional activity of the individual C component.

In the present review, acquired abnormalities and inborn deficiencies will be discussed in relation to human disease. A detailed review of inborn deficiencies of the complement system has been given in Chapter 12.

2. Acquired Abnormalities

2.1. Complement in Allergic Diseases

2.1.1. Asthma

In a recent report (Kay *et al.,* 1974) it has been suggested that C4 measurements may be of value in the classification of asthma, since they correlate better with various asthma-associated clinical features than levels of IgE. Adults whose

IRMA GIGLI • Departments of Dermatology and Medicine, New York University Medical Center, New York, New York.

disease originated in childhood show changing patterns in the clinical features in relation to the duration of the disease that correlated with levels of C4, but not with levels of IgE. In particular, the wheeze pattern changed from episodic to chronic, and the levels of C4 were correspondingly lower. A similar but less significant pattern was found with C2 and C3, but not with C1q, C6, C7, or factor B.

Complement levels were also measured daily in hospitalized patients with acute asthma. In older nonallergic asthmatics, the levels of C1 and C4 fell during the course of the acute illness, whereas the levels remain unchanged in subjects with allergic asthma.

2.1.2. Serum Sickness-like Syndrome

This term is used to denote the syndrome occurring several days after the administration of serum, penicillin, sulfonamides, or other drugs, and characterized by fever, arthralgias, urticaria, and angioedema. This syndrome has been considered the prototype of acute immune-complex disease. During the course of the disease, the whole serum complement (CH_{50}) is lowered, Dixon (1965) has examined the C profile during serum sickness in rabbits. The lowering of serum C included all components, and occurred at the time when circulating immune complexes were present in the circulation. The clearance of the immune complexes and the fall in C in serum coincided with the development of glomerulitis. In man, there is much less information than exists in animal models.

2.2. Complement in Connective Tissue Diseases

2.2.1. Systemic Lupus Erythematosus

Although depressions of whole C activity are occasionally observed in patients with SLE who have a relatively benign course, complement abnormalities are most often associated with increased severity of the disease (Schur and Sandson, 1968), Antigen–antibody (DNA protein–anti-DNA antibody) complexes activate complement, and these complexes may be responsible for many of the features of this disease (Agnello et al., 1971). In active disease, depressed serum levels of C1, C1q, C4, C2, C3, and C9 have been demonstrated (Hanauer and Christian, 1967), Serial measurements of C components have revealed decreased levels preceding clinical exacerbations (Kohler and ten Bensel, 1969).

The detection of immune complexes in serum that precipitate with C1q, and the deposition of immunoglobulins, DNA, C1q, C4, and C3 in the glomerulus and the dermal–epidermal junction in skin lesions (Tan and Kunkel, 1966) are consistent with the presence of immune complexes that fix complement (Koffler et al., 1967). Turnover studies have demonstrated an increased catabolic rate of these proteins, suggesting their utilization in immunopathologic reactions (Carpenter et al., 1969).

Recently, the C levels in the CSF of patients with SLE have been examined (Petz et al., 1971a; Hadler et al., 1973). The level of C4 in patients with active CNS lupus disease was found to be depressed.

Although the depression of the early components, C1, C4, and C2, indicates activation of the classical pathway, alternate pathway activation has been demonstrated by depressed serum levels of properdin and Factor B, and by the deposition of these components and IgA immunoglobulin in the glomeruli (Westberg *et al.*, 1971) and the skin (Jordan *et al.*, 1975b).

2.2.2. Rheumatoid Arthritis

In this disease, abnormalities of C are for the most part restricted to the synovial fluid, where the total hemolytic activity is significantly depressed compared with the serum level (Zvaitler, 1973; Ruddy and Austen, 1970). In contrast, the joint fluid of patients with arthritis secondary to gout, ankylosing spondylitis, Reiter's syndrome, and osteoarthritis is not altered in comparison with the serum level (Pekin and Zvaitler, 1964; Hedberg, 1967). In general, there is a correlation between the severity of the C depression and the severity of the disease. Levels of C1 are variably depressed, and reduction of C4, C2, Factor B, and C3 is seen in synovial fluid from patients with seropositive rheumatoid arthritis. The intra-articular utilization of C3 is accompanied by the appearance in the fluid of free C3d (Zvaitler, 1969), a cleavage product of C3b produced by C3b inactivator. Chemotactic factors C5a and C$\overline{5}$67 were found in approximately 50% of rheumatoid arthritis joint fluids. Inclusions of immunoglobulins, C1q, C4, and C3 were found in leukocytes from the synovial fluid of patients with more severe C depletions (Britton and Schur, 1971). The inflammatory cells within the synovium have been shown to synthesize C components (Ruddy and Colten, 1974).

Aggregates of IgG in rheumatoid synovial fluid have been recognized by precipitation with IgM rheumatoid factor (Winchester *et al.*, 1970) or with isolated C1q (Winchester *et al.*, 1969). The reduction of complement is thought to reflect its intra-articular utilization by these aggregates (Zvaifler, 1973; Ruddy *et al.*, 1971).

Serum C levels in rheumatoid arthritis are usually normal or elevated. Low C levels are associated with severe disease, a high titer of rheumatoid factor, Felty's syndrome, and cutaneous vasculitis. Increased catabolism of serum C3 has been demonstrated in rheumatoid vasculitis (Soter *et al.*, 1974a; Franco and Schur, 1971).

2.3. Complement in Dermatologic Diseases

2.3.1. Bullous Diseases of the Skin

Pemphigus and bullous pemphigoid are chronic blistering skin diseases in which immunoglobulins and C are present in the epidermis (Beutnor *et al.*, 1970). With the use of immunofluorescence techniques, these immunoreactants have been shown in the intercellular substance of the epidermis in the skin and mucosa of patients with all forms of pemphigus (Beutner *et al.*, 1966), whereas in bullous pemphigoid, the deposits are present in the basement membrane zone (Beutner *et al.*, 1970). Deposits of C1q, C4, and C3 are present in early acantholytic lesions of pemphigus, suggesting that the C system may contribute to the pathogenesis of the disease. Basal membrane antibodies may also fix properdin and Factor B (Jordan, 1976), in addition to C1q, C4, and C3 (Jordon *et al.*, 1975a). Both properdin and

Factor B have been demonstrated in bullous pemphigoid, indicating the participation of the alternative pathway. On the other hand, only alternative pathway components have been found in herpes gestationis, a rare blistering disease seen during pregnancy (Provost and Tomasi, 1973), and in dermatitis herpetiformis (Provost and Tomasi, 1974). In the latter, IgA is deposited in the skin in a granular pattern, but no C components were found in skin biopsies of patients free of skin eruptions as a result of dapsone treatment. Additional C3 deposits and appearance of skin lesions followed discontinuation of therapy (Seah *et al.,* 1973). These observations suggest that C activation via the alternate pathway might be responsible for initiation of skin lesions.

Serum C components have been found to be normal or elevated in these conditions despite the consistent finding of local activation.

2.3.2. Cutaneous Necrotizing Angiitis

Cutaneous necrotizing angiitis may be present as either palpable purpura, nodules, ulcers, or, less commonly, recurrent urticaria, and each clinical presentation may be associated with hypocomplementemia or a normal C system (Soter *et al.,* 1976).

Analysis of the C system im patients with palpable purpura and concomitant collagen vascular disease or cryoglobulinemia reveals an abnormality that reflects the associated disease or the existence of a cryoglobulin (Soter *et al.,* 1974a; Asghar *et al.,* 1975). For example, in patients with rheumatoid arthritis and vasculitis in whom the level of rheumatoid factor is high, low levels of C1, C4, and C2 were observed. This serum profile is consistent with activation of the classical pathway, and is similar to the utlization profile observed in the synovial fluid of patients with rheumatoid arthritis without vasculitis (Ruddy and Austen, 1970). In patients with SLE and vasculitis, there was activation of the classical pathway, with marked depletion of C1q and recruitment of the alternative pathway, with utilization of the terminal C sequence identical to the C abnormalities seen in patients with SLE and active renal disease without vasculitis.

In patients with Sjögren's syndrome, the C profile in serum reflected the type and nature of the underlying cryoglobulin. In patients with IgG–IgM cryoglobulin, there were low levels of C4 and C2 consistent with activation of the classical pathway. In a patient with an IgG–IgA cryoglobulin, there were low levels of C3 and C9, and properdin and Factor B fluctuated at the lower limit of normal (Soter *et al.,* 1974a). The levels of C1, C4, and C2 remained in the normal range consistent with activation of the alternative pathway. In one patient with Sjögren's syndrome and vasculitis without a cryoprotein, the C system was normal. Therefore, the C profile in serum was distinctly different, and reflected the presence and type of cryoglobulin, rather than a uniform picture for the clinical and histological presentation.

In addition to those individuals with concomitant collagen vascular diseases, other groups of patients with cutaneous necrotizing angiitis and hypocomplementemia exist. A unique patient with C1q depression associated with vasculitis and presenting with urticaria and angioedema has been reported (Marder *et al.,* 1976). C1 hemolytic activity was reduced, but C1s protein was within the normal range. C4 and C3 were only moderately decreased. This example of vasculitis and angioedema with hypocomplementemia may be part of a syndrome. Other presentations following within this syndrome may include the patients with recurrent urticaria (Soter *et al.*, 1974b), occasionally purpura, and arthralgia in the presence of hypocomplementemia in whom biopsy studies of the skin lesions have revealed necrotizing angiitis (McDuffie *et al.*, 1973; Ballow *et al.*, 1975b; Sissons *et al.*, 1974). Serologic evidence of SLE is lacking in this patient.

2.4. Complement in Hematologic Diseases

2.4.1. Autoimmune Hemolytic Anemias

Cold agglutinin hemolytic anemia is characterized by the presence of IgM autoantibodies with specificity for the I antigen present on the surface of erythrocytes. Erythrocytes carrying C4 and C3 are routinely found in cold agglutinin disease in the absence of detectable antibody (Evans *et al.*, 1968), the IgM presumably having dissociated from the cell. Cold agglutinins are thought to become attached to the erythrocytes and to activate complement in peripheral vessels and to dissociate in a warmer environment, leaving the activated C components. Cold agglutinins appear transiently following certain infectious illnesses, but these patients rarely develop clinically significant hemolysis. In the cold agglutinin syndrome, C activation seems to be responsible for the anemia observed (Atkinson and Frank 1974). The attachment of C3 to the erythrocyte surface appears to enhance the sequestration of erythrocytes by the reticuloendothelial system through the C3b receptor site present on macrophages (Abramson and Lee, 1974). If sufficient numbers of C molecules attach to the erythrocyte membrane, the patient will develop intravascular hemolysis. The demonstration that unsequestered erythrocytes from patients with cold agglutinin hemolytic anemia are relatively resistant to C-induced lysis, and do not react in immune adherence although the immunologically detectable C3 is present on their surfaces, may be explained by the action of the C3b inactivator (Ruddy and Austen, 1971). In support of this hypothesis is the fact that erythrocytes from patients with cold agglutinin syndrome commonly have C3d on their circulating erythrocytes (Petz *et al.*, 1971b).

Most cases of hemolytic anemia involve an autoantibody of the IgG class. This antibody has anti-Rh specificity and reacts with an antihuman IgG. C proteins have been found on the sensitized erythrocytes in numbers ranging from less than 10% to more than 50% of cases reported in series (Dacie, 1962; Leddy and Swisher, 1971). Cases in whom bound C components can be demonstrated or in whom C3 hypercatabolism is present (Petz *et al.*, 1968) may reflect quantitatively larger amounts of IgG antibody on the erythrocyte membrane. The role of C in warm antibody-mediated hemolytic anemia is probably to amplify or augment the effect of IgG in the clearance of the erythrocytes in the spleen, or sometimes the liver (LoBuglio *et al.*, 1967).

2.4.2. Paroxysmal Nocturnal Hemoglobinuria

In paroxysmal nocturnal hemoglobinuria (PNH), there is a population of erythrocytes with membrane alterations reponsible for a marked susceptibility to the lytic effect of the terminal C components in the absence of specific antierythrocyte antibody (Rosse, 1971). Experiments with C3-convertase generated with purified components indicate that cells of these patients are unusually sensitive to terminal components activated via the classical pathway (Götze and Müller-Eberhard, 1970), and experiments with inulin or cobra factor activation of the alternative pathway produce similar results. Though the mechanism of C activation in these patients is not clear, it has been shown *in vitro* that minor changes in the balance between calcium and magnesium concentrations, with a relative increase in magnesium, may allow activation of the alternative pathway and lysis of the PNH cells (May *et al.*, 1973).

2.4.3. Drug-Induced Anemia and Thrombocytopenia

Lysis of erythrocytes and platelets has been described as a result of treatment with a number of drugs, including *p*-amino salicylic acid, phenacetin, quinidine, quinine, stibophen, and penicillin. These drugs are capable of binding to the surfaces of both cell types, and agglutinate in the presence of a specific IgG antibody in the serum. In some cases, it appears that the immune complexes formed between the drug and the antibody are bound to the cell surfaces after the formation of the complexes. These cells are lysed by C, but more commonly, C3b is deposited on the erythrocytes or platelets or both leading to sequestration by fixed macrophages (Dacie, 1962).

2.4.4. Acquired Deficiency of CĪ INH in Lymphoid Syndromes

Activation of the first component of C and depletion of CĪ INH has been observed in association with different types of lymphoproliferative disorders. The first description of this association was in two patients with lymphosarcoma and circulating 7S IgM (Caldwell *et al.*, 1972), who were found to have unusual C component profiles, in which C1, C4, C2, and CĪ INH were diminished in the presence of normal C3 and an elevated C9. One of these patients experienced attacks of angioedema that could be distinquished from HAE by the absence of any C system defect in other family members and by the reduced level of C1 in the patient's serum. The CĪ INH deficiency in these patients is acquired, most likely as a result of interaction with CĪ. The capacity of the patients' sera to diminish C1 when mixed with normal serum suggested the presence of a material that fixed and activated this C protein. The presence of an appreciable concentration of 7S IgM introduces the possibility that this abnormal immunoglobulin plays a role. Since this initial report, six additional cases with angioedema and lymphoproliferation disorders have been reported (Oberling *et al.*, 1975). In three of the patients, recurrent angioedema preceded a clinically recognizable lymphoproliferative disorder. In one case, C activation was due to a circulating complex of lymphocyte surface antigen and specific antibody, as demonstrated by the presence of a cold-reactive IgM antilymphocyte antibody in the serum (Day *et al.*, 1975). In another case, C1 activation was due to interaction with peripheral blood monocytes, or with cells obtained from tumor masses (Schrieber *et al.*, 1975).

2.5.1. Tropical Diseases

Activation of the C system in malaria has been known for many years. Recently, detailed studies on adults and children with acute *Plasmodium falciparum* malaria infections have demonstrated activation of the classical C pathway, with sharp drops in C1, C4, and C2. Reduction of serum C3 levels was found in 83% of the patients, while Factor B levels were only slightly depressed. A correlation was found between reduction of C3 and the degree of anemia and thrombocytopenia (Srichaibul *et al.*, 1975). An immune reaction associated with C activation is believed to contribute to injury of red blood cells and platelets, and to promote the development of systemic intravascular coagulation (Greenwood and Brueton, 1974).

Dengue hemorrhagic fever is accompanied by extremely low C protein levels in serum and increased catabolism of C3 and C1q, especially during the period of hemorrhagic shock (Bokisch *et al.*, 1973). In view of the known effects of C on the vasculature and release mechanisms of vasoactive amines, these observations strongly implicate C activation as an important factor in the development of shock syndrome in dengue hemorrhagic fever.

2.5.2. Infectious Hepatitis with Arthritis

In acute viral hepatitis, depressed C levels are commonly found in patients with prodromal symptoms of arthralgia or arthritis and an urticarial skin rash (Alpert *et al.*, 1971). Serum C4 is markedly reduced, while C1q and C3 are minimally decreased or unchanged. Hepatitis-associated antigen (HAA) has been found in the serum. In the joint fluid of these patients, there is reduction in the total hemolytic activity, and HAA is present (Onion *et al.*, 1971). In one patient with diffuse vasculitis, immunofluorescent studies showed deposits of HAA antigen, IgG, and C3 in the vascular endothelium (Gocke *et al.*, 1970). As the disease progresses from its prodromal stage to frank hepatitis, HAA may disappear and the C levels may return to normal. Many of the clinical findings, as well as laboratory studies, are suggestive of a serum-sickness-like syndrome.

2.6. Complement in Renal Diseases

Depression of serum C in glomerulonephritis following scarlet fever was first described early in this century (Gunn, 1914–1915). Depressions of total C activity are the rule early in the course of acute poststreptococcal glomerulonephritis (AGN), with transient depressions of C4 and more persistent depressions of C3 and C5 (Kohler and ten Bensel, 1969). In the patients with chronic glomerulonephritis who have reduced C levels, C3 remains low, while C1, C4, and C2 are normal (Gewurz *et al.*, 1968b). Hypocomplementemia is most commonly associated with membranoproliferative glomerulonephritis (MPGN), and these patients usually experience a slowly progressive diminution in renal function. Hypercatabolism of C3 has been observed in some patients with hypocomplementemic chronic glomerulonephritis (Michael *et al.,* 1969), but in other studies, the catabolic rate was normal (Alper and Rosen, 1967). The finding of circulating products of C3 activation in the serum of some of these patients and of C3 deposits in the glomeruli suggests that *in vivo* utilization of C3 may account for the depressed levels of this component. The observation of depressions of both properdin (Rothfield *et al.,* 1972; Gewurz *et al.,* 1969) and Factor B (Perrin *et al.,* 1973) supports the view that activation of the alternative pathway is responsible for the changes in the serum C activity. Furthermore, although deposits of immunoglobulins are often not found in the glomeruli in either type of glomerulonephritis, deposits of properdin, corresponding in location to deposits of C3, have been observed (Westberg *et al.,* 1971). Although the mechanism that leads to activation of the alternative pathway remains unclear, the role of C3Nef (West *et al.,* 1973) is of obvious interest in view of the apparent ability of this serum factor to initiate the alternative activation mechanism.

In contrast to the findings in AGN and MPGN, depressed serum levels of all components of the classical C activation have been reported in glomerulonephritis in SLE and the evidence for involvement of the alternative pathway is less impressive (Kohler and ten Bensel, 1969). In SLE and AGN, changes in the serum levels of C correlate well with the clinical course of the disease (Ruddy *et al.,* 1972b; Lewis *et al.,* 1971), while little correlation is apparent between the serum abnormalities and the clinical progress in MPGN. Extensive reviews in this area have been published (West *et al.,* 1973; Ruddy *et al.,* 1972b).

3. Genetic Abnormalities

3.1. Complement Component Deficiencies

3.1.1. C1q Deficiency Associated with Immunologic Deficiency Syndrome

Association of hypogammaglobulinemia with partial C1q deficiency was first described by Müller-Eberhard and Kunkel (1961). The C1q levels are in the range of one-half to two-thirds of the normal mean values; C1 hemolytic activity is variably depressed (Kohler and Müller-Eberhard, 1969; Stroud *et al.,* 1970). Because C1 activity depends on the combined function of C1q, C1r, and C1s, the discrepancy among C1 hemolytic activity (Gewurz *et al.,* 1968a), depressed C1q protein, and a relatively normal C1s concentration suggests that only a portion of the C1q in human serum is contained in the intact C1 molecule and that the metabolism or synthesis of C1s, C1r, and C1q is not linked (Stroud *et al.,*, 1970). Since C1q and certain immunoglobulins interact in free solution, it is possible that immunoglobulins may have a stabilizing or protective effect on C1q catabolism. In the absence of normal amounts of IgG, C1q leaves the intravascular space and is subject to degradation. This hypothesis is supported by direct measurements of the metabolism and distribution of purified and radiolabeled C1q in 2 patients with the Bruton X-linked type of immune deficiency in whom the depressed levels of C1q were associated with hypercatabolism of this protein, rather than with impaired synthesis (Kohler and Müller-Eberhard, 1972). In addition, an intravenous injection of an IgG preparation free of C1q into a patient with the sporadic form of hypogammaglobulinemia was followed by a gradual increase of the C1q protein, reaching normal levels over the course of 24 hr (Frank, and Atkinson, 1975).

Severe C1q depressions have been described in patients with combined immunodeficiency who had both lymphopenia and hypogammaglobulinemia inherited in an autosomal recessive pattern (Müller-Eberhard and Kunkel, 1961). Those with X-linked inheritance have serum C1q levels resembling patients with the common Bruton type of agammaglobulinemia. The differences in C1q levels between these two forms of severe immunodeficiency may indicate an additional synthetic defect in the autosomal form of the disease. Three of four patients with low C1q who have received successfully bone marrow grafts (Ballow *et al.*, 1973) have shown a rise to normal C1q level. It is possible that the grafted tissue may have restored the cell type responsible for C1q synthesis (Day *et al.*, 1970).

3.1.2. C1r Deficiency

Initially, this defect was described in a young girl with proteinuria and chronic glomerulonephritis who had abnormally low levels of C1r, C2, and C4. A renal biopsy demonstrated C3 deposits in the glomerular membranes (Pickering *et al.*, 1970). The patient developed renal insufficiency and underwent renal transplantation. Despite clinical improvement, her C1 titer remained below 1% of normal. Family studies were not possible. The finding of two additional cases in a brother and sister from a second family suggests an autosomal basis for this disorder (Moncada *et al.*, 1972).

The second case of C1r deficiency was found in an 18-year-old boy who had had painless ulcerations of the skin, atrophy, scarring, and painful "erythemano-dosum" like lesions. He had arthralgias without joint deformity, fever, nausea, and vomiting (Day *et al.*, 1972). Biopsy of the skin lesions showed vasculitis without the characteristic C3 deposition seen in systemic lupus erythematosus (SEL). Renal biopsy showed a mild focal glomerulitis with C3 and IgG deposition in a coarse granular pattern compatible with SLE. His 24-year-old sister had had recurrent otitis media and infections of the upper respiratory tract and skin. More recently, she had had bronchitis and transient nondeforming polyarthritis. Neither patient had positive LE preparations or antinuclear antibodies. Five other siblings were well, but three others died early in life—two in infancy from G.I. problems and one at the age of 12 of an illness similar to that of the brother. Four generations have been studied in this large family (Abramson *et al.*, 1971). The CH_{50} in the two affected individuals is undetectable. Hemolytic C1 activity is less than 0.5% of normal, and immunodiffusion measurements of C1 subunits demonstrate undetectable C1r, normal C1q, and C1s levels approximately 50% of normal. C1r levels in the heterozygous members are detectable at approximately 60–80% of normal.

The association of a mild C1s deficiency in the two homozygous individuals of this family, as well as in the first patient described, suggests that it may be a linkage of C1r and C1s synthesis (Stroud, 1974).

3.1.3. C1s Deficiency

Deficiency in the C1s subunit has been reported in two families in which the propositus presented with a clinical picture of lupus erythematosus (Leddy *et al.*, 1974; Pondman *et al.*, 1969). As in the C1r-deficient patients, the LE preparations were negative; however, one of the patients, a 6-year-old girl, developed anti-DNA antibodies during the time of the study. The second patient presented with, in addition to the absence of C1s, a low C1q level, thought to be due to fixation by antigen–antibody complexes. Two sisters and a brother were also deficient in C1s (Blum *et al.*, 1976); however, the parents had normal levels. No further details are presently available for these families.

3.1.4. C4 Deficiency

This serum defect has been recognized in an 18-year-old girl with a lupus-like syndrome. She had no LE cells antinuclear factor, or IgG deposition in the skin, despite a typical molar eruption and arthralgias. Her serum was totally deficient in C4 by functional and immunochemical analysis. Her mother's serum contains half the normal levels of C4 (Hauptman *et al.*, 1974). A second individual homozygous for C4 deficiency has been identified (Alper and Rosen, 1976).

3.1.5. C2 Deficiency

Isolated deficiencies of this component of complement have been described in one or more members of 14 kindred (Agnello *et al.*, 1975). The pattern of inheritance of this defect is characterized by a deficiency of a pair of autosomal codominant alleles, each of which codes for half the normal synthesis of C2.

Although in the originally described pedigrees (Klemperer *et al.*, 1967), the subjects were clinically normal, there are now several examples of connective tissue diseases associated with the C2 deficiency. Skin lesions resembling discoid lupus erythematosus (Agnello *et al.*, 1972) or Henoch-Schonlein purpura (Friend *et al.*, 1975) have been noted. Rheumatic disease, lupus-like syndrome, glomerulonephritis, and polymyositis are frequency found. The mechanism of these associations is unknown, but is statistically an unlikely coincidence. It has been suggested that the absence of C2 may predispose these individuals to latent virus infections. Though there is no direct evidence in these patients for latent or chronic viruses, mycoplasma-like structures were found in the serum of one patient.

3.1.6. C3 Deficiency

A 15-year-old girl from South Africa was found to have no detectable C3 in her serum. She had a disease characterized by repeated pyogenic infections, including pneumonia, bacterial meningitis, otitis media, and septicemia (Alper *et al.*, 1972a). By immunochemical analysis, her serum C3 level was less than 0.25 mg/100 ml (normal values: 100–200 mg/100 ml), and functional evaluation detected less than 0.1% of the normal concentration. All the other components were present at normal levels. Her serum was unable to opsonize bacteria adequately (Stossel *et al.*, 1974), or to mobilize leukocytes in response to a chemotactic stimulus. Other C-mediated functions such as hemolytic and bactericidal activity, were also markedly depressed or absent (Alper *et al.*, 1970).

Two additional C3-deficient children have been studied in the United States. One is a 4-year-old girl of English extraction who had had several episodes of pneumonia, arthritis, (probably septic), and otitis media (Ballow *et al.,*, 1975a). The child's mother, grandfather, and several uncles have half-normal levels of C3; the father is unknown. The other patient too has also had numerous episodes of infection and serological defects, as described in the other C3-deficient children.

Another patient with C3 deficiency has been identified recently: a 3-year-old child whose serum contained about 1% of the normal C3 levels (Alper and Rosen, 1976). This patient, in contrast to the other three, has not as yet had severe infections, although the serological abnormalities were similar to those reported for the other C3-deficient subjects.

Pedigree analysis in the original family is consistent with the inheritance of a nonexpressed allele at the C3 locus, for which no gene product appears in the serum.

3.1.7. C5 Deficiency and C5 Dysfunction

C5 deficiency has been reported in two individuals in a single family. The proposita in this family was a black female with SLE, with mild renal disease, a positive LE preparation, and anti-DNA antibodies. Both she and a healthy sister lacked hemolytic and antigenic C5. There was a defect in the patient's serum ability to generate chemotactic factors in response to stimuli, but this defect was not associated with repeated infections. Family studies in three generations demonstrated an autosomal recessive transmission (Rosenfield and Leddy, 1974).

A familial humoral abnormality resulting in deficient opsonization has been related to a functional defect of C5 (Miller and Nilsson, 1970; Nilsson et al., 1974). The probent, an 18-month-old infant with Leiner's syndrome, presented with recurring infections due to gram-negative bacteria and failure to thrive. His serum did not enhance the phagocytosis of yeast or of staphylococcus aureus to the same extent as does normal plasma. Although the patient's C5 appeared normal in amount, mobility, and antigenicity, the opsonic defect in vitro could be overcome by the addition of normal rodent serum, but not by the addition of C5-deficient rodent serum. The patient was treated with fresh frozen plasma in order to supply normal C5, and showed marked improvement. A discrete defect of C5 that impairs its ability to enhance the phagocytosis of only certain antigens and leaves intact its antigenicity and function in immune hemolysis has been postulated.. The possibility exists, however, that there may be an additional, as yet undisclosed abnormality in the serum.

3.1.8. C6 Deficiency

The defect in C6 was noted in an 18-year-old woman with gonococcal arthritis and a mild Raynaud's phenomenon. C6 was found absent by function and immunochemical tests. This patient has normal clotting parameters; this observation is of interest because of the retarded coagulation of blood reported in C6-deficient rabbits (Leddy et al., 1974; Heusinkveld et al., 1974). A second patient with a deficiency of C6 has been reported: a 6-year-old boy with repeated episodes of meningococcal meningitis (Lim et al., 1976).

Both sera were deficient in hemolytic and bactericidal activity and lysis of PNH cells. These activities were restored by purified human C6.

3.1.9. C7 Deficiency

Autosomal recessive transmission of C7 has been found in two families (Boyer *et al.*, 1975; Wellek and Opferkuch, 1975). One patient has severe Raynaud's phenomenon, sclerodactyly, and telangiectasia. Symptoms began in late childhood with swelling and stiffness of her hands, blanching on exposure to the cold, and gangrene of the terminal phalanx. Partial deficiency was found in the serum of the patient's parents, brother, and children. The patient's serum was deficient in opsonizing yeast particles and in the generation of chemotactic factor by antigen–antibody complexes and endotoxin. The patient does not have recurrent bacterial infections, but further details of the case have not been reported.

The second C7-deficiency individual is an 18-year-old boy who is presently healthy.

3.1.10. C8 Deficiency

A female with prolonged disseminated gonococcal infection was found to be C8-deficient following the demonstration of absent hemolytic and bactericidal activity in serum (Petersen *et al.*, 1975).

Several patients with deficiencies of late-acting C components have been ascertained because of systemic neisserial infections. This finding may implicate the serum bactericidal mechanism as an important feature of host defense against these organisms.

3.2 Inhibitor Deficiencies

A series of regulators of C exist that act to modify the rate of activation or to inhibit function. Two clinically important deficiencies of C inhibitors have been described, and are discussed in this section.

3.2.1. C$\overline{1}$ INH Deficiency

Hereditary angioedema (hereditary angioneurotic edema) results from a genetically determined deficiency of the C$\overline{1}$ INH (Donaldson and Evans, 1963; Landerman *et al.*, 1962). It is characterized by recurrent, circumscribed subepithelial edema of the skin and the mucosa of the gastrointestinal and upper respiratory tracts. A faint macular or serpiginous erythema occasionally precedes cutaneous angioedema. Cutaneous angioedema may develop over several hours at any given site, lasting for 48–72 hr. It does not pit and is not pruritic. Local trauma may precipitate an attack in an extremity, and dental extraction or a tonsillectomy has resulted in oropharyngeal edema, progressing to airway obstruction. Although cutaneous involvement tends to be well circumscribed, labial edema may progress to involve the contiguous mocosa. There can be concurrent or isolated involvement of the gastrointestinal tract, with nausea, vomiting, severe abdominal cramps, and watery diarrhea.

The disease is transmitted as an autosomal dominant without sex preference.

Most patients have 10–30% of the normal inhibitor level, raising the question whether these individuals are heterozygous for the trait of whether true homozygosity has been observed. Approximately 15% of patients have normal or elevated levels of a nonfunctional inhibitor protein that differs among the different kindred with respect to its electrophoretic mobility and functional acitvity (Rosen et al., 1965, 1971). Demonstration of absence of a functional serum inhibitor (Gigli et al., 1968) of $C\bar{1}$ affords the genetic marker that delineates hereditary angioedema (HAE), and introduces the possibility that uninhibited $C\bar{1}$ is involved in the pathogenesis of the attacks. Patients with HAE are continuously subjected to the action of low levels of C1, as evident from chronically reduced levels of C4 (Donaldson and Rosen, 1964) and a markedly increased catabolism of radiolabeled C4 (Carpenter et al., 1969). Two observations indicate that attacks are associated with a further activation of endogenous uninhibited $C\bar{1}$: (1) increased serum esterase activity against N-acetyl L-tyrosine ethyl ester, inhibitable by purified $C\bar{1}$ INH; (2) disappearance of functional C2 and C4 activities and C4 protein. In addition, evidence for local activation of C1 has been obtained by demonstrating that the levels of the $C\bar{1}$ substrates were lower in the involved extremity than in the control. The reason for the activation of uninhibited $C\bar{1}$ accompanying the attacks is unknown. Incubation of plasma obtained from patients with HAE during asymptomatic intervals spontaneously generates smooth muscle–contracting activity, and generation of this activity is inhibited in the presence of antibody to C4 or to C2 (Donaldson et al., 1969). A heat-stable polypeptide has been isolated from the incubated plasma, and is clearly distinguishable from bradykinin. In vitro combinations of purified $C\bar{1}$s, C4, and C2 have produced low-molecular-weight fragments similar in amino acid composition to this polypeptide, but as yet this material has not been fully characterized (Lepow, 1971).

Other mediators of vascular permeability have also been implicated in HAE. Urinary histamine levels are increased during attacks of angioedema (Granerus et al., 1967). This increase may reflect the release of C3a anaphylatoxin by $C\overline{42}$. Histamine itself does not appear to have a central role, since antihistaminics do not affect the course of the disease.

3.2.2. C3b Inactivator Deficiency

A second defect of C component regulation has been recognized in a patient with a lifelong history of infections (Abramson et al., 1971; Alper et al., 1970) by such organisms as diplococcus pneumonia, Haemophilus influenzae, and B-hemolytic streptococci. These infections have included septicemia, repeated episodes of pneumonia, meningitis sinusitis, and otitis media. The patient's serum did not support C-dependent phagocytosis enhancement, chemotactic-factor generation, or bactericidal activity for smooth gram-negative organisms. C-component levels were normal, with the exception of C3, which was markedly lowered, and it was present mostly as the conversion product, C3b. The catabolic rate of C3 in vivo was elevated, confirming that C3 was being cleaved in vivo. C5 was lowered to about 40% of the normal mean value.

The patient's serum not only was deficient in C3, but also had a markedly lowered concentration of Factor B. Addition of purified Factor B to the patient's serum resulted in cleavage of this component *in vitro,* the cleavage being inhibited by small amounts of normal serum. Deficiency of an inhibitor of the alternate pathway was thought to be responsible for the multiple C abnormalities observed (Alper *et al.,* 1972b). This suggestion was confirmed by the infusion of normal plasma in to the patient, which caused prompt disappearance of C3 conversion products and a rise in concentration of native C3 and C5, Factor B rose transiently and fell again. All C-mediated functions were restored. These observations indicated that C3, C5, and Factor B were being consumed *in vivo,* and that the patient's missing inhibitor of the alternative pathway was being supplied by the plasma. This was confirmed when all the effects of whole plasma were mimicked by an infusion of purified C3b inactivator.

Confirmation that the patient was probably homozygous for C3b inactivator deficiency was obtained by the study of this protein in the serum of his family (Abramson *et al.,* 1971). His mother, three of his six siblings, and two nephews had approximately 40–50% of the normal concentration of this protein.

References

Abramson, N., and Lee, D. P., 1974, Immune hemolytic anemias, in: Disease-A-Month, Year Book Medical Publishers, Chicago.

Abramson, N., Alper, C. A., Lachman, P. J., *et al.,* 1971, Deficiency of C3b inactivator in man, *J. Immunal.* **107**:19.

Agnello, V., Ruddy S., Winchester, R. J., *et al.,* 1975, Hereditary C2 deficiency in systemic lupus erythematosus and acquired complement abnormalities in an unusual SLE-related syndrome, in: *Immunodeficiency in Man and Animals*, (D. Bergsma, R. A. Good, and N. W. Paul, eds.), Birth Defects Original Article Series, Vol. 11, No. 1, p. 312, The National Foundation March of Dimes.

Agnello, V., Koffler, D., Eisenberg, J. W., Winchester, R. J. and Kunkel, H. G., 1971, C1q precipitins in the sera of patients with systemic lupus erythematosus and other hypocomplementemic states: characterization of high and low molecular weight types, *J. Exp. Med.* **134**:2285.

Agnello, V., deBracco, M., and Kunkel, H. G., 1972, Hereditary C2 deficiency with some manifestations of systemic lupus erythematosus, *J. Immunol.* **108**:837.

Alper, C. A., and Rosen, F. S., 1967, Studies on the *in vivo* behavior of human C3 in normal subjects and patients, *J. Clin. Invest.* **46**:2021.

Alper, C. A., and Rosen, F. S., 1976, Genetics of the complement system, *in: Adv, Hum. Genet.* (J. Disk, ed.), **7**:141.

Alper, C. A., Abramson, N., Johnston, R. B., Jandl, J. H., and Rosen, F. S., 1970, Increased susceptibility to infection associated with abnormalities of complement mediated functions and of the third component of complement (C3), *N. Engl. J. Med.* **282**:349.

Alper, C. A., Colten, H. R., Rosen, F. S., Rabson, A. S., Macnag, G. M., and Gear, J. S. S., 1972a, Homozygous deficiency of the third component of complement in a patient with repeated infections, *Lancet* **2**:1179.

Alper, C. A., Rosen, F. S., and Lachmann, P. J., 1972b, Inactivator of the third component of complement as an inhibitor in the properdin pathway, *Proc. Nat. Acad. Sci. U.S.A.* **69**:2910.

Alpert, E., Isselbacher, K. J., and Schur, P. H., 1971, The pathogenesis of arthritis associated with viral hepatitis; complement component studies, *N. Engl. J. Med.* **285**:185.

Asghar, S. S., Faber, W. R., and Cormane, R. H., 1975, C1q precipitin in the sera of patients with allergic vasculitis (Gougerot-Ruiter syndrome), *J. Invest. Dermatol.* **64**:113–118.

Atkinson, J. P., and Frank, M. M., 1974, Studies on the *in vivo* effect of antibody: interaction of IgM antibody and complement in the immune clearance and destruction of erythrocytes in man, *J. Clin. Invest.* **54**:339.

Ballow, M., Day, N. K., Biggar, W. D., *et al.,* 1973, Reconstitution of C1q after bone marrow the immune clearance and destruction of erythrocytes in man, *J. Clin. Invest.* **54**:339.

Ballow, M., Day, N. K., Biggar, W. D., *et al.,* 1973, Reconstitution of C1q after bone marrow transplantation in patients with severe combined immunodeficiency, *Clin. Immunol. Immunopathol.* **2**:28–35.

Ballow, M., Yang, S. Y., and Day, N. K., 1975a, Complete absence of the third component of complement, *J. Clin. Invest.* **56**:703.

Ballow, M., Ward, G. W., Gershwin, M. E., and Day, N.K., 1975b, C1 bypass complement activation pathway in patients with chronic urticaria and angioedema, *Lancet* **2**:248.

Beutner, E. H., Lever, W. F., Witebsky, E., *et al.,* 1966, Autoantibodies in pemphigus vulgaris, *J. Amer. Med. Assoc.* **192**:682.

Beutner, E. H., Chorzelski, T. B., and Jordon, R. E., 1970, in *Autosensitization in Pemphigus and Bullous Pemphigoid,* p. 194, Charles C. Thomas Co., Springfield, Illinois.

Blum, L., Lee, K., Lee, S., Barone, R., and Wallace S.. L., 1976, Hereditary C1s deficiency, *Fed. Proc. Fed. Amer. Soc. Exp. Biol.* **35**:655.

Bokisch, V., Top, F.H., Russell, P. K., Dixon, F. J., and Müller-Eberhard, H. J., 1973, The potential pathogenic role of complement in dengue hemorrhagic shock syndrome, *N. Engl. J. Med.* **289**:996.

Boyer, J. T., Gall, E. P., Norman, M. E., Nilsson, U. R., and Zimmerman, T. S., 1975, Hereditary deficiency of the seventh component of complement, *J. Clin. Invest.* **56**:905–913.

Britton, M. C., and Schur, P. H., 1971, The complement system in rheumatoid synovitis. II. Intracytoplasmic inclusions of immunoglobulins and complement, *Arthritis Rheum.* **14**:87–95.

Caldwell, J. R., Ruddy, S., Schur, P. H., and Austen, K. F., 1972, C1̄ inhibitor deficiency in lymphosarcoma, *Clin. Immunol. Immunopath.* **1**:39–52.

Carpenter, C. B., Ruddy, S., Shehadeh, I. H., Müller-Eberhard, H. J., Merrill, J. P., and Austen, K. F., 1969, Complement metabolism in man: hypercatabolism of the fourth (C4) and third (C3) component in patients with renal allograft rejection and hereditary angioedema, *J. Clin. Invest.* **48**:1495.

Dacie, J. V., 1962, *The Haemolytic Anaemias, Congenital and Acquired. Part II, The Auto-Immune Anaemias,* 2d Ed., Grune & Stratton, New York.

Day, N. K., Gewurz, H., Pickering, R. J., and Good, R. A., 1970, Ontogenic development of C1q synthesis in the piglet, *J. Immunol.* **104**:1316.

Day, N. K., Geiger, H., Stroud, R. M., deBracco, M., Moncado, B., Windhost, D., and Good, R. A., 1972, C1r deficiency: an inborn error associated with cutaneous and renal disease, *J. Clin. Invest.* **51**:1102.

Day, N. K., Winfield, J. B., Winchester, R. J., and Kunkel, H. G., 1975, Evidence for immune-complexes involving anti-lymphocyte antibodies associated with hypocomplementemia in chronic lymphocytic leukemia (CLL), *Clin. Res.* **23**:410a.

Dixon, F. J., 1965, Experimental serum sickness, *in: Immunological Diseases* (M. Samter and H. L. Alexander, eds.), p. 253, Little, Brown & Co., Boston.

Donaldson, V. H., and Evans, R. R., 1963, Biochemical abnormality in hereditary angioneurotic edema: absence of serum inhibitor of C′1-esterase, *Amer. J. Med.* **35**:37.

Donaldson, V. H., and Rosen, F. S., 1964, Action of complement in hereditary angionedurotic edema: role of C′1-esterase, *J. Clin. Invest.* **43**:2204.

Donaldson, V. H., Ratnoff, O. D., Dias da Silva, W., and Rosen, F. S., 1969, Permeability increasing activity in hereditary angioneurotic edema plasma. II. Mechanisms of formation and partial characterization, *J. Clin. Invest.* **48**:642.

Evans, R. S., Turner, E., Bingham, M., *et al.,* 1968, Chronic hemolytic anemia due to cold agglutinins. II. The role of C′ in red cell destruction, *J. Clin. Invest.* **47**:691–701.

Franco, A. E., and Schur, PH., 1971, Hypocomplementemia in rheumatoid arthritis, *Arthritis Rheum.* **14**:231–238.

Frank, M., and Atkinson, J. P., 1975, Complement in clinical medicine, *Disease of the Month—January* Yearbook Publication, Chicago.

Friend, P., Repine, J. E., *et al.,* 1975, Deficiency of the second component of complement with chronic vasculitis, *Ann. Intern. Med.* **83**:813–817.

Gewurz, H., Pickering, R. J., Christian, C. L. Synderman, R., Margenhagen, S. E., and Good, R. A., 1968a, Decreased C1q protein concentration and agglutinating activity in agammaglobulinemia syndromes: an inborn error reflected in the complement system, *Clin. Exp. Immuol.* **3**:437.

Gewurz, H., Pickering, R. J., Mergenhagen, S. E., *et al.,* 1968b, The complement profile in acute glomerulonephritis systemic lupus erythematosus and hypocomplementemic chronic glomerulonephritis: contrasts and experimental correlations, *Int. Arch. Allergy Appl. Immuol.* **34**:556–570.

Gewurz, H., Pickering, R. J., Naff, G., *et al.,* 1969, Decreased properdin activity in acute glomerulo-nephritis, *Int. Arch. Allergy Appl. Immunol.* **36**:592–598.

Gigli, I., Ruddy, S., and Austen, K. F., 1968, The stoichiometric measurement of the serum inhibitor of the first component of complement by inhibition of immune hemolysis, *J. Immunol.* **100**:1154.

Gocke, D. J., Hsu, K., Morgan, C., *et al.,* 1970, Association between polyarteritis and Australia antigen, *Lancet* **2**:1149–1153.

Götze, O., and Müller-Eberhard, H. J., 1970, Lysis of erythrocytes by complement in the absence of antibody, *J. Exp. Med.* **132**:898–915.

Granerus, G., Hallberg, L., Laurell, A. B., and Wetterqvist, H., 1967, Studies on the histamine metabolism and the complement system in hereditary angioneurotic edema, *Acta Med. Scand.* **182**:11–22.

Greenwood, B. M., and Brueton, M. J., 1974, Complement activation in children with acute malaria, *Clin. Exp. Immunol.* **18**:267–272.

Gunn, W. C., 1914—1915, The variation in the amount of complement in the blood in some acute infectious diseases and its relation to the clinical features, *J. Pathol, Bacterial,* **19**:155.

Hadler, N. M., Gerwin, R. D., Rank, M. M., Whitaker, J. N., Baker, M., and Decker, J. L., 1973, The fourth component of complement in the cerebrospinal fluid in systemic lupus erythematosus, *Arthritis Rheum.* **16**:507.

Hanauer, L. B., and Christian, C. L., 1967, Clinical studies of hemolytic complement and the 11S component, *Amer. J. Med.* **42**:882–890.

Hauptman, G., Grosshans, E., Heid, E., Mayer, S., and Basset, A., 1974, Lupus erythmateux aigu avec deficit complet de la fraction C4 du complement, *Nouv. Presse Med.* **3**:881.

Hedberg, H., 1967, Studies on synovial fluid in arthritis. I. The total complement activity. II. The occurrence of mononuclear cells with *in vitro* cytotoxic effect, *Acta Med.* Scand. *Suppl.* **479**:1–137.

Heusinkveld, R. S., Leddy, J. P., Klemperer, M. R., and Breckeridge, R. T., 1974, Hereditary deficiency of the sixth component of complement in man. I. Immuno-chemical, biologic and family studies; II. Studies on hemostasis. *J. Clin. Invest.* **53**:544–558.

Jordon, R. E., 1976, Complement activation in pemphigus and bullous pemphigoid, *J. Invest. Dermatol.* **67**:366–371.

Jordon, R. E., Nordby, J. M., and Milstein, H., 1975a, The complement system in bullous pemphigoid. III. Fixation of C1q and C4 by pemphigoid antibody, *J. Lab. Clin. Med.* **86**:733–740.

Jordon, R. E., Schroeter, A. L., and Winkelmann, R. K., 1975b, Dermal–epidermal deposition of complement components and properdin in systemic lupus erythematosus, *Br. J. Dermatol.* **92**:263–272.

Kay, A. B., Bacon, B., Mercer, B. A., Simpson, H., and Crofton, J. W., 1974, Complement components and IgE in bronchial asthma, *Lancet* Oct. 19, 916.

Klemperer, M. R., Austen, K. F., and Rosen, F. S., 1967, Hereditary deficiency of the second component of complement (C2) in man: further observations in a second kindred, *J. Immunol.* **98**:72.

Koffler, D., Schur, P. H., and Kunkel, H. G., 1967, Immunological studies concerning the nephritis of systemic lupus erythematosus, *J. Exp. Med.* **126**:607–624.

Kohler, P. F., and Müller-Eberhard, H. J., 1969, Complement immunoglobulin relation: deficiency of C'1q associated with impaired immunoglobulin G synthesis, *Science* **163**:474.

Kohler, P. F., and Müller-Eberhard, H. J., 1972, Metabolism of human C1q: studies in hypogrammaglobulinemia, myeloma and systemic lupus erythematosus, *J. Clin. Invest.* **51**:868.

Kohler, P. F., and ten Bensel, R., 1969, Serial complement component alterations in acute glomerulonephritis and systemic lupus erythematosus, *Clin. Exp. Immunol.* **4**:191–202.

Landerman, N. S., Webster, M. E., Becker, E. L., *et al.,* 1962, Deficiency of inhibitor for serum globulin permeability factor and/or plasma kallikrein, *J. Allergy* **33**:330.

Leddy, J. P., and Swisher, S. N., 1971, Acquired immune hemolytic disorders, in: *Immunological Diseases* (M. Samter and H.L. Alexander, eds.), p. 1083, 2d Ed., Little, Brown & Company, Boston.

Leddy, J. P., Frank, M. M., Gaither, T., Baum, J., and Klemperer, M. R., 1974, Hereditary deficiency of the sixth component of complement in man. I. Immuno-chemical, biologic and family studies, *J. Clin. Invest.* **53**:544.

Lepow, I. H., 1971, Permeability-producing peptide by-product of the interaction of the first, fourth and second components of complement, in: *Biochemistry of the Acute Allergic Reactions, Second International Symposium* (K. F. Austen and E. L. Becker, eds.), pp. 205–215, Blackwell Scientific Publications, London.

Lewis, E. J., Carpenter, C. B., and Schur, P. H., 1971, Gamma G globulin subgroup composition of the glomerular deposits in human renal diseases, *Ann. Intern. Med.* **75**:555.

Lim, D., Gewurz, A., Lint., T. F., *et al.,* 1976, Absence of the sixth complement component in a patient with repeated episodes of meningococcal meningitis, *J. Pediatr.* **89**:42.

LoBuglio, A. F., Cotran, R. S., and Jandl, J. H., 1967, Red cells coated with immunoglobulin G: binding and sphering by mononuclear cells in man, *Science* **158**:1582–1585.

Marder, R. J., Rent, R., Choi, E. J., and Gewurz, H., 1976, Selective C1q deficiency associated with urticaria-like lesions and cutaneous vasculitis, *Amer. J. Med.* **61**:560–565.

May, J. E., Rosse, W., and Frank, M. M., 1973, Paroxysmal nocturnal hemoglobinuria: alternate-complement pathway mediated lysis induced by magnesium, *N. Engl. J. Med.* **289**:705.

McDuffie, F. C., Sams, W. M., Jr., Maldonado, J. E., Andreini, P. H., Conn, D. L., and Sarnayoa, E. A., 1973, Hypocomplementemia with cutaneous vasculitis and arthritis. Possible immune complex syndrome, *Mayo Clin. Proc.* **48**:340.

Michael, A. F., Herdman, R. C., Fish, A. J., *et al.,* 1969, Chronic membranoproliferative glomerulonephritis with hypocomplementemia, *Transplant. Proc.* **1**:925–932.

Miller, M. E., and Nilsson, U. R., 1970, A familial deficiency of the phagocytosis-enhancing activity of serum related to a dysfunction of the fifth component of complement (C5), *N. Engl. J. Med.* **282**:354.

Moncada, B., Day., N. K.B., Good, R. A., and Windhorst, D.B., 1972, Lupus erythematosus-like syndrome with a familial defect of complement, *N. Engl. J. Med.* **286**:689.

Müller-Eberhard, H. J., 1975, Complement, in: *Annual Review of Biochemistry* Vol. 44 (E.E. Snell, P. D. Boyer, A. Meister, and C. C. Richardson, eds.), p. 697, Annual Reviews, Palo Alto, California.

Müller-Eberhard, H. J., and Kunkel, H. G., 1961, Isolation of a thermolabile serum protein which precipitates globulin aggregates and participates in immune hemolysis, *Proc. Soc. Exp. Biol. Med.* **106**:291.

Nilsson, U. R., Miller, M. E., and Wyman, S., 1974, A functional abnormality of the fifth component of complement from human serum of individuals with a familial opsonic defect, *J. Immunol.* **112**:1164–1176.

Oberling, F., Hauptmann, G., Lang, J. M., *et al.,* 1975, Acquired deficiency in C1 esterase inhibitor in lymphoid syndromes, *Presse Med.* **4**:2705–2708.

Onion, D. K., Crumpacker, C. S., and Gilliland, B. C., 1971, Arthritis of hepatitis associated with Australia antigen, *Ann. Intern. Med.* **75**:29–33.

Pekin, T. J., Jr., and Zvaifler, N. J., 1964, Hemolytic complement in synovial fluid, *J. Clin. Invest.* **43**:1372–1382.

Perrin, L. H., Lambert, P. H., Nydegger, U. E., and Miescher, P. H., 1973, Quantitation of C3PA (properdin factor B) and other complement components in diseases associated with a low C3 level, *Clin. Immunol. Immunopathol.* **2**:16.

Petersen, B. H., Graham, J. S., and Boroks, G. F., 1975, Human deficiency of the eighth component of complement, *Clin. Res.* **23**:294A.

Petz, L. D., Fink, D. J., Letsky, E. A., *et al.,* 1968, *In vivo* metabolism of complement. I. Metabolism of the third component (C'3) in acquired hemolytic anemia, *J. Clin. Invest.* **47**:2469–2484.

Petz, L. D., Sharp, G. C., Cooper, N. R., and Irvin, W. S., 1971a, Serum and cerebral spinal fluid complement and serum autoantibodies in systemic lupus erythematosus, *Medicine* **50**:259.

Petz, L., Fudenberg, H. H., and Fink, D., 1971b, Immune adherence reactions of human erythrocytes sensitized with complement *in vitro* and *in vivo*, *J. Immunol.* **107**:1714.

Pickering, R. J., Naff, G. B., Stroud, R. M., Good, R. A., and Gewurz, H., 1970, Deficiency of C1r in human serum: effects on the structure and function of macro-molecular C1, *J. Exp. Med.* **141**:803.

Pondman, K. W., Stoop, J. W., Cormane, R. H., and Hannema, A. J., 1969, Abnormal C'1 in a patient with systemic lupus erythematosus, presented at the Third Complement Workshop.

Provost, T. T., and Tomasi, T. B., Jr, 1973, Evidence for complement activation via the alternate pathway in skin disease. I. Herpes gestationis, systemic lupus erythematosus and bullous pemphigoid, *J. Clin. Invest.* **52**:1779.

Provost, T. T., and Tomasi, T. B., Jr., 1974, Evidence for activation of complement via the alternate pathway in skin diseases. II. Dermatitis herpetiformis, *Clin. Immunol. Immunopathol.* 3:178.

Rosen, F. S., Charache, P., Pensky, J., and Donaldson, V., 1965, Hereditary angioneurotic edema: two genetic variants, *Science* **148**:957.

Rosen, F. S., Alper, C. A., Pensky, J., Klemperer, M. R., and Donalson, V. H., 1971, Genetically determined heterogenicity of the C1 esterase inhibitor in patients with hereditary angioneurotic edema, *J. Clin. Invest.* **50**:2141.

Rosenfield, S. I., and Leddy, J. P., 1974, Hereditary deficiency of fifth component of complement (C5) in man, *J. Clin. Invest.* **53**:67 (abstract).

Rosse, W. F., 1971, The life-span of complement-sensitive and-insensitive red cells in paroxysmal nocturnal hemoglobinuria, *Blood* **37**:556–562.

Rothfield, N., Ross, H. A., Minta, J. O., and Lepow, I. H., 1972, Glomerular and dermal deposition of properdin in systemic lupus erythematosus, *N. Engl. J. Med.* **287**:681.

Ruddy, S., and Austen, K. F., 1970, The complement system in rheumatoid synovitis. I. An analysis of complement component activities in rheumatoid synovial fluids, *Arthritis Rheum,* **13**:713–723.

Ruddy, S., and Austen, K. F., 1971, C3b inactivator of man. II. Fragments produced by C3b inactivator cleavage of cell-bound or fluid phase C3b, *J. Immunol.* **107**:742–750.

Ruddy, S., and Colten, H. R., 1974, Rheumatoid arthritis. Biosynthesis of complement proteins by synovial tissues, *N. Engl. J. Med.* **290**:1284.

Ruddy, S., Müller-Eberhard, H. J., and Austen, K. F., 1971, Direct measurement of intra-articular hypercatabolism of third complement component (C3) in rheumatoid arthritis (RA) and systemic lupus erythematosus (SLE), *Arthritis Rheum.* **14**:410.

Ruddy, S., Gigli, I., and Austen, K. F., 1972a, The complement system of man, *N. Engl. J. Med.* **287**:489.

Ruddy, S., Hunsicker, L. G., Schur, P. H., *et al.,* 1972b, Abnormality of alternate pathway in systemic lupus erythematosus and hypo-complementemic chronic glomerulonephritis, *J. Clin. Invest.* **51**:82a.

Schreiber, A. D., Abdou, N., Atkins, P., Goldwein, F., Loyue, T., Cerbi, C., McDermott, P., and Zweiman, B., 1975, Pseudo-hereditary angioedema: report of a second case, *Clin. Res.* **23**:296a.

Schur, P. H., and Sandson, J., 1968, Immunologic factors and clinical activity in systemic lupus erythematosus, *N. Engl. J. Med.* **278**:533–538.

Seah, P. P., Mazaheri, M. R., and Fry, L., 1973, Complement in the skin of patients with dermatitis herpetiformis, *Br. J. Dermatol.* **89** (Suppl.):12.

Sissons, J. G. P., Peters, D. K., Gwyn Williams, D., and Boulton-Jones, M. J., 1974, Skin lesions, angio-oedema, and hypocomplementaemia, *Lancet* **2**:1350.

Soter, N. A., Austen, K. F., and Gigli, I., 1974a, The complement system in necrotizing angiitis of the skin (vasculitis), *J. Invest. Dermatol.* **63**:483.

Soter, N., Austen, K. F., and Gigli, I., 1974b, Urticaria and arthralgias as manifestations of necrotizing angiitis (vasculitis), *J. Invest. Dermatol.* **63**:485.

Soter, N. A., Mihm, M. C., Gigli, I., Dovrak, H. F., and Austen, K. F., 1976, Two distinct cellular patterns in cutaneous necrotizing angiitis, *J. Invest. Dermatol.* **66**:344.

Srichaibul, T., Puwasatien, P., *et al.,* 1975, Complement changes and disseminated intravascular coagulation in plasmodium falciparum malaria, *Lancet* **1** (April 5):770–772.

Stossel, T. P., Alper, C. A., and Rosen, F. S., 1973, Serum dependent phagocytosis of paraffin oil emulsified with bacterial lipopolysaccharide, *J. Exp. Med.* **137**:690.

Stroud, R. M., 1974, Genetic abnormalities of the complement system in man associated with disease, *Transplant. Proc.* **6**:59.

Stroud, R. M., Nagaki, K., Pickering, R. J. *et al.,* 1970, Subunits of the first component of complement in immunologic deficiency syndromes: independence of C1s and C1q, *Clin. Exp. Immunol.* **7**:133.

Tan, E. M., and Kunkel, H. G., 1966, An immunofluorescent study of the skin lesions in systemic lupus erythematosus, *Arthritis Rheum.* **9**:37–46.

Wellek, B., and Opferkuch, W., 1975, A case of deficiency of the seventh component of complement in man. Biological properties of a C7 deficient serum and description of a C7 inactivating principle, *Clin. Exp. Immunol.* **19**:223–236.

West, C. D., Ruley, E. J., Forristal, J., and Davis, N. C., 1973, Mechanisms of hypocomplementemia in glomerulonephritis, *Kidney Int.* **3**:116.

Westberg, N. G., Naff, G. B., Boyer, J. T., *et al.,* 1971, Glomerular deposition of properdin in acute and chronic glomerulonephritis with hypocomplementemia, *J. Clin. Invest.* **50**:642–649.

Winchester, R. J., Agnello, V., and Kunkel, H. G., 1969, The joint-fluid γ G-globulin complexes and their relationship to intraarticular complement diminution, *Ann. N. Y. Acad. Sci.* **168**:195–203.

Winchester, R. J., Agnello, V., and Kunkel, H. G., 1970, Gamma globulin complexes in synovial fluids of patients with rheumatoid arthritis: partial characterization and relationship to lowered complement levels, *Clin. Exp. Immunol.* **6**:689–706.

Zvaifler, N. J., 1969, Breakdown products of C′3 in human synovial fluids, *J. Clin. Invest.* **48**:1532–1542.

Zvaifler, N. J., 1973, The immunopathology of joint inflammation in rheumatoid arthritis, *Adv. Immunol.* **16**:265.

Abbreviations

A—Amboceptor (Forssman antibody)
Ab—antibody
Ag—antigen
AFC—antibody-forming cell
AFCP—antibody-forming cell precursor
ATC—activated thymus cells

B cells—bone-marrow-derived cells
BSA—bovine serum albumin

C_{na}, C_{nb}, C_{nc}, C_{nd}—fragments of complement components produced by enzymatic cleavage mostly during the activation process
C—complement
C1 . . . C9—complement components
$\overline{C1}$, etc.—the overbar indicates an activated component that has acquired enzymatic or other biological activity
Con A—concanavalin A

DMBA—dimethylbenzanthracene
DNCB—dinitrochlorobenzene
DNP—2,4-dinitrophenol
DNP-6L—2,4-dinitrophenyl conjugated with L-glutamic acid and L-lysine copolymer
DPFC—direct plaque forming cells
DTH—delayed thymus hypersensitivity

E—erythrocytes (sheep red blood cells)
EA—sensitized erythrocytes
EDTA—ethylenediaminetetraacetate

Fab—fraction ab of the immunoglobulin molecule

Fc—fraction c of the immunoglobulin molecule
FLV—Friend leukemia virus

GH—growth hormone
GVH—graft versus host

I—the immune region of the major histocompatibility complex
Ia—immune region associated
IBS—immunologic burst size
Ig—immunoglobulin
IgA—immunoglobulin A
IgG—immunoglobulin G
IgM—immunoglobulin M
IgT—immunglobulin on T cells
IO—immunocompetent precursor
IR—immune response

LPS—lipopolysaccharides
Ly—designation of a T cell subset

MCA—methylcholanthrene
MHC—Major histocompatibility complex
MLC—mixed lymphocyte culture

NIP 4—hydroxy-3-iodo-5-nitrophyenylacetic acid

OVA—ovalbumin

PHA—phytohemagglutinin
PFC—plaque forming cells
PTU—propylthiouracil

RBC—red blood cells
RFC—rosette-forming cells
RS—Reed–Sternberg cells

S–Con A—succinyl–concanavalin A

SRBC—sheep red blood cells

T cells—thymus-derived cells

TL—thymus lymphocyte antigen

TL−—thymus lymphocyte antigen (negative)

TL+—thymus lymphocyte antigen (positive)

TXB—thymectomized, irradiated, and bone marrow reconstituted

TXB-NT—TXB mouse with new born thymus graft

TXB-3T—TXB mouse with three-month-old thymus graft

TXB-33T—TXB mouse with 33-month-old thymus graft

Index